CARING *for* KIDS

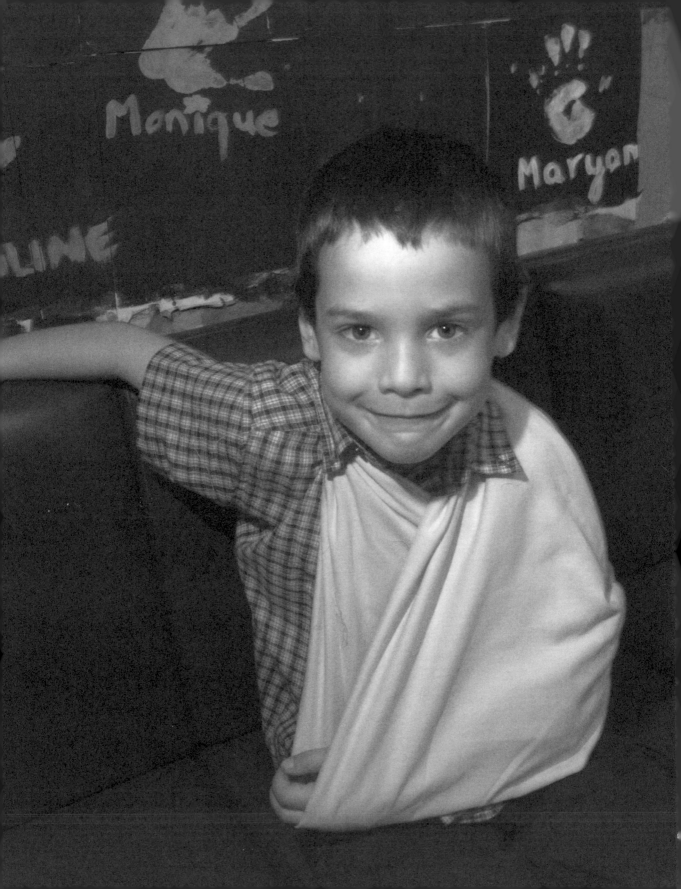

THE COMPLETE GUIDE TO CHILDREN'S HEALTH

CARING *for* KIDS

General *editors:* NORMAN SAUNDERS, MD, FRCPC,
and JEREMY FRIEDMAN, MB.ChB, FRCPC

FIREFLY BOOKS

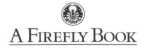

A FIREFLY BOOK

Published by Firefly Books (U.S.) Inc. 2006

First printing

Publisher Cataloging-in-Publication Data (U.S.)

Caring for kids : the complete guide to children's health / edited by Norman
Saunders and Jeremy Friedman.
[448] p. : col. ill., photos. ;   cm.
Includes bibliographical references and index.
Summary: A comprehensive reference to health and wellness in children aged
zero to ten, written by a team of physicians from the Hospital for Sick Children,
Toronto, Canada. Topics covered include common infections and diseases, growth
and nutrition, allergic disorders, and accidents and emergencies
ISBN-13: 978-1-55407-160-9
ISBN-10: 1-55407-160-7
1. Children--Health and hygiene. 2. Child care.   3. Pediatrics--Popular works.
I. Saunders, Norman.   II. Friedman, Jeremy. III. Title.
618.92 --dc22   RJ61.C37 2006

Published in the United States by
Firefly Books (U.S.) Inc.
P.O. Box 1338, Ellicott Station
Buffalo, New York 14205

Published in Canada by Key Porter Books Limited.

Text design: Ingrid Paulson
Additional text formatting: Brian Lehen Graphic Design Ltd.
Medical illustrations: John Lightfoot
Cover design: Ingrid Paulson
Cover photograph: © Royalty-free/Corbis

Printed in Canada

Contents

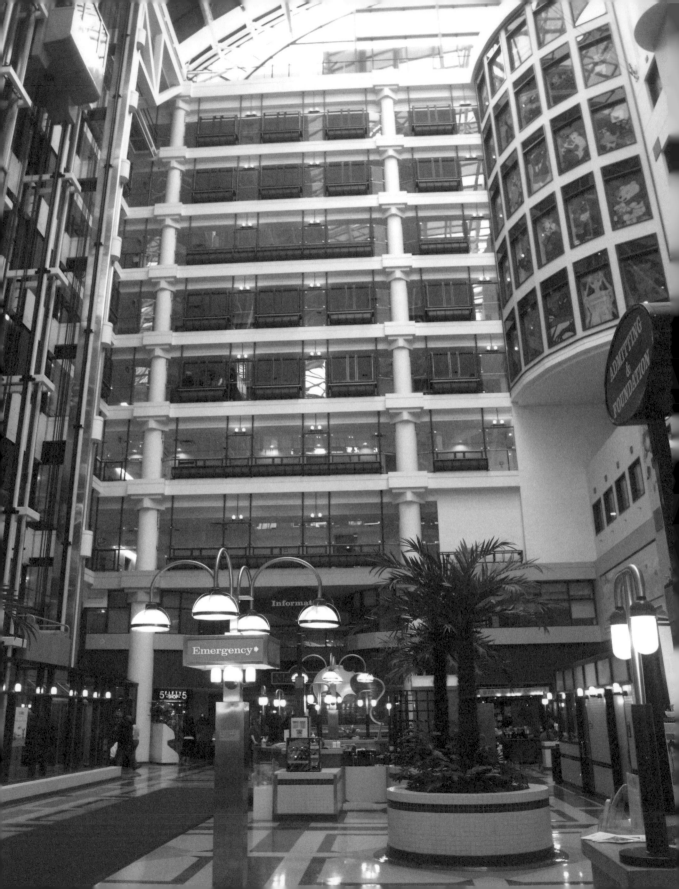

Introduction

Every parent wants to succeed at parenting. In fact, of the many things that people strive to do well, caring for their children pretty well tops the list. This book has been written with the belief that parents will always do the right thing for their children—if only they know what that right thing is! In the pages that follow, you will find the information you need to better understand and deal with the health problems that your children can face.

Bookstore shelves are crammed with hundreds of volumes that offer parenting advice. What's so special about this book? Lots. First, *Caring for Kids: The Complete Guide to Children's Health* has been written in partnership with The Hospital for Sick Children. The hospital is more than an excellent health sciences center; it's an institution that's also world renowned. "Sick Kids," as the hospital is frequently and affectionately called, is one of the world's best known health care facilities. It is regarded as a place where children will receive the highest level of care—regardless of background or means— simply because this is what our children deserve. Sick Kids serves not only today's generation of youngsters; its research and teaching programs are dedicated to serving future generations as well. Each year, the faculty at Sick Kids continues to train tomorrow's caregivers while producing literally hundreds of research papers in order to better understand and deal with the problems children may face.

We have recruited an extraordinary group of contributors to help write *Caring for Kids*. These authors are all experienced pediatricians on the staff of The Hospital for Sick Children. They also serve as members of the Faculty of Medicine at the University of Toronto, Canada. Several of them conduct busy pediatric practices and, therefore, appreciate both the theoretical and practical aspects of children's problems. The pediatricians whom we have selected to write this guide are all respected for their knowledge of both the art and the science of caring for children and their health. Collectively, these contributing authors have distinguished themselves by winning numerous teaching, citizenship and clinical awards. We think you will notice that they understand kids, relate to parents and know about the problems of childhood.

The Hospital for Sick Children, affectionately called "Sick Kids," is one of the largest pediatric academic health science centers in the world, with an international reputation for excellence in health care, research and teaching.

Another very important aspect of this guide is its content. Wherever possible, the information and advice that we have provided is based on the best available scientific evidence. This approach is sometimes called evidence-based pediatrics and, where possible, we have followed this philosophy. Most of the illnesses that kids must deal with are minor and self-limiting. Other problems can be much more serious and complex and capable of permanently altering family life. Yet, regardless of the nature or scale of any given challenge, the management of these should always remain thoughtful, compassionate and informed.

The first chapter of this book deals with some of the more important symptoms that parents must deal with. It will inform you what needs to be considered and how best to approach that particular problem. The rest of the chapters are divided by the appropriate body system or age group and describe the nature of many specific conditions that affect children. They seek to answer the following questions: What is the condition? What can parents normally expect to happen? How should the problem be treated? The final chapter provides a reference guide to help cope with some of the common accidents and emergencies that can occur in childhood.

We hope that you will find this book useful. Few things are more gratifying than meeting a child's needs. If this guide helps you, even slightly, to better serve the family you love, then our efforts will have been worthwhile.

—Jeremy Friedman, MB.CHB, FRCP(C) and Norman R. Saunders MD, FRCP(C)

*Editor's note: Terms set in **bold** in the text are defined in the glossary on pages 423–30.*

Contributors

Without the invaluable work of these men and women, this book would not have been possible. All contributors come from the Division of Paediatric Medicine, The Hospital for Sick Children, and the Department of Paediatrics, University of Toronto, Canada.

Dr. Tara Baron
Dr. Stacey Bernstein
Dr. Mark Feldman
Dr. Beth Gamulka
Dr. Marvin Gans
Dr. Saul Greenberg
Dr. Moishe Ipp
Dr. Sheila Jacobson
Dr. Sanjay Mahant
Dr. Patricia Parkin
Dr. Michael Peer
Dr. Elena Pope
Dr. Adam Rappoport
Dr. Michelle Shouldice
Dr. Michael Weinstein

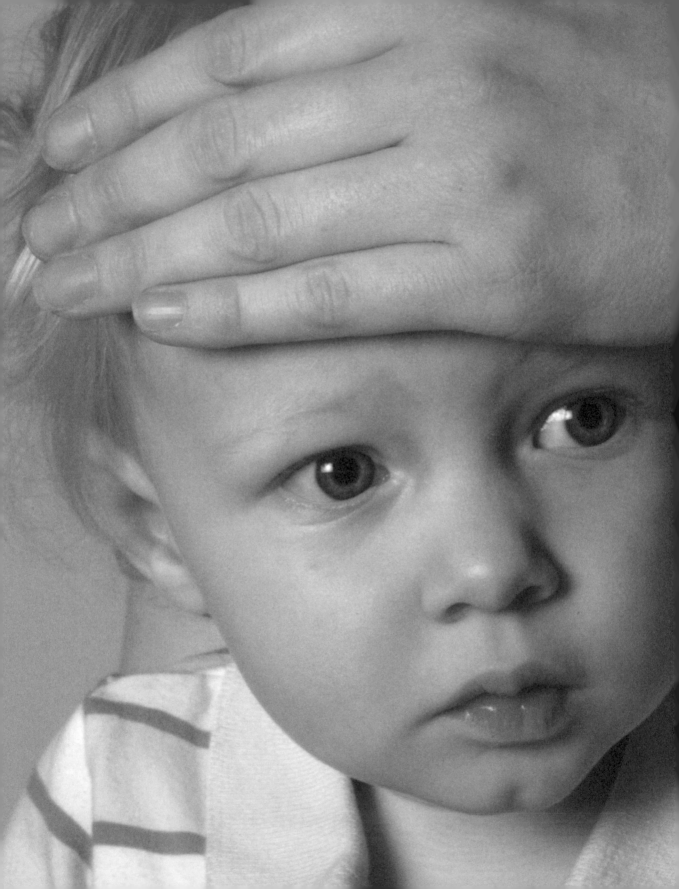

Common Symptoms

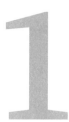

Abdominal Pain

ACUTE ABDOMINAL PAIN

What is acute abdominal pain? Most parents will be faced at some point with the dilemma of deciding what to do with their child who has a stomach ache. Actually, the term "stomach ache" is not usually correct because the pain could be coming from anywhere in the belly, from the bottom of the rib cage down to the groin, including the stomach, intestines, kidneys, bladder, liver and other organs. It could even be **referred pain** from pneumonia at the base of the lung causing irritation of the diaphragm and giving the impression that the pain is coming from the abdomen. Remember that children in the first two years of life will probably not be able to tell you where the pain is and may just cry and pull up their legs.

When medical people talk about "acute" pain, we mean that it has been present for a short period of time, usually hours or days. Abdominal pain that has been present for months has a very different set of causes and is dealt with in a separate section on pages 20–22 (Recurrent Abdominal Pain). The difficulty with acute abdominal pain is deciding which child might have a serious problem—such as appendicitis

requiring immediate medical attention—versus the many others with a more benign and self-limited cause that may not require any treatment at all.

What causes acute abdominal pain? There are a number of causes requiring surgery that generally need immediate attention. It is the possibility of these conditions that tends to provoke concern in parents when their child has acute abdominal pain.

- Appendicitis almost always begins with pain around the navel and moves from there down to the lower right side of the abdomen. The pain is sharp and steady, continuing to get worse over time. Any movement—coughing, jumping or pressing down over the affected area—tends to be very painful. Children will often have a **low-grade fever,** poor appetite, nausea and vomiting. Appendicitis is uncommon in the first few years of life.
- Intussusception occurs when a piece of intestine telescopes into the next part of the bowel and then becomes stuck. This condition causes acute abdominal pain and is most common between the ages of 6 months and 3 years. Two clues that this unusual problem is occurring are first,

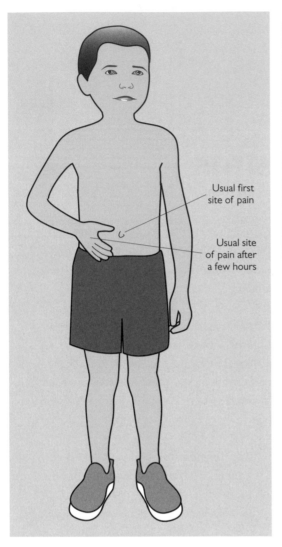

Usual first
site of pain

Usual site
of pain after
a few hours

PAIN PATTERN IN APPENDICITIS

Abdominal pain usually begins around the navel. The pain gradually becomes more severe and migrates to the lower right-hand side of the abdomen during the next few hours. In some children, the pain is in the lower right abdomen from the beginning.

the appearance of bloody stools that look like red current jelly and, second, the episodic nature of the pain. Your child's behavior will alternate between being comfortable, even playful, and having periods of inconsolability due to spasms of severe, crampy pain.

- Another very rare but important cause of pain requiring surgery is the twisting of the small intestines on its stalk, called midgut volvulus. These children will have severe pain and vomit dark green bile-containing material, as will most children with a blockage of their intestines. Unlike adults, gallstones and kidney stones are very uncommon in previously healthy children.

There are a number of less serious and much more common reasons why children complain of acute abdominal pain.

- Frequently, a child will complain of a stomach ache after eating too much, eating too quickly or eating something that didn't "agree" with him. These pains settle down rapidly within a few hours.
- Constipation can cause quite severe abdominal cramps and is a very common cause of stomach aches. A child with constipation will generally have a history of infrequent, very hard stools that can also be painful to pass. There may be some blood on the paper after wiping or in the toilet bowl.
- Infections can also cause acute abdominal pain. Pain that is associated with vomiting of stomach contents and often followed the next day by watery, foul-smelling diarrhea is usually due to viral gastroenteritis. These children will generally not feel well and might have a low-grade fever (below 101.3°F/38.5°C) and a poor appetite. There could be a friend or family member with similar symptoms as it is quite contagious.
- Bacterial infections that cause inflammation of the large intestine, called colitis, can cause

cramping that is often associated with high fevers and bloody stools in a sick-looking child. This is more common in returning travelers or those exposed to potentially contaminated food (food poisoning) or water.

- Kidney and bladder infections should also be considered as the source of abdominal pain. Kidney infections can be accompanied by fever, vomiting and lower back pain, while bladder infections can cause pain on urination, increased frequency of urination and new onset bedwetting at night. Sometimes children with strep throat or otitis media (ear infection) complain of a stomach pain in addition to their sore throat or earache.

- Other inflammations of the bowel, not directly caused by infection, can also produce abdominal pain. Inflammatory bowel disease (IBD), either Crohn's disease or ulcerative colitis, tends to produce symptoms in teenagers but can occur at any age. Children with these conditions can first come to the doctor because of poor growth and weight loss with intermittent episodes of severe abdominal cramps, often accompanied by diarrhea that is sometimes bloody. Children with Crohn's disease can also have mouth ulcers, joint pains and rashes.

- One condition that most parents haven't heard about but is an important cause of severe acute abdominal pain is called Henoch-Schonlein purpura (HSP). In this disease, there is inflammation of the blood vessels that produces a characteristic rash and, often, crampy abdominal pain, frequently with bloody stools. The rash is usually most

WHEN SHOULD I WORRY ABOUT MY CHILD'S ACUTE ABDOMINAL PAIN?

SYMPTOM	CONDITION
Sharp, steady and increasing over the course of the day	Appendicitis
Moving from navel to right groin	
Worse with movement	
Paroxysms of severe pain in child under 3 years	Intussusception
Well between episodes	
Bloody stools	
Dark green "bilious" vomiting	Intestinal obstruction
Bloody stools	Bacterial infection
With poor growth and weight loss over months	IBD
With rash over legs and buttocks	HSP
Fever, vomiting, dysuria, frequent urination	Urinary tract infection

prominent on the legs and buttocks, and resembles bruising (purpura). These children can also have joint pains and swelling, decreased urine production or blood in the urine due to kidney inflammation.

- Lactose intolerance is a popular diagnosis that is actually quite uncommon in young children, especially those of Caucasian ethnicity. Children who cannot tolerate lactose tend to have abdominal cramps, bloating, gas or diarrhea following exposure to the lactose sugar that is found in milk and dairy products.

- Food allergy can occasionally cause gastro-intestinal symptoms. The most common would be an allergy to the protein in cow's milk that usually causes diarrhea and cramping in young babies.

How is acute abdominal pain treated? If your child has any of these worrisome symptoms, fairly urgent medical attention is required. However, the tummy aches that the vast majority of children have are not accompanied by any of these characteristics and will likely settle down after a few hours with some reassurance and distraction. If your child's pain seems different or more severe than usual, it is always safest to discuss this with your physician. The management of viral gastroenteritis and constipation is discussed in the sections devoted to those topics.

RECURRENT ABDOMINAL PAIN (RAP)

Not every illness—the perception of feeling unwell—is caused by a known disease that can be proven by medical testing. Many individuals have symptoms for which no illness can be identified. Such is the case in that common pediatric problem: recurrent abdominal pain (RAP). About 15 percent of school-aged children, more often girls, suffer from this condition and only a very small percentage of the abdominal pain is due to a specific and recognizable disease. Yet, because of the discomfort and your understandable concern about a possible underlying disease, the problem of RAP in childhood is significant and worth understanding.

There are three broad types of functional (that is, not caused by a distinct identifiable disease) recurrent abdominal pain in childhood: irritable bowel syndrome (IBS), dyspepsia and

the third is simply referred to as functional recurrent abdominal pain, or functional RAP. There is frequently some overlap in these but their diagnoses are based on distinct features: they are not diagnoses of exclusion made only after extensive testing.

Irritable Bowel Syndrome (IBS)

What does irritable bowel syndrome look like? There are different criteria that have been used to define IBS yet the key features are common to most definitions. Basically, the condition is associated with recurrent or persistent abdominal discomfort that is relieved by a bowel movement (defecation). Typically, there is a sense your child's tummy is swollen and his stools are occasionally accompanied by the passage of mucus. The stools are either loose and frequent (about or more than three per day) or else they are infrequent (fewer than three per week). After the movements, the child may also feel that evacuation was not complete.

How is irritable bowel syndrome treated? The treatment for IBS is imperfect. A medical examination can provide an explanation of the problem, give reassurance and exclude serious disease. If constipation is a feature, a high fiber diet is often helpful. The recommended amount of dietary fiber in grams is calculated by adding five to the child's age. (For example, a 6-year-old should get 5 + 6 = 11 grams of fiber daily.) Laxatives, such as mineral oil or milk of magnesia, can also improve symptoms. If soft, frequent stools are present, eliminating excess sugar, such as fructose and lactose, may help. You should also avoid using the sweetener sorbitol. Various medications have been tried for IBS, particularly in adults, but their role in childhood IBS is less well studied. You should talk with your child's doctor before using them and then discuss when to use them.

Dyspepsia

What is dyspepsia? Dyspepsia refers to a recurrent or persistent pain or discomfort that is most noticeable above the belly button (umbilicus). It can be caused by an ulcer, which is relatively rare in children, by gastroesophageal reflux disease (GERD), which produces heartburn when the stomach's contents regurgitate back up the esophagus, or by a disease such as Crohn's that involves the upper bowel. Finally, it can be functional with no known cause.

What does dyspepsia look like? Two patterns of dyspepsia have been described but there can be so much overlap that the distinction often lacks value. The first pattern is ulcerlike with pain as the major symptom. The second kind of dyspepsia is called the dysmotility type, so called because it seems to be caused by disordered bowel muscle coordination. Your child can have nausea or vomiting, bloating and a sense of having had enough to eat early in the meal. It can be difficult to distinguish functional dyspepsia from the other causes of upper abdominal pain and discomfort. Heartburn and the refluxing of food obviously suggest GERD, but ulcer disease and functional dyspepsia are often indistinguishable.

How is dyspepsia treated? Your child needs a careful medical examination and even that may not be enough. Sometimes, your child will be referred to a pediatric gastroenterologist who is an expert in bowel disease. Occasionally, examining the esophagus, stomach and duodenum with a scope will be necessary to rule out an ulcer or another serious condition.

Symptoms can often be reduced by avoiding

RED FLAGS IN RECURRENT ABDOMINAL PAIN

- The further the pain is from the belly button, the more likely there is a disease causing the symptoms.
- Pain that wakens a child in the night is more likely to have a cause.
- Weight loss, vomiting, unexplained fevers, joint pains and blood in your child's stool are causes for concern.
- A family history of inflammatory bowel disease increases the chance that your child's abdominal pain is also due to IBD.

---

aggravating foods, often spicy or fatty ones. Medications known to upset the stomach, such as ibuprofen, can also be eliminated. Smaller, more frequent meals may relieve the sense of bloating and early satiety. Often, your child's physician will prescribe a trial of medication that reduces stomach acidity, such as ranitidine or omeprazole.

Functional Recurrent Abdominal Pain

What is functional recurrent abdominal pain (functional RAP)? The majority of children with recurrent or persistent abdominal pain will have functional RAP. More often, the patient is female with symptoms beginning between age 5 and 10 years. The prevalence of functional RAP peaks between the ages of 8 and 10 years.

Once again, it is important to realize that, although there is no distinct disease present, there still is illness. In other words, functional RAP is a symptom-based diagnosis rather than a pathological one. It has distinctive features although the exact cause or causes have yet to be found.

What does functional RAP *look like?* Classically, the pain is located around the belly button and is quite variable in its intensity. Although it can be severe enough to disrupt activity, often it is present as a low-grade discomfort. Meals, exercise and the time of day don't appear to influence the pain. Often, there are other symptoms, such as headache and limb pain. Yet, in spite of all the complaining, the child appears physically healthy. Many of the children are described as intense, conscientious or "highly strung." There is also a tendency for other family members to suffer from functional painful symptoms, such as tension headaches.

How is functional RAP *treated?* Once again, a review of the symptoms and a complete physical examination are needed. Obtaining a typical history and finding nothing physically wrong during the exam are usually sufficient to establish the diagnosis. The reassurance that nothing serious is causing the pain is often enough to reduce the severity of the problem with no additional therapy. Laboratory testing has little value in identifying unsuspected disease. Except when actual disease is suspected, tests are probably unnecessary. Medication is of little proven value in treating functional RAP. Constipation or lactose intolerance, if it coexists, can be treated appropriately.

Once the diagnosis of functional RAP has been made, the goal of therapy is to attain as normal a lifestyle as possible. Your child should be encouraged to not allow the pain to control events. Rather, the child should control events. He needs to attend school regularly. Obvious stressors should be eliminated or, at least, reduced.

Reassurance and lifestyle adjustments seem to help. Within a few weeks of diagnosis, 30 percent to 50 percent of children will notice that their pain has disappeared or significantly decreased, so that it no longer disrupts activities. Unfortunately, many who suffered from RAP as children will develop functional pain as adults.

Backache

The spine is a truly remarkable anatomical structure. This flexible column consists of 24 bones (vertebrae), separated by shock-absorbing disks of cartilage, fastened together by numerous ligaments, and all moved purposefully by an array of muscles. However, like any complex arrangement, things have a tendency to go wrong. Over 80 percent of human beings will complain of significant back pain at some point in their lives, costing society billions of dollars. Although backache tends to be more common in adults, 30 percent of children, particularly adolescents, suffer from the problem too.

COMMON BACKACHE

What causes backache? The majority of back pain in children is the result of straining some of the 200 muscles that allow us to move our back or maintain our posture. Usually the cause can be identified as overdoing some physical activity or lifting a heavy object awkwardly. A number of factors have been implicated in causing back pain: carrying backpacks, excessive time spent at a computer, low physical activity level, personality type and underlying mood.

The widespread use of backpacks to carry books has been suggested as a source of backache. About three-quarters of teenaged backpack users do complain of some backache but studies have failed to demonstrate a connection between the degree of back pain and the weight of the bag. It seems that if carrying a backpack does contribute to recurrent backache, the pain produced is mild and transient. Very few children whose back pain is severe enough to be referred to a pediatric orthopedic clinic are diagnosed with backpack-induced muscle strain.

Physical inactivity and computer usage have also been implicated in backache. There is an association between the number of hours spent at a computer and the frequency of back pain. It seems that active children are less likely to complain of common backache than sedentary ones, but competitive athletes are more prone to back injury.

Recurrent backache is more likely to occur in children who have previously complained of other pain symptoms, particularly tension headache or nonspecific recurrent abdominal pain. Such individuals just seem to respond more intensely to their bodies' signals.

What does backache look like? Common backache is usually described as an aching or stiffness in the middle or lower back that becomes abruptly painful with lifting or arching the back. Unlike more serious problems, the pain does not radiate down the leg to the calf. It tends to resolve gradually after a week or two. Unfortunately, recurrences tend to be common.

What do I do about backache? Many people have different ideas about how to best manage backache. Unfortunately, there seem to be more strong opinions than actual facts about dealing with backache. Certainly, the pain of muscle strain is often relieved by simple painkillers, like ibuprofen or acetaminophen. Local heat using a hot water bottle or heating pad is often comforting and helps reduce the muscle spasm. A firm mattress, reinforced with a board if necessary,

may help with sleep. Complete bed rest is not usually necessary but your child should avoid activities that aggravate the pain, especially heavy lifting and jarring sports. Chiropractic treatment has been shown to help many adults with recurrent back pain but its effectiveness for younger patients is less established. In one of the few available studies, 40 percent of children seeking chiropractic care for backache rated their pain as "much improved" after seven days of treatment. Massage certainly can provide short-term pain relief but is unlikely to resolve the problem or prevent recurrence.

The best way to prevent recurrent backache is to maintain good overall physical fitness. Children who repeatedly complain of back strain should try a routine of simple but specific exercises that can be obtained from your child's health care provider, coach or physiotherapist.

OTHER CONDITIONS THAT CAUSE BACK PAIN

Although most back pain is caused by temporarily strained muscles, a few more serious conditions can produce backache in children.

Spondylolysis
What is spondylolysis? This refers to the presence of a defect in the bony structure of a vertebra, usually the one just above the sacrum in the lower spine. It essentially means that a part of the vertebra attaching to the bone below is in two pieces rather than one. Usually, spondylolysis is thought of as a form of stress fracture caused by repetitive overuse and bone fatigue. Less often, it follows sudden injury. Although not present at birth, spondylolysis seems to occur in individuals with a genetic predisposition to it.

What does spondylolysis look like? About 4 percent of children have spondylolysis but suffer no symptoms from it. When it does cause backache, the pain tends to occur in the lower spine, worsens with extension and is relieved by rest. The hamstring muscles may appear tight. Simple x-rays of the spine can show the defect, although bone scans or computerized tomography (CT) scans of the spine are often more sensitive.

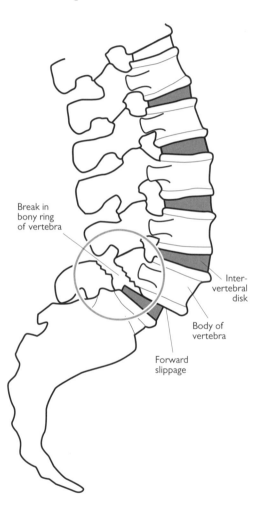

Break in
bony ring
of vertebra

Inter-
vertebral
disk

Body of
vertebra

Forward
slippage

SPONDYLOLISTHESIS
Spondylolisthesis is a condition in which a break in both sides of the ring allows the body of the vertebra to slip forward.

How is spondylolysis treated? The treatment is "conservative." Although bed rest is unnecessary, restricting athletic activity to comfortable walking or cycling is recommended. Sports involving hyperextension of the spine should be avoided, usually for four to six weeks. Pain relievers can be used when necessary to control significant discomfort. An exercise program designed to strengthen the abdominal muscles and increase flexibility in the hamstrings can reduce the recurrence of backache.

Spondylolisthesis

What is spondylolisthesis? Don't worry if you struggle pronouncing this condition: you are not alone. It refers to the horizontal forward slippage of a vertebra. Spondylolisthesis is most likely to happen where the fifth, or lowest, lumbar vertebra slides forward on the sacrum. This slippage is the result of a pre-existing spondylolysis that makes the attachment of the vertebra to the sacrum unstable and usually occurs during the growth spurt of adolescence.

What does spondylolisthesis look like? Children with spondylolisthesis complain of low back pain that seems worse with activity. When the vertebra slides forward enough, the nerve root will be pressed. This causes the pain to radiate down the leg to the calf or foot. There may numbness or weakness in the affected lower limb.

How is spondylolisthesis treated? If the slippage is minor, the conservative treatment described for spondylolysis is usually advised. Progression usually stops in late adolescence. Children should avoid contact sports. In the more pronounced cases of spondylolisthesis, it is necessary to stabilize the vertebra. These children will require surgery.

Diskitis

What is diskitis? Diskitis is an inflammation of the disks between the vertebrae. Usually the inflammation is caused by an infection, most commonly due to the bacteria *Staphylococcus aureus*. Typically, diskitis afflicts a younger age group than the other causes of backache: the two peaks in occurrence happen at 6 months to 4 years of age and then from 10 to 14 years.

What does diskitis look like? Children with diskitis might complain of back pain or they might limp, refuse to bear weight or, in infants, appear irritable. There is usually local tenderness in the middle of the back over the spine at the site of the affected disk. They usually have a fever and, sometimes, leg weakness. Their white blood count can be raised and the blood tests that suggest inflammation tend to be abnormal. Staphylococcus might be grown on blood culture. A CT scan of the spine is better at detecting diskitis than simple x-rays.

How is diskitis treated? If bacterial infection is found, your child will be given intravenous antibiotics for a few weeks. The inflammation is controlled with non-steroidal anti-inflammatory drugs (NSAIDs), such as ibuprofen and naproxen, that also relieve the pain. Additional painkillers may be needed. In severe cases, bed rest and even immobilization are necessary.

SPINAL DEFORMITIES: SCOLIOSIS AND KYPHOSIS

Scoliosis is an abnormal spinal curvature that exists in the frontal plane; in other words, the spine bends to one side when viewed head

OTHER CONDITIONS THAT PRODUCE BACK PAIN

The list of disorders associated with back pain is quite lengthy. Sometimes, backache can be due to very unusual causes. Rarely, spinal or other tumors cause back pain. So can kidney infection or even inflammatory bowel disease when it begins as an inflammation of the sacroiliac joint. Remember, these conditions are very rare and backache isn't. Most of the time, muscle strain will be the problem. When in doubt, have your child examined by your health care provider. Here are some guidelines:

Seek help immediately, if:
- Your child can't walk.
- Your child's pain seems extreme or unrelieved at all by medicine.
- Your child has a fever.
- Your child seems very sick.
- Your child's pain is the direct result of trauma or injury.

Otherwise, if:
- Pain is no better after three days of treatment.
- Pain persists after two weeks.
- Pain travels down the back of the leg below the knee.
- The child is younger than 10 years old.
- The problem recurs regularly.
- You have a general concern about the problem.

on. Thus, it may appear as if the child's shoulders are uneven or hips are not level. The condition is common, especially in preadolescent and adolescent females. It is very unusual for simple scoliosis to cause back pain, particularly when the curve is not great.

Kyphosis is the term that describes the forward curve of the spine in the thorax, or chest region. Normally, most people have a flexible curve ranging from 20 degrees to 40 degrees when viewed from the side. Parents of teenagers are often exasperated with their children when poor posture amplifies this roundness. But a flexible round back seldom creates pain. There is another kind of kyphosis that does cause backache, although usually of low intensity. It is called Scheuermann's disease and is indicated by an inflexible kyphosis and back pain in previously normal children. The vertebrae appear wedge-shaped on spinal x-rays because the condition is created by a difference in growth rates between the front part of the vertebra and the back. If the curvature is severe, the spine can be braced temporarily, which can reduce the curve or prevent any further progression to unacceptable levels. Otherwise, simple pain relief when the discomfort is bothersome is all that is needed to treat the problem.

Chest Pain

What is chest pain? When most people think of pain in the chest, they usually worry about the presence of a serious heart problem. While this might sometimes be appropriate for an adult, it is almost never the case in children. Chest pain in children is rarely due to serious illness. Nevertheless, the complaint should be taken seriously as the symptom can be very disturbing, especially in younger children. On occasion, it can be caused by something that requires treatment.

Chest pain can originate from the muscles and bones of the chest wall, the lungs, the esophagus or the heart, or it may even be caused by a problem located in the abdomen. This complaint becomes more common after the age of 12, but is not uncommon in younger children as well. In about a quarter of the children with chest pain, it will tend to recur for more than six months. Interestingly, about half of these children will have a family member with similar complaints.

What causes chest pain? There are a number of problems involving the chest wall that can lead to pain.

- After overuse of muscles with excessive or new exercise, children can have muscle strain.
- Costochondritis, or inflammation of the rib's cartilage, is characterized by a very sharp pain in the front of the chest wall. The diagnosis is confirmed by tenderness when pushing over the area where the ribs join onto the breastbone. This problem is sometimes preceded by a cold or exercise.
- Obviously a direct blow, or similar trauma to the chest, can cause bruising and pain as well.
- At the onset of puberty, both boys and girls can have some tenderness of the breasts.
- Persistent cough can cause pain due to overuse of the chest muscles.
- In addition, infection of the lung (pneumonia) or an air leak from the bronchial tubes, called a pneumothorax, may cause pain, and both are accompanied by other signs of breathing difficulty.
- Indigestion due to esophagitis, an inflamed

esophagus from acid reflux, can cause a burning pain behind the breastbone. Your child will often complain of "heartburn" after meals, particularly if he has eaten spicy foods.

- Rarely, in young children, the ingestion of a foreign body, for example, a penny, can lead to pain if the object becomes stuck in the esophagus. This can develop after a choking episode.
- As mentioned, heart disease is an uncommon cause of childhood chest pain, comprising less than 5 percent of the cases. Abnormal heart rhythms, structural defects, heart valve abnormalities and infections of the heart can all cause some discomfort in the chest. This generally happens in a child who is known to have heart disease or who appears significantly unwell at the time. Fainting (syncope), palpitations and pain with exertion can also suggest that your child's doctor should do a thorough heart exam.
- Anxiety and emotional stress can be a factor, particularly in adolescent girls. It is often seen in conjunction with school problems, family stress and social problems. They might hyperventilate (breathe rapidly) and their hands and feet could tingle as well.

However, probably up to half of all children complaining of chest pain will have no specific diagnosis. Even after appropriate testing, your child's doctor will not be able to give you a definitive cause for the pain. The good news is that in most of these children the pain will ultimately disappear without any serious illness ever developing.

What do I do about chest pain? The treatment will depend on the likely cause. Reviewing your child's situation with the above possibilities in mind

WHEN TO SEE A DOCTOR URGENTLY IF YOUR CHILD HAS CHEST PAIN:
- young age, sudden onset
- looks unwell, especially if any significant breathing difficulty
- associated with fainting or palpitations
- concern about possible swallowing of a foreign body
- high fever
- consistently wakes him up from sleep

can help to clarify where the pain is coming from. You will need to decide whether to seek medical attention and, if so, how urgently. The younger your child and the shorter the duration of the symptoms (not lasting for months), the more likely there will be something significant that could require testing or treatment.

If your child has had a direct injury to the chest or there are sufficient clues pointing toward a lung or heart problem, a chest x-ray will likely be necessary. In the rare cases where the heart is potentially the problem, an electrocardiogram (ECG) may be helpful. In the majority of cases your child's doctor will need a thorough description of the problem followed by a physical examination and no further testing will be required.

Treatment for musculoskeletal problems involving the chest wall include rest, heat and analgesics such as ibuprofen. Chest infections causing chest pain will often need antibiotics. And, if indigestion is suspected, a trial of antacids is useful. In the latter case, improvement of the indigestion would help confirm your suspicion of esophagitis.

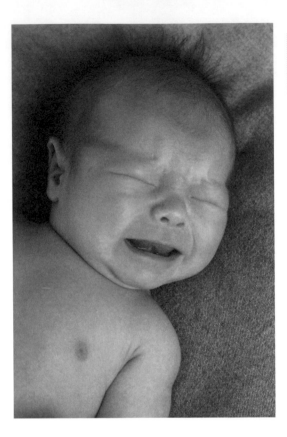

Colic

What is colic? All babies cry. It is nature's way of alerting parents that their infant has unmet needs. However, some babies cry much more than others. When a healthy baby repeatedly has episodes of intense crying for no apparent reason, the condition is referred to as infantile colic. Typically, colic begins in the first weeks of life, peaks by 2 months of age and ends at 4 or 5 months. Often, these episodes occur most frequently in the late afternoon or early evening and the baby may be inconsolable and appear to be in pain. Understandably, for parents, colic can be frustrating, exhausting and demoralizing.

What causes colic? Many theories have been proposed but no one really knows for sure. Probably, there are many different causes of colic, all of which lead to excessive crying. In some children, colic is due to a digestive difficulty, such as an intolerance to cow's milk protein. In others, it may result from an intense infantile temperament. For most, the cause is never found. Yet, one thing is certain: colic is no one's fault.

What do I do about colic? Few situations will open a parent's mind to treatment suggestions more than colic. If your baby is crying constantly, you may be willing to try anything. But not everything works. Here is what you can do.

First, get rid of those nagging concerns that something must be wrong with your child. Have the baby checked by your doctor. Second, try to appreciate that you are dealing with a phase that will eventually pass but must be dealt with for now. Coping means sharing the burden. For example, if the baby generally cries from 6 until 10 p.m., let one parent become the prime caregiver from 6 until 8 and the other can look after things from 8 until 10, perhaps with a feeding dividing the two periods. Thus, a four-hour problem is reduced to two. You won't feel guilty reading the newspaper or resent your spouse's insistence on taking a break from parenting.

Another successful coping strategy is scheduling your week so that a trusted relative or friend can look after your child for a few hours. It's okay to arrange time just for you. Parenting, after all, is a tough job and no one should be expected to work 24 hours a day, 7 days a week. Try to ensure that you and your spouse get out as a couple at least once a week. Even a quick bite alone together can help retain the romantic component to your partnership. Rest if you feel exhausted and try to exercise regularly when you can. In short, by sharing the load, scheduling relief pre-emptively and restoring some control to your own life, you can keep your personal batteries charged before they become completely drained.

Will changing my baby's diet help? Sometimes. Studies have shown that colicky infants fed cow's milk-based formulas frequently improve when switched to a hypoallergenic formula, such as Nutramigen or Alimentum. The advantage of using a soy-based formula is less clearly established. Removing lactose from his diet or adding fiber does not appear to reduce excessive crying. Thus, if your baby is colicky and formula-fed, switching to a hypoallergenic formula for a week is worth a try. Similarly, if you are nursing you can try removing cow's milk protein from your own diet for a while to see if your child's colic is triggered by allergy.

Can changing how my baby is handled improve colic? Increased carrying does not reduce crying. Nor do specific management techniques such as an early response to crying, gentle motion, trying pacifiers or using infant carriers. Still, parents with a colicky infant will probably try all these methods, either on the advice of friends and relatives or out of desperation. Unfortunately, the fact remains that most behavioral intervention seems to make little difference to colic. So, if the cries of a colicky baby become intolerable, it is probably best to let him cry and try not to feel too guilty about doing so.

What about using medication to treat colic? Some drugs, such as dicyclomine, clearly can improve colic. But dicyclomine can also produce very serious side effects and is no longer recommended for use in infants. Simethicone drops probably work no better than a placebo. Finally, in one study,

herbal tea was demonstrated to improve colic in some babies but has not become standard therapy. Some herbal preparations, called gripe water, may even contain some alcohol. Be aware, when herbs are used as medicine, the same caution you use with all medications should apply to them.

Constipation

What is constipation? Constipation in children refers to a pattern of infrequent bowel motions (BMs) associated with straining and discomfort. Although the stools of children with constipation tend to be large and firm, such BMs should not automatically be equated with constipation if they are painless and regular. Rather, this is just a normal variant. Similarly, healthy, comfortable breast-fed infants often have infrequent stools that are still quite soft. This situation, too, is not really constipation in spite of the infrequency of BMs. So whether your child has four bowel motions a day or only one every fourth day, this can be normal as long as the stool is not hard and difficult or painful to pass.

Because normal stool patterns are often seen as a sign of health, parents seem to display quite an interest in their children's stools. Thus, when a child becomes constipated, you might become concerned, and then frustrated. Yet constipation, particularly beyond early infancy, is seldom caused by serious disease. In fact, constipation is actually quite common: in one study, 16 percent of toddlers were reported by their parents to be constipated.

What causes constipation? Most childhood constipation, over 95 percent, is due to chronic functional constipation, which means that no identifiable disease is at fault. Rather, a number

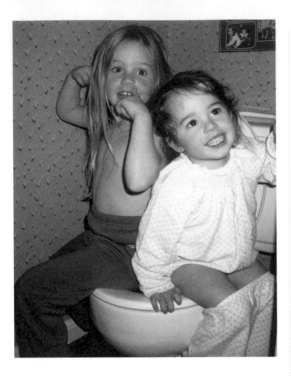

of factors can be involved. These include an inherited tendency toward slow fecal passage, your child's diet (too little fiber or fluid), psychological issues (for example, too much pressure to become toilet trained) and an understandable tendency to avoid the painful defecation caused by huge BMs, which only causes further stool retention.

Rarely, a true pathological condition may be causing a child's constipation. Hirschsprung's disease, which is associated with faulty neurological development in the large bowel, can produce constipation from birth. One of the clues that suggests this condition is when a newborn does not pass meconium in the first 24 to 48 hours of life. Congenital abnormalities of the spinal cord or anus, and some endocrine disorders, such as hypothyroidism, also can cause constipation.

What does constipation look like? The great majority of children who are constipated appear quite healthy. There usually is no history of weight loss, unexplained fever, vomiting or diminished appetite. If present, they are "red flags" that can indicate the presence of an underlying disease. On the other hand, your child might have a history of withholding his stool. This strongly suggests functional constipation.

Occasionally, constipation is associated with overflow leakage. This involuntary stool passage is called encopresis. It is very disturbing to the family faced with the problem. To treat the encopresis, the constipation must first be taken care of. You can find more detailed information about encopresis on pages 37–38.

Your child's physical examination tends to be normal. His doctor may well feel stool as a soft, squishy lump in the lower abdomen. There are occasionally signs of an anal tear (fissure). This can result in a little bleeding, often seen on the tissue after wiping. A rectal examination, if done, reveals normal anal sphincter (opening) tone and lots of stool in the rectum. An empty rectum suggests Hirschsprung's disease.

How is constipation treated? Constipation is best managed when treatment is individualized. Mild constipation that follows a child's brief illness, during which there was fever and diminished oral intake, is obviously a different situation than dealing with the child who defiantly withholds stools and then experiences overflow soiling. Yet, the main components of therapy are fairly consistent. First, for all but the mildest cases, your child's doctor should assess the contributing factors, both physical and psychological. Possible causative diseases can be excluded and the problem better understood. Demystifying the constipation is followed by a treatment plan that provides a clear framework for approaching the problem. Next, the accumulated stool must

MEDICATIONS USED TO TREAT CONSTIPATION

MEDICATION	DOSE	MODE OF ACTION	PRECAUTIONS
Mineral oil	$\frac{1}{10} - \frac{1}{3}$ tsp/lb (1–3 mL/kg) per day orally	Lubricant laxative	Not for young infants and never force feed: it can cause **aspiration pneumonia.** Unwanted oily seepage in underwear.
Lactulose	$\frac{1}{10} - \frac{1}{3}$ tsp/lb (1–3 mL/kg) per day orally	Increases stool water content	Safe and well tolerated.
Sorbitol	$\frac{1}{10} - \frac{1}{3}$ tsp/lb (1–3 mL/kg) per day orally	Increases stool water content	Safe and well tolerated.
Senna (Senokot)	1–5 yr: 1 tsp (5 mL) with breakfast 5–12 yr: 1 tsp (5 mL) twice daily	Stimulant laxative	Used for disimpaction. Don't use if severe cramping present.
Bisacodyl (Dulcolax)	5 mg orally or 5–10 mg rectally	Stimulant laxative	Used for disimpaction. Give at bedtime to reduce cramps.
Ducosate Na (Colace)	$\frac{1}{5} - \frac{1}{3}$ tsp/lb (2–3 mL/kg) per day in divided doses	Stool softener	Safe but don't use in combination with mineral oil as oil absorption is increased.
Glycerin suppository	1 infant suppository/d for < 2–3 days	Lubricant	Used for disimpaction.
Phosphate enema (Fleet)	2–12 yr: 4 tbs (60 mL) as single dose	Increases stool water content	For disimpaction only. Use only with medical advice.

be emptied (disimpaction). Usually, this can be accomplished by oral laxatives but enemas may be needed. Eliminating the impacted stool helps restore normal muscle tone in the rectum and the appropriate urge to defecate. Finally, a maintenance plan is needed to preserve bowel regularity. Usually, this strategy involves changing your child's diet, modifying his behavior and judicious laxative usage.

Behavior modification includes scheduling regular, unhurried toileting times. A diary or calendar combined with a reward system can provide motivation if your child is mature enough to participate in this training format. Family conflict over toileting issues should stop. Encourage your child to take control of his own toileting. There can be no battle of wills once the battlefield is removed.

Although the scientific evidence for dietary modification to help constipation is not strong, dietary change is commonly used to treat the problem, often with apparent success. A high-fiber diet and increased fluid intake are recommended. This can easily be achieved by adding bran cereals, whole wheat bread, prunes or figs, baked beans, peas, lentils and corn to the diet. Dietary carbohydrates, especially sorbitol, are also encouraged to increase stool frequency. These are found in prune and apple juices and in pears. You should encourage your child to eat a balanced diet that includes all the food groups, including fruits and vegetables, but not to the point of conflict.

Medication is a major component in the treatment of chronic constipation, both for disimpaction and maintenance. Usually, the thought of several months of laxatives is not pleasing for either parents or child, but their use is both appropriate and beneficial. There are different types of laxatives. Some, like mineral oil, are lubricants. Others, such as lactulose and sorbitol, increase stool water content. There are also stimulant laxatives that help restore normal rectal tone and stool evacuation. Suppositories and enemas are sometimes needed to achieve adequate stool emptying. They are best used after medical consultation, as the potential side effects can be serious and most children are disturbed by their use.

Cough

What is a cough? Technically, a cough is the reflex response of a person's airways to irritation. A child's cough is one of the most common symptoms parents must learn to manage. Fortunately, most of the time, a cough is merely the result of an innocuous viral illness that soon passes. As such, it should be accepted as part of growing up because few remedies effectively reduce the cough of the common cold. Occasionally, however, a cough signifies a more serious and potentially treatable disease. It helps to know what conditions can produce a persistent or recurring cough and how parents can better identify them.

What can a cough look like? Determining which particular cough should cause concern is an important challenge. This is best done by assessing the characteristics of the cough. There are three basic features to consider: the duration of the cough, its quality and the associated symptoms.

Duration. Coughs can either be acute, that is, lasting less than three weeks, or chronic. Those coughs of brief duration are generally due to respiratory tract infection, usually the common cold. Rarely, an acute cough will suddenly follow a choking episode that suggests that food or even a foreign body has entered the respiratory system. When a cough persists for a longer period of time or recurs frequently, an underlying disorder must be considered.

Quality. The nature of the cough can provide a clue to its cause. For example, a hoarse, barky cough is associated with croup. An intense coughing spasm that ends in a high-pitched sound (whoop) as the child takes air in, suggests **pertussis** (whooping cough). The dry honking and incessant cough that disappears during sleep is typical of a habit cough. Wet coughs producing green sputum suggest infection.

Associated features. Like most things in life, a specific concern such as a cough is best considered in context.

- Your child with allergies whose productive cough is accompanied by a wheeze probably has asthma.
- Children whose colds always go to the chest with lots of coughing may have asthma. In asthma the cough is often worse at night or after exertion.
- An ill-looking child with a fever who seems to be breathing quickly may well have pneumonia.
- The cough that begins with a cold but persists and is associated with facial pain and green nasal discharge suggests **sinusitis**.
- Poor weight gain and recurrent chest infections may indicate an underlying condition, such as cystic fibrosis or an immune deficiency.

What do I do about a cough? Most coughs are due to simple upper respiratory tract infections that must run their course. Little can or, for that matter, should be done to reduce a cough caused by the common cold. Codeine and dextromethorphan (DM), the two most commonly used cough suppressants, do work—but only as well as a placebo. The same goes for expectorants or echinacea. They're pretty well useless. You might as well offer your child chicken soup or a cup of tea. There are literally dozens of so-called doctor-recommended cough syrups that are available without prescription but that can cause side effects, particularly in young infants. As they are of little help and may occasionally cause harm, we generally don't recommend their use, particularly in the first year of life.

Treating the underlying condition is the key.

WHEN SHOULD YOU SEEK HELP?

- For all newborns and young infants who cough.
- For any child who looks ill or seems to be working hard to breathe.
- If the cough begins after a choking spell.
- If there is no improvement in the cough after a week or if there seems to be a worsening of the symptoms.
- If there is an associated whoop, dusky (blue) spell or significant wheeze.
- Whenever your instincts tell you to.

The cough of asthma needs no cough suppressant, just good anti-asthma therapy. Pneumonia or a sinus infection needs antibiotics. And foreign bodies obviously must be removed.

What is my role? Essentially you need to identify those conditions that require investigation or a specific treatment. If the characteristics of the cough (duration, quality and associated features) are causing you concern, seek medical advice. Similarly, if your instincts warn you that the problem is more than a cold, get it checked. Most of the time, parents respond very reasonably when their children develop respiratory symptoms.

Often, a doctor's physical examination of the child will provide the right diagnosis. Sometimes, simple blood tests and/or a chest x-ray are needed. On rare occasions, more extensive investigation will be required to identify the cause of a cough. These tests are targeted to identify a suspected condition. For example, sweat chloride may be measured to detect cystic fibrosis. A bronchoscopy, which allows the airways to be seen directly, may be necessary to exclude a foreign body. A CT scan of the chest, tuberculin testing or pulmonary function tests may occasionally be appropriate.

Diarrhea

What is diarrhea? Diarrhea is the passage of bowel movements that are more frequent and looser than usual. In order to decide whether or not your child has diarrhea, it is necessary to know what his typical bowel patterns have been in the past. For example, the typical mustard-colored, watery, seedy stool of a breast-fed infant is entirely normal. Some healthy breast-fed babies may have 10 stools a day while others are equally happy producing one or two stools per week. By the age of 18 months, most children have one or two formed stools a day.

The consistency of a person's stool is largely determined by its water content. Normally, much of the liquid present in stool is reabsorbed through the lining of the intestines resulting in a formed bowel motion. However, when the intestines are irritated, for example during an infection, the stool rushes through the bowel quickly, taking more of the liquid material with it. In some bowel diseases, body water is actually secreted into the gut. The result is looser stools: diarrhea.

Many parents are very impressed by the color of their children's diarrhea. This is generally not very helpful as a green stool simply means that the material is passing through the intestines very rapidly. The presence of blood in the stool is more helpful. Fresh red blood suggests that the source of bleeding is in the lower part of bowel, or colon, as opposed to a blacker bloody stool that may look like tar, called melena. This suggests that the bleeding is coming from high up in the bowel, closer to the stomach or duodenum.

What is acute diarrhea and what are its causes? Diarrhea can be described as either acute or chronic, depending on its duration. Anything less than two weeks is referred to as acute diarrhea. By far the most common cause of acute diarrhea is an infection of the gastrointestinal tract, called gastroenteritis or, commonly, stomach flu. This is usually indicated by a **low-grade fever** and vomiting that then goes on to diarrhea after about 24 to 48 hours. The stools are usually very watery, often green and foul smelling. Diarrhea usually lasts less than a week. Most cases of gastroenteritis are caused by a highly contagious virus such as rotavirus or Norwalk virus. Therefore, other family members and friends may also have symptoms around the same time. The actual infection tends to be harmless and self-limiting, but the combination of vomiting and diarrhea place the child at high risk for dehydration. To prevent this, parents are advised to give the child lots of liquid in frequent, small amounts.

Acute diarrhea can also be caused by bacteria, such as salmonella, shigella, E. coli or campylobacter. These infections are more likely to be picked up while traveling in developing countries or by eating foods or drinking water that is contaminated. Children with these bacterial infections tend to be sicker than those with viral gastroenteritis. They often have higher fevers and frequently there is blood mixed in with the stool, which is very unusual in viral gastroenteritis. Parasitic infections can also be acquired by ingesting contaminated food or water. **Giardiasis** (see pages 98–99) is the most common. Many infected children have no symptoms but it can cause diarrhea with pale, floating, foul-smelling stools. This should be suspected, for example, in children who drink well water or who develop symptoms after a camping trip (beaver fever).

Food poisoning is a form of stomach flu caused by certain chemicals, called toxins, that are produced by bacteria, often staphylococcus. Food or water contaminated with these toxins are ingested, which produces profuse vomiting and diarrhea about two to six hours afterward. A clue that food poisoning is the cause of an outbreak of acute diarrhea would be the presence of similar symptoms in other people who ate the same food.

Diarrhea can occur as a side effect of medication, particularly certain antibiotics. When this happens, it does not mean that the child is necessarily allergic to the medicine or that the drug must be stopped, especially if the diarrhea is quite mild.

What produces chronic diarrhea in kids? It is easiest to look at the causes of chronic diarrhea by the age of the child. Remember, for babies in the first few months of life, frequent mushy stools are usually normal. The most common true problem would be some intolerance to the cow's milk protein present in many formulas. Even breast-fed babies can have this disorder because these proteins can be in their mother's breast milk. These babies may seem uncomfortable feeding and might even vomit. Babies with cow's milk protein intolerance tend to lose microscopic amounts of protein and blood in the stools. If severe, it can cause them to look pale from anemia and a bit puffy if the protein loss is large. Many of the children allergic to cow's milk also cannot tolerate soy protein. Therefore, they may require a special hypoallergenic

formula, free of both milk and soy, in order to thrive. Fortunately, for the great majority of affected children, this intolerance seems to settle by 2 or 3 years of age.

Lactose intolerance can also produce chronic or persistent diarrhea. Here's how: The sugar in milk and dairy products is called lactose. In order for it to be absorbed, lactose must first be partially broken down by an enzyme, lactase, that is found on the microscopic tips of the intestinal wall. If the amount of lactase is reduced, the result is an inability to digest the lactose in milk products. The undigested lactose passes into the large intestine and ferments, resulting in abdominal cramps, bloating and diarrhea. Permanent lactose intolerance is an uncommon condition in young children. It is most prevalent among children of Asian and African descent but, even in them, it is very rare for symptoms to show up until they are at least 2 to 3 years old. Teenagers and adults tend to have more symptoms. Lactose intolerance is much more common after a bout of diarrhea due to viral gastroenteritis. In this case, microscopic damage to the intestinal wall reduces the amount of available lactase and results in the frequent passage of watery stools whenever milk is consumed. This problem is temporary and tends to clear up after a few weeks. If there is any question that lactose intolerance is causing diarrhea, then you might try lactose-free formula for infants or avoid dairy products for older children.

Celiac disease or gluten sensitive enteropathy occurs when the small intestine is extremely sensitive to a particular protein, called gluten, that is found in wheat, rye, barley and oats. This gluten sensitivity eventually damages the lining of the intestine resulting in malabsorption (difficulty in absorbing food). A clue to the diagnosis is that symptoms don't start until some time after

SEEK IMMEDIATE MEDICAL ATTENTION	CONCERNED ABOUT
Vomiting and refusing to drink	dehydration
Unexplained drowsiness, dry tongue and sunken eyes	dehydration
The stools are mixed with fresh blood or are black and tar-like	bleeding
The stools are pale and oily and do not flush	malabsorption
Severe abdominal cramps	inflammatory bowel disease

the infant is fed cereals, usually toward the end of the first year. Most children with a gluten sensitivity are very irritable, have poor weight gain and energy levels, and their stomach might stick out. Celiac disease can sometimes be a difficult diagnosis to make: not every case is a fussy infant with diarrhea and poor weight gain. It might not even be diagnosed until adulthood. Yet, whatever the age or how it shows up, celiac disease responds very well to the removal of gluten from the diet.

Other forms of food allergy can also produce diarrhea but this is relatively unusual. If children are truly allergic to foods, such as eggs or nuts, they are more likely to react with rashes, hives, swelling of the lips and breathing difficulties, although they might also have diarrhea and vomiting.

Other causes of malabsorption can result in diarrhea and abnormal stools. Cystic fibrosis is an inherited disease, one of the signs of which is malabsorption. The ducts in the pancreas become blocked up, preventing the pancreatic digestive enzymes from entering the bowels. As a result, the child has difficulty digesting fat: the stools tend to look oily and are difficult to flush as they tend to float. In addition to the diarrhea, children with cystic fibrosis often suffer frequent chest infections. Parents of young babies may notice that their skin tastes salty. Children with cystic fibrosis seem to feed very well but, because of malabsorption, gain weight slowly.

Inflammatory bowel diseases, such as Crohn's disease and ulcerative colitis, can also produce chronic diarrhea. These conditions are rare in younger children and mainly affect teenagers. Inflammatory bowel disease often runs in families and results in inflammation of the intestines. Children with Crohn's disease usually have diarrhea, abdominal cramping or just poor growth and weight gain. Ulcerative colitis is characterized by diarrhea, typically bloody, and over time is associated with weight loss and poor growth. When we see children with bloody diarrhea we usually think of an acute bacterial infection, but if it does not settle down and the stool cultures do not grow any bacteria, inflammatory bowel disease should be considered, especially in a teenager.

Many healthy toddlers produce frequent watery stools, sometimes containing undigested food particles. These youngsters don't complain of any abdominal pain and they gain weight appropriately. Such children are said to have "toddler's diarrhea." This may be related to a high intake of fluids, especially fruit juice, because the sugar causes excess fluid to be poured into the intestine. Reducing sugar in the diet and increasing fiber content will improve stool frequency and consistency.

Paradoxically, severe constipation can be another cause of chronic diarrhea. Children who have very large stools blocking the rectum may leak liquid stool around the hard stool, usually resulting in soiled underwear. These children will have a history of infrequent very hard stools or anal fissures. Aggressively treating the constipation, under medical supervision, will bring the situation under control.

How can I treat diarrhea? The treatment of diarrhea depends on making the right diagnosis. Acute diarrhea is usually treated with fluid and electrolyte (salt) replacement. Infants should be offered special electrolyte solutions (called **oral rehydration solutions**) but you don't have to stop breast-feeding. Older children can be given soup, tea, soft drinks and diluted fruit juice. As for solids, let the child's appetite determine food intake. In the past, doctors recommended restricting solid intake but, unless your child is vomiting nonstop, it is better to continue offering light, tasty meals. Some of the bacterial and parasitic causes of gastroenteritis might require treatment with antibiotics, but only after the organism has been cultured in the stool and the symptoms persist. Antidiarrheal medications are not recommended for children because they don't cure the problem and can mask the diagnosis.

If the diarrhea continues for more than a week, you should see your regular physician who will work through the possible causes based on your child's age, history, physical examination and laboratory tests.

Encopresis (Fecal Soiling)

What is encopresis? As much as parents love their children, most feel that by the time their toddler turns 2 or 3, they have changed enough diapers. It's time for toilet training. In many families, however, the task is not that simple. About 3 percent of 4-year-olds, mainly boys, are not bowel trained. This condition is called encopresis.

From a practical standpoint, there are two patterns of encopresis. The most common is soiling associated with constipation and fecal retention. In this situation, the rectum is so continually stretched that your child has difficulty sensing the need to defecate. Overflow leakage also tends to occur. A number of factors may have predisposed your child to constipation. Some healthy children seem normally predisposed to infrequent stools. It's just how their bowel works. Other contributors to constipation include diet, stool retention to avoid a painfully large bowel movement, toileting fears and ineffective toilet training. Only very rarely is a child's constipation due to an unsuspected medical condition involving the gut or nervous system.

The second pattern of encopresis occurs without constipation. Typically, a battle of wills has developed between the parents who want their child bowel trained and the child who, for whatever reason, defiantly resists being told what to do.

What does encopresis look like? Most often there has been a prior history of hard and/or infrequent bowel motions. The child with constipation-induced encopresis typically produces small, poorly formed stools and has leakage day or night.

In the unconstipated group, the stools tend to be large and well formed. They can be deliberately deposited in annoying places that can infuriate parents. The child tends to be strong willed and resists instruction. Another scenario is the youngster with attention deficit hyperactivity disorder (ADHD) who impulsively responds to the urge "to go" whether or not a toilet is nearby.

How is encopresis treated? The problem of encopresis is simply too charged with emotion to be managed without assistance. Your child's doctor can review the situation, exclude any possible medical cause for the condition and offer a treatment plan that will provide the framework for ending the soiling.

Dealing with any constipation is a priority. Only when the rectum is no longer stretched with excess stool will normal bowel sensation be restored and overflow soiling ended. Although a healthy, high-fiber diet will eventually help, by the time encopresis has developed, laxatives are needed. There are different types. Some laxatives soften the stool and lubricate its passage, some add bulk to the stool, which is not needed in this situation, and some stimulate the bowel to contract. The choice of laxatives should be individualized according to the situation. When things improve, your child can be weaned slowly from laxative use.

Behavioral management is also an important part of treating encopresis. The emphasis should be positive, not punitive.

- Praise and reward work best.
- Encourage regular toilet sitting for at least a few minutes. Often after meals or first thing in the morning are the most productive times.
- Once the constipation improves, begin a "star chart," a calendar that records successful days with a star or sticker.
- When a particular target has been reached, a suitable reward (not necessarily material) can follow.

If your child's encopresis is the result of a battle of wills, end the battle. When confrontation over toileting stops, so will your child's need for resistance. You can discuss the matter with your child either by yourselves or with mediation provided by your child's doctor. Essentially, declare a truce. Transfer responsibility for bowel control to your child. Let him decide when to use the toilet without reminders. The only assistance offered should be help in disposing of stools. This task should be viewed as unpleasant but not earth-shattering. If the situation shows no improvement after a month or so, review the problem again with your child's doctor. Sometimes, more intense counseling or psychiatric assistance is needed.

Although managing encopresis tends to be a challenge for everyone involved, things do eventually get better. Less than 1 percent of children have a problem by age 11. It's highly unlikely that your child will get married in diapers.

Enuresis (Bedwetting)

What is enuresis? Nocturnal enuresis refers to wetting the bed at night while your child is asleep. Diurnal enuresis, on the other hand, refers to wetting during the day while awake. Doctors may talk about primary enuresis, referring to children who have never been "dry," or secondary enuresis, which begins at least six months after the child is dry.

Most children will become toilet trained between 2 and 4 years of age. Night wetting still occurs in about 40 percent of 3-year-olds, and this decreases to 20 percent by the age of 5 years. Boys are affected with primary nocturnal enuresis more than girls. Interestingly, there seems to be a tendency for bedwetting to run in families. If you were a bedwetter (you will likely need to ask your own parents about this), your child has a 45 percent chance of following in your wet footsteps. If both you and your spouse were bedwetters, then this likelihood goes up to 77 percent!

When should I consider enuresis to be a problem? Most parents become concerned about nighttime bedwetting after the age of 5 or 6 years, although children themselves aren't usually concerned about the issue until 7 or 8 years of age. Daytime wetting may be considered a problem in a child older than 4 years who wets on most days. A child who was previously trained and begins wetting during the day or night has secondary enuresis. A child with this should always be taken to his doctor because the enuresis could indicate an underlying problem.

What causes enuresis? In most cases, bedwetting results from a delayed maturation of parts of the nervous system that control the bladder. Different children are ready for this at different ages. Think of how some babies are walking at 9 months while other normal infants only start at 15 months: each individual develops at a different pace. Also, the bladder may not be developed enough to hold urine for a full night. Clues to this lack of readiness include:

frequent small amounts of urine passed during the daytime or wetness several times during the night. In addition, the child may not be capable of recognizing that the bladder is full, waking and going to the washroom.

Secondary enuresis can result from a new stress in the child's life, for example, the arrival of a new sibling, illness or a death in the family, even divorce. Very rarely, in about 1 percent of cases, there are conditions such as diabetes, sickle-cell disease, constipation and various bladder problems that can contribute to the bedwetting. Many of these children display additional symptoms that provide clues to the source of the problem. For example, excess urine production (polyuria) is seen in diabetes. Children with bladder infections might also have pain and frequent urination. They usually need to urinate urgently and the urine passed may be cloudy and smelly. Constipated children will have very hard infrequent stools and may also leak some liquid stool (encopresis).

Diurnal enuresis (daytime wetting) can be caused by problems with the nerve supply to the bladder, for example cerebral palsy. If there is a spinal cord problem then walking and bowel motions can also be affected. Other possible causes of daytime wetting include constipation, urinary tract infection and diabetes.

How is enuresis treated? Children almost always outgrow their bedwetting, so that many will manage well without any specific treatment at all. Only 5 percent of 10-year-olds and 2 percent of 16-year-olds will still be bedwetters.

The most important thing for you to remember is that enuresis is unconscious and involuntary. Your child is not trying to make things difficult for or torture you. Most parents do not appreciate having to constantly change and wash the

WHEN SHOULD YOU GO TO THE DOCTOR?

- Nighttime wetting: when it bothers. the child, usually by 7 or 8 years.
- Daytime wetting: from the age of 5.
- Wetting in a previously dry child (secondary enuresis).
- If there are other symptoms: polyuria, frequency, dysuria, constipation.

WHAT CAN I DO TO HELP?

- Do not blame or punish.
- Support and reassure.
- No drinking just before bed.
- Go to the washroom before bed.
- Use a star chart (positive reinforcement).
- Try a bedwetting alarm.

- Use a plastic cover on the mattress.
- If your child wets the bed, you might want to encourage one who is old enough to help with changing the bedding. This should not be seen as a punishment but more as a form of self-sufficiency. Make sure that the other children are also given chores so that one child doesn't feel singled out.
- A calendar on which your child sticks a star after each dry night provides extra motivation. This is successful in about 20 percent of children, although some of them do relapse.
- Encouraging your child to go without diapers overnight when he is not ready is unlikely to help.

Bedwetting alarms are often recommended, particularly for older children who are highly motivated to achieve dryness. There are many different types of alarms. They usually consist of a device for sensing wetness, which is attached to the child's pajamas close to the groin, and a buzzer close to the child's ear. The first drops of urine will set off the alarm, which wakes the child and stops the urination. The child then takes off the alarm and goes to the washroom. If the child is sufficiently motivated and willing to use the alarm for a month or two, the success rate is as high as 70 percent to 90 percent. About 20 percent relapse when they stop using the alarm.

Some doctors may recommend bladder stretching exercises, such as encouraging the child to hold on for a few minutes after the initial urge to urinate. This is theoretically helpful in a child with a small functional bladder capacity. The evidence as to how helpful these exercises are is inconclusive.

There are a number of medications that are prescribed for the treatment of bedwetting. Because this is a developmental problem that

bedding, but resist your feelings of frustration and anger. You need to make sure that your child understands that it is not his fault, that you do not blame the child or think he is lazy and that it will get better with time.

There should be no teasing by other family members: they should be sensitive to the problem. Enuresis is usually embarrassing for the child and may lead to a reluctance to sleep over at a friend's home or camp. Some common sense, simple rules can help.

- Your child should not drink, especially anything containing caffeine, just before bedtime, although do not send a child to bed thirsty.
- Expect your child to go to the washroom just before bedtime.

tends to get better with time, the risks and benefits of these options should be carefully discussed before starting medication. The most frequently recommended medicine is called DDAVP (desmopressin), a form of antidiuretic hormone. This hormone occurs naturally in the body to help you retain water and decrease urination. It can be given by nasal spray or tablets. It is effective in up to 70 percent of children, but many of them will relapse once they stop the drug. Desmopressin is particularly useful for short-term concerns, such as ensuring dryness on overnight stays with friends or at overnight camp. An older medicine called imipramine has also been shown to be effective in some cases. It is more commonly used as an antidepressant and can have some serious side effects. It should not be considered as a first choice for therapy. Imipramine is particularly dangerous if an overdose is taken, so you would need to keep it well out of reach of any children.

Fainting (Syncope)

What is fainting? The medical term for fainting is syncope. It is defined as a temporary but complete loss of consciousness that is accompanied by a loss of postural tone and followed by spontaneous recovery. Syncope is common: 15 percent of individuals faint at least once during childhood, usually in adolescence.

As you will read, there are many different causes for syncope; some are serious but most are not. Yet, the basic mechanism for fainting remains the same: the occurrence of a sudden decrease of blood supply to the brain.

Circulation to the brain is maintained by a complex control system that requires adequate amounts of blood, good cardiac (heart) output

and sufficient tone in the blood vessels to maintain blood pressure. This latter component, the maintenance of vessel tone, is important as it allows adjustments for various changes in posture, such as sitting up or standing. The process is controlled by certain tone sensors that cause the muscles in the blood vessels to contract or relax as needed, using the nerve pathways of the sympathetic nervous system.

What can cause fainting? Most fainting spells are due to something called neurocardiogenic syncope which is the medical term for a simple faint. In some individuals, the reflexes that control postural tone are very sensitive, making them susceptible to fainting. Fear, real or imagined, or an unpleasant stimulus such as the sight of blood, provokes a response that can rapidly lower blood pressure. The blood supply to the brain drops and the individual faints. The typical scenario is an adolescent who is standing, often in hot or close quarters for some time. Before consciousness is lost, there is usually a feeling of light-headedness, weakness, blurred vision or nausea. The teen usually looks pale or sweaty. Consciousness and body tone are then lost, usually only briefly. Prolonged unresponsiveness and muscle jerks can occur in a simple faint but they are quite rare. After the faint, there is no state of confusion but symptoms return if he sits or tries to stand too soon. The occurrence of an occasional simple faint is seldom a sign of serious disease.

Another cause for fainting is called orthostatic hypotension. In this situation, blood pressure falls abruptly when a person stands up without sufficient compensation of an increased heart rate. Blood flow to the brain becomes inadequate followed by events similar to the simple faint. Orthostatic hypotension is most

WARNING SIGNS IN SYNCOPE

- Simple fainting in a child under the age of 10 years is unusual. Seek a cause.
- Fainting that occurs with exercise may be due to a heart problem.
- A history of palpitations or prior heart surgery also suggests a cardiac cause.
- If the child is diabetic or appears clammy, shaky or weak, and/or it has been several hours since he ate, consider low blood sugar (hypoglycemia).
- If the fainting comes on suddenly without warning signs and is associated with muscle jerking and drowsiness afterwards, think seizure.
- If the fainting occurs repeatedly, always in front of an audience, in an adolescent girl, has no "aura" and causes little anxiety and no injury from the fall, consider a conversion reaction.

likely to occur in susceptible individuals who have been standing for long periods, particularly if conditions exist that reduce their blood volume. Dehydration from diarrhea or sweating excessively from heat and exercise are common examples of this. Certain medications, alcohol and poor muscle tone can also contribute to orthostatic hypotension.

A number of heart conditions can lead to fainting. These are much less common than simple faints but extremely important to identify because, if undiagnosed and untreated, sudden death can be the tragic result. The three groups of cardiac conditions that are associated with syncope are: obstructive defects that prevent adequate blood flow on exertion, coronary artery abnormalities that can deprive the heart muscles of enough oxygen, and arrhythmias, which are abnormalities in the heart's electrical conduction system that controls the beating of the heart.

The defects prevent the heart from increasing its rate when required, ultimately leading to inadequate cerebral blood flow. Examples of these include heart block and an inherited condition, called prolonged Q-T syndrome. Two clues that suggest a cardiac cause for a child's syncope are a history of palpitations or fainting during exertion. Obstructions are usually accompanied by a readily detected heart murmur and conduction defects are often, but not necessarily, associated with a history of previous heart surgery. Yet some cardiac causes of syncope present no clues that warn us of their presence. Therefore, anyone who faints deserves an electrocardiogram (ECG) and anyone who faints on exertion warrants a detailed cardiac evaluation, including monitoring heart rate for a prolonged period using a Holter monitor.

Psychological causes for fainting must also be considered. Some individuals can become so anxious that they hyperventilate, which, if severe enough, results in a brief loss of consciousness. Usually, a classical history makes this diagnosis obvious. Some cases of syncope are conversion reactions, which are dramatically acted out, fake fainting spells. These are most likely to occur in adolescent girls. Their presence is suggested by a history of recurrent bouts of fainting without initial light-headedness, weakness, nausea or pallor. Conversion reactions always seem to happen in front of witnesses; the teen shows little of the anxiety expected from a faint and any fall is protected so it never produces injury.

There are a number of other medical conditions that can be associated with a loss of consciousness. A coughing spasm can actually be so severe that too little oxygen reaches the brain. This is frequently seen in pertussis (whooping cough). Low blood sugar (hypoglycemia) can produce syncope. An intoxicated teen can pass out if he drinks enough. And, of course, a seizure can produce unconsciousness. Usually, convulsions differ from syncope because they have few or no preliminary symptoms, there are usually associated convulsive movements and the child appears drowsy when consciousness is restored.

What do I do about fainting? Although 80 percent of all syncope is due to a simple faint (neurocardiogenic syncope), anyone who faints for the first time should be evaluated. The treatable causes of syncope must be identified through appropriate testing. Therefore, you should consult a health care professional.

Recurrences of syncope are more often seen in those with psychological or cardiac causes.

Fever

What is a fever? Fever is a sign. It is not an illness. Fever means that the body's temperature is elevated, usually in response to an infection or inflammation. Therefore, fever should not necessarily be seen as a bad thing but rather as an appropriate immune reaction. Generally, finding the cause of a child's fever is the problem, not the fever itself.

The body's normal temperature ranges from 96.8°F to 100°F (36°C to 37.8°C). There is a natural rhythm to body temperature: it is lower in the morning and increases in the early evening. A child is considered to be febrile (have a fever) if the temperature is above this range but the exact number will vary depending on where the

temperature is taken. The usual definition of fever is a temperature over 100.4°F (38°C), if taken rectally. If measured in the mouth (orally) or the ear (tympanic), fever is a temperature over 99.5°F (37.5°C) while under the arm (axillary), it is over 99°F (37.2°C).

Where and how should I take the temperature? When a child is very feverish it is often easy to tell by the age-old method of touching the forehead with the back of the hand, but this is not at all reliable and is not recommended. The forehead strips that change color on contact with the skin are also too inaccurate to be useful. The older glass mercury thermometers have to some extent been replaced by the newer plastic digital thermometers that are cheap, easy to use and give a much quicker reading. Some authorities do not recommend using mercury thermometers because the glass can break leading to accidental exposure to mercury. Both glass and digital thermometers can be used to measure the temperature in the mouth, rectum or armpit.

Rectal temperatures are the most accurate but least convenient and practical. In order to use a rectal thermometer, place some petroleum jelly on the tip of the thermometer, insert the tip into the anus no farther than 1 inch (2.5 cm) and leave it in place for three minutes. Oral temperatures are obtained by placing the tip of the thermometer in the mouth under the tongue and are quite difficult to use in younger children due to lack of cooperation. The child needs to press his lips together without biting the thermometer for two to three minutes in the case of mercury thermometers, less time with digital models. Taking the temperature in the ear is easier and much quicker, but the tympanic thermometer is

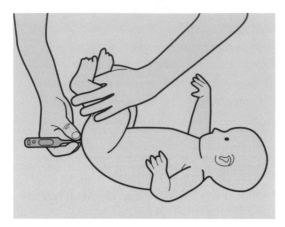

TAKING A RECTAL TEMPERATURE
When taking a child's temperature rectally, pinch the lubricated thermometer 1 inch (2.5 cm) from the end to avoid inserting too far.

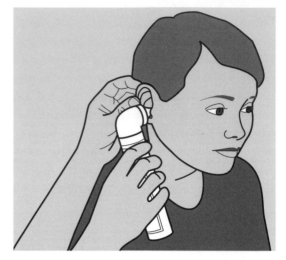

USING A TYMPANIC THERMOMETER
Gently pull the ear backward and upward, then apply the thermometer tip to seal the ear canal.

more expensive and can be inaccurate to within 0.9°F (0.5°C) of the rectal temperature. It is sometimes difficult to fit the ear piece well in younger babies, and so some authorities don't recommend its use in the first year or two of life. Taking the temperature with an oral thermometer under the arm is easiest but also least accurate. The thermometer needs to stay high in the armpit for about five minutes with the arm tightly against the child's side.

Ultimately the exact temperature may not be as important as how the child looks and is behaving: treat the child and not the thermometer! An accurate temperature reading is very important in the first three months of life and, therefore, a rectal temperature is the only reliable method to use. Thereafter, families may choose a tympanic or axillary route until the child is about 4 years old, at which time an oral temperature becomes practical. In one study the majority of children between 5 and 16 years of age preferred to have their temperature taken in the ear rather than under the arm.

What could be causing the fever? You should be asking, "What is causing the fever?" not "What can I do to stop the fever?" The most common cause of fever is some sort of infection. In children, viral illness tends to be much more common than more serious bacterial infections. For example, if your child has cold symptoms, the fever is likely secondary to a viral upper respiratory tract infection. If he is vomiting and has diarrhea, the fever is likely caused by a viral stomach flu. If the fever stays up and he has a cough with some difficulty breathing then he may have a more serious problem, such as a chest infection (pneumonia). To tell the difference between a mild viral infection and a more serious bacterial infection you need to look not so much at the fever but more at your child's behavior in general. Very rarely, the first sign of more serious problems, such as inflammatory conditions, for example, arthritis, or even malignancy, can be a fever, but these children will generally have other worrisome symptoms and fever that lasts longer than just a few days.

When should I worry? The majority of fevers are likely to be caused by viral infections for which there is no specific treatment. If your child is generally healthy and looks well despite the fever, still has an appetite and is playful and active, it is not necessary to seek medical attention in the first 48 hours. If you feel that the child is uncomfortable as a result of the fever, you can give fever control medication (antipyretics), and it is somewhat reassuring if the child perks up as the fever breaks. If your child is under 6 months, or you are having difficulty controlling the fever after 48 hours, or the child looks unwell in other ways, it may be advisable to seek medical advice.

There are certain scenarios where a fever needs to be dealt with by seeking medical attention immediately. In the case of children whose immune system is compromised—for example, children with cancer or sickle-cell disease—a fever may be the first sign of a life-threatening infection. Their bodies may be unable to fight off the infection without medication. A more common problem would be the infant who develops a fever in the first three months of life. In this case, the immune system is still developing: the signs and symptoms of a very serious infection, such as **meningitis,** can be very nonspecific. Fever might be the only clue that something serious is brewing. It is not safe to assume that the higher the temperature the more serious the illness, as children with mild viral infections can have fevers of 104°F (40°C), while those with serious bacterial infections can have a temperature of 101.3°F (38.5°C) or, occasionally in younger infants, subnormal temperatures.

How do I treat the fever? Medication is only necessary if your child appears to be uncomfortable or irritable as a result of the fever, which is often not

YOUR CHILD HAS A FEVER IF THE TEMPERATURE IS:

LOCATION	TEMPERATURE
In the armpit	>99°F (37.2°C)
In the mouth	>99.5°F (37.5°C)
In the ear	>99.5°F (37.5°C)—may vary slightly depending on the manufacturer
In the rectum	>100.4°F (38°C)

the case. The evidence from studies suggests that antipyretic (antifever) medication will not alter the course of the illness. The most commonly used antipyretic drug is acetaminophen, which is available in drops, syrup, chewable tablets, capsules and suppositories (good for use in children who are vomiting or refuse to take medication by mouth). The dosage will depend on the weight of the child, 5 mg to 7 mg per pound (10 to 15 mg per kg) given every four hours if necessary. Another commonly used option is ibuprofen, which studies have shown to be equally effective and as safe as acetaminophen. It is only required every six to eight hours at a dose of 2.5 mg to 5 mg per pound (5 mg to 10 mg per kg). Acetylsalicylic acid (aspirin) is not recommended for children because of the risk of them developing Reye's syndrome, which is a serious condition affecting the brain and liver. Antipyretic medications should not be used in the first three months of life without first checking with your doctor.

We generally recommend dressing your child lightly and not bundling him up, because this can prevent the escape of the body's excess

MOST COMMON CAUSES OF CHILDHOOD FEVER BY AGE:

AGE	CAUSE	SUSPECT IF
Newborns (0–2 m)	– infections are usually viral but very difficult to distinguish from more serious bacterial infections – dehydration and overbundling can cause a very low-grade fever in the first few weeks	
Infants (2–12 m)	– upper respiratory viral infections (colds) – ear infections (especially after 6 m) – teething does not cause fever	– runny nose, congested – irritable, pulling on ear
Toddlers, preschoolers (1–6 yrs)	– upper respiratory viral infections – otitis media (ear infection) – sore throat/tonsillitis – gastroenteritis (stomach infections) – respiratory infections (pneumonia/bronchitis)	– runny nose, congested – irritable, pulling on ear – sore throat, red pusy tonsils – vomiting, diarrhea – cough, breathing difficult
Schoolchildren (>6 yrs)	– respiratory infections (pneumonia/bronchitis) – urinary tract infections (especially in girls)	– cough, breathing difficult – pain with urination, foul-smelling urine

heat. If your child is feeling cold and is shivering, it is acceptable to cover him with a light blanket until the shivering stops. It is important that children stay well hydrated and be offered plenty of liquids. Tepid water sponging when combined with antipyretics has shown a slight advantage in trials over medication alone in bringing the fever down in the first 30 minutes after treatment. Avoid using water so cold as to make your child shiver and generate more body heat. Sponging with rubbing alcohol is definitely not recommended.

Since most fevers are viral in origin, no specific treatment is available to treat the infection. Antibiotics do not work against viruses, so they should not be used for children with colds, flu or sore throats not caused by strep. If the fever has a bacterial cause, as for example in urinary tract infections, strep throat and some ear infections, then it is likely that your child will require antibiotics.

Can the fever do any harm? Fever on its own is not dangerous to the child unless it reaches extremely high levels (over 104.9°F/40.5°C), which is very unusual. Children between the ages of 6 months and 6 years can occasionally have a convulsion with the fever, called a febrile convulsion. This occurs in about 4 percent of all children. Although it is an extremely frightening and distressing experience for the parents, febrile convulsions are not dangerous and do not lead to any brain damage. Studies have shown that 97 percent of these children tend to grow out of the seizures by the age of 6 years and will function normally at school and university. There is no evidence to suggest that lowering the fever with acetaminophen will decrease the likelihood of the child having a febrile convulsion. That said, most physicians and parents do treat fevers more readily with acetaminophen in children with a past history of febrile convulsions.

Headache

Headaches are quite common in children. They tend to worry parents because most people recognize that headaches can indicate the presence of serious disease. Although it is possible for a headache to signal the existence of a brain tumor or suggest **meningitis,** fortunately these

situations are very rare. How then should you react when your child complains of a headache? The best approach is to evaluate the problem in the context of the entire situation. Headaches tend to occur in distinctive patterns that help define their nature and suggest the best treatment. Because children are often incapable of describing their symptoms precisely, it is generally wise to consult a physician when the cause of a child's headache seems in doubt.

MIGRAINE

What is migraine? Migraines are recurrent headaches caused by a transient spasm and the subsequent dilatation of arteries supplying the brain. The reasons why some people, about 5 percent to 7 percent of school-aged children, possess this tendency for blood vessel instability is unclear but there is often a family history of migraines. A number of migraine triggers have been implicated, such as food intolerance (cheddar cheese, nitrites, MSG), stress, disordered sleep, bright lights and even weather changes.

Typically, children with migraine experience a throbbing pain that begins on one side of the head or pounds at the temples. Sometimes the discomfort is preceded by the presence of abnormal sensations, such as blurred vision, flashing light, numbness of the extremities or even distortions of body images. These sensations are called "auras" and appear less commonly in children than adults. Migraine headache is frequently accompanied by abdominal pain, nausea and vomiting. Often the child appears pale and complains of feeling lightheaded or is bothered by lights (**photophobia**). The entire episode can last a few hours or even a day or so. Sleep frequently brings relief and the end of the headache. One noteworthy feature of migraine is that between attacks, sufferers are symptom-free.

Not all migraine is typical. Some children with migraine have severe cyclical vomiting rather than a headache. Another type of migraine, basilar migraine, involves the artery that supplies the lower part of the brain. These children tends to have double vision (diplopia), unsteadiness (ataxia), ringing in the ears (tinnitus), dilated pupils and pain at the back of the head. Very rarely, migraine can even manifest itself as temporary weakness or numbness on one side.

How should migraine be managed? An **acute** episode of migraine can often be managed simply by providing pain relief with nonprescription medicine like acetaminophen or ibuprofen. Some studies suggest that ibuprofen is the better of the two for treating migraine. Prescription analgesics, especially ones that are specifically designed to treat migraine, might be administered to children with more severe headaches. Older children who can recognize migraine attacks early sometimes do well with an ergotamine preparation or sumatriptan. When vomiting is a significant problem, antiemetics, such as dimenhydrinate are frequently required. Of course, the best treatment is prevention. Often the use of a diary will help identify the initiating stimuli for migraine attacks and, once discovered, eliminating these triggers will significantly reduce the problem. A number of studies have suggested that behavior management can help migraine sufferers. Biofeedback and relaxation through self-hypnosis can be effective in children old enough to be taught the methods. Occasionally, the frequency and severity of the

FEATURES OF MIGRAINES

- Strong family history of migraine.
- Headache occasionally preceded by a warning sensation or aura.
- Pain often starts on one side of head.
- Pain feels like a throbbing or pounding.
- Nausea, vomiting, abdominal pain and pallor often accompany the pain.
- Child seems well between attacks.

migraine attacks are sufficient to justify taking preventative medicine on a daily basis.

TENSION HEADACHES

Can children get "tension headaches"? You bet they can. A number of children, particularly older girls, experience frequent headaches that appear stress related. Their pain is produced by unconscious contractions of the muscles in the neck, jaw and face. Usually, the pain is described as an aching or pressure sensation rather than the pounding described by migraine sufferers. It is often not really at one specific location, although the back of head and forehead areas are common sites. Tension headaches tend to be steady in nature and low grade in intensity. They often occur daily, but seldom disrupt activities and almost never wake the child up from sleep. Unlike migraine, tension headaches are uncommonly associated with vomiting or pallor. They are often said to occur later in the day or after a stressful activity. However, because being at school is often the stressful trigger, tension headaches can also begin in the morning. Often the factors provoking headache are obvious: scholastic difficulty, peer group conflict, family discord. In other children the cause seems less related to a specific trigger than the child's intense personality and need to be perfect. In fact, the term, "intensity headache" is often more accurate than "tension headache."

How are tension headaches treated? A thorough medical history and physical examination will help to exclude serious disease as a cause of your child's headache. It will also provide an opportunity to start a dialogue on the identification and reduction of stressful triggers. Relieving tension remains the most important treatment of tension headaches. Most of the time, the actual headache can be controlled by simple analgesics, such as acetaminophen or ibuprofen. Drugs are not the only treatment for tension headaches: relaxation exercises and yoga, stress-relieving activities, such as sports or dance, and even enjoying some down time watching television can help children deal with their discomfort.

Is there any overlap between migraine and tension headaches? Certainly. About 20 percent of children with recurring headaches have features of both migraine and tension headaches. This, of course, is not surprising as migraine is often brought on by anxiety or tension. Furthermore, there is no reason why tension headaches should provide immunity from migraine. Thus, a mixed pattern of recurrent headaches can exist, characterized by frequent, low-intensity, pressure-type pain punctuated from time to time by more intense, throbbing headaches associated with nausea and pallor. You can best help your child with a combination of pain

WARNING SIGNS

- Headaches that progressively worsen over a few weeks.
- Headaches that wake a child from sleep.
- Vomiting early in the morning.
- Headaches that occur in preschool-aged children.
- A fever or stiff neck accompanies the headache.

relievers, relaxation techniques and the reduction of identified stressors.

Which headaches suggest serious disease? Headaches that progressively increase in severity over a short period of time and that are associated with either night waking or early morning vomiting should concern you greatly. This picture suggests an elevation in the pressure inside the head that can be due to a brain tumor or hemorrhage. Headaches in preschool children are rare enough to warrant investigation when they occur. Equally alarming are headaches associated with seizures or localizing symptoms or when your doctor detects a neurological abnormality. All these situations require careful medical evaluation and probably neurological imaging, such as computerized tomography (CT) or magnetic resonance imaging (MRI) of the head.

THE INITIAL HEADACHE

How should I respond to a headache in a previously well child? When a child complains of a headache for the first time, the situation poses a diagnostic problem. It can be difficult to determine what is going on and what, if anything, should be done. You must use common sense. First, exclude those conditions that, if present, would demand urgent attention.

- Thus, if your child has both a fever and headache, make sure that he seems alert and can flex his neck without pain, otherwise meningitis becomes a real concern.
- Likewise, if your child has a head injury, seems dazed and complains of a headache, go to your nearest emergency department immediately. Most situations will not be that urgent but still warrant a medical evaluation to assess the problem.
- The relatively well child with a sore throat and a headache may well have strep throat.
- One with persistent nasal discharge could have **sinusitis** that needs treatment.
- In the short term, pain relief with simple analgesics will provide comfort for the child.

Limping

What is limping? Limping refers to an abnormal walking pattern resulting from pain, weakness or structural abnormalities. It is never normal and should not be ignored. There are many possible causes for a limp that range in severity from poorly fitting shoes or a splinter in the foot to serious cancers of the bone. The list of causes is long because children are at increased risk of muscle, bone and joint problems. They tend to be active and their bones are still immature and growing.

What causes limping? The causes vary depending on the age of the child and whether the limp has started suddenly or been gradually getting worse over the course of weeks or months. There are a wide range of possibilities to consider, including inherited and developmental problems, infections, inflammations, injuries, tumors and other illnesses.

If your child has no pain with the limp, this could suggest a discrepancy in the length of the two legs or developmental **dysplasia** of the hip (DDH). A difference in leg lengths could have been present from birth or can occur as the result of damage to the leg. DDH used to be called congenital dislocation of the hip and doctors routinely look for it as part of their examination of newborn babies and at well-baby checkups. You may have noticed extra skin creases on one thigh or that the one hip didn't open as much as the other when you change the diaper. You usually notice the limp when the child starts to walk.

The joints (septic arthritis) or the bones (osteomyelitis) in the legs can become infected resulting in a limp, or more often a complete refusal to walk. The infection is usually caused by bacteria that spread through the bloodstream from elsewhere in the body. The child often has a fever and poor appetite and may look unwell. Depending on which joint or bone is infected, the pain and loss of function may be restricted to that area, or may affect the whole leg. The pain is usually quite severe. There may be swelling and redness over the sore area. Septic arthritis is a medical emergency, because the pus can cause permanent damage to the joint. If infection is suspected then immediate medical attention is necessary.

Inflammation of the joints, that is, juvenile rheumatoid arthritis, can occur in children. Symptoms will vary depending on the type of arthritis. The inflammation can come and go, and affects different joints throughout the body.

The limp can be worse at the beginning of the day rather than at the end of the day, as seen with muscle weakness such as muscular dystrophy. A joint, often the knee, can appear swollen or puffy. Particularly in some types of arthritis, young children can have a fever, **swollen glands** and a rash as well.

It is important to review what the child was doing before you noticed the limp, because injury to the muscles or bones may be responsible. Ankle sprains are common in older children and usually result from a fall when the foot is twisted onto its outside edge. This causes the ankle to swell up and movement in any direction is painful. In young children, a "toddler's fracture" can occur after jumping or twisting and the child might have minimal swelling and a mild limp.

Tumors of the blood (leukemia) and of the bone (osteosarcoma and Ewing's sarcoma) can both result in a limp. Children with leukemia are often under 5 years of age. They might complain of bone pain and look pale and tired and have lost weight. Bone tumors are more common in the teenage years and these children often complain of a persistent deep pain at night and when they are at rest.

There are a number of conditions affecting the hips that could cause your child to limp. They are generally more common in boys. Problems in the hip can cause pain in the knee, which may be misleading. **Transient synovitis** (inflammation of the synovial membrane covering the joint) of the hip is the most common of these hip disorders, and its cause is unknown. It is most often seen in children between 3 and 10 years of age and sometimes occurs one to two weeks after a cold. The child generally feels well. Usually he does not have a fever and, if present, it will be low grade (below 100.4°F/38°C). The hip joint is painful to move and the child may refuse to walk. Perthes

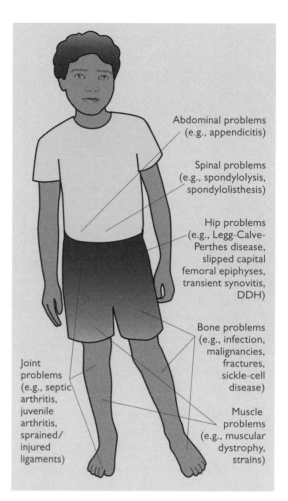

CAUSES OF LIMPING

When a child is limping, the actual site of pain can be misleading; for example, an abnormality in the hip may cause pain in the thigh or knee.

disease is a softening of the growing end of the femur, or thigh bone (see page 219). It occurs in the same age group as transient synovitis. There may or may not be any pain associated with the limp, which begins gradually. Slipped capital femoral **epiphyses** describes a condition where the top part of the femur "slips" into an abnormal position. This usually is diagnosed in overweight teenagers who have sought medical help because of a limp and pain in the hip joint.

Spinal problems (for example, spondylolysis, where a vertebra is defective, or spondylolisthesis, where a vertebra slips forward) and abdominal problems (for example, appendicitis) can also cause a limp. Children with sickle-cell disease may be taken to the doctor because of a crisis in the bones causing pain and refusal to bear weight. The toes (or fingers) can become swollen as the first sign in a previously undiagnosed case.

Swollen or Painful Scrotum

A variety of conditions can cause a boy's scrotum to enlarge or be painful. Although some of these problems are rare, others are not. Collectively, the diseases that produce a painful or swollen scrotum are common and important to identify. You should be aware of what the possibilities are in this situation and how to respond properly to them. All cases of a swollen or painful scrotum will require a medical assessment but some causes demand urgent attention.

What is a scrotum? In order to best understand the potential problems, a little knowledge of anatomy is required. The scrotum is a bag or sac beneath the penis that contains two testicles. These are the glands that produce sperm and the hormone testosterone. Capping each testicle is a structure called the epididymis that is essentially a collection of little spermatic ducts. Both the testes and the epididymis may have little remnant tags or appendices that can occasionally twist on their stalks, producing pain and swelling. Finally, each testicle needs a blood supply, the testicular artery, veins and a tube to transport the sperm (the vas deferens). These structures are held together in a wrapping, the spermatic cord.

What problems cause the scrotum to swell and hurt? Probably, the most critical one to identify is torsion of the testicle. This condition occurs when the spermatic cord twists tightly, interfering with the blood supply to the testicle. Typically, torsion occurs either in the newborn period or in early puberty. In the latter age group, sudden severe testicular pain is present and is frequently accompanied by nausea or vomiting. Initially, there is swelling and later redness of the scrotum. Observant examiners might notice the affected testicle seems higher than its counterpart. Also, touching the inner thigh no longer elevates the affected testicle, because the cremaster muscle that acts to elevate the testicle (the cremasteric reflex) cannot do so. Torsion of the testicle is an emergency! In order to save the testis, rapid surgical treatment is required. A child with suspected testicular torsion should be taken immediately to an emergency department where the diagnosis can be confirmed by physical examination and an evaluation of the testicular blood flow using a color Doppler ultrasound test.

Testicular torsion also occurs in newborn males. Here, the problem shows up as a painless scrotal swelling. There may be a bluish swelling and a solid mass that doesn't transilluminate (allow light to pass through it). Unfortunately, urgent surgery is unlikely to save the testis. Electively, the scrotum can be surgically explored to ensure that no tumor is present and that the remaining testicle is properly anchored.

Small structural remnants of tissue, the appendix of either the testicle or the epididymis, can also twist on their stalks. When this happens, the situation is called torsion of the testicular appendages. Usually boys aged 7 to 11 years are the ones affected. They will have pain but it is not as severe or rapid in onset as the pain of testicular torsion. Although swelling and redness of the scrotum eventually may appear, initially, there may only be a blue dot of discoloration apparent beneath the scrotal skin. The symptoms of appendiceal torsion settle down after about a week, during which time rest and pain relievers will help comfort the boy. It may take a little longer for the swelling to completely subside.

Epididymitis is the inflammation of the epididymis, the tubular structure attached on top and behind the testicle. Epididymitis can be associated with a urinary tract infection or it can be caused by a viral illness, particularly adenovirus. In adolescent boys, epididymitis can even be the result of sexually transmitted disease. The symptoms of epididymitis may include painful or frequent urination followed by slowly

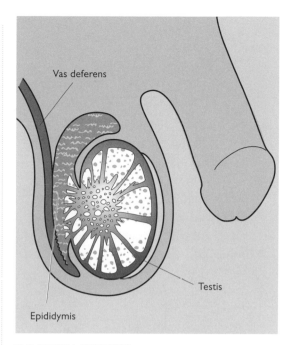

THE SCROTAL CONTENTS

increasing scrotal discomfort often localized to the upper pole of the testicle. The scrotum may be swollen or red. Because epididymitis can closely mimic testicular torsion, the diagnosis needs to be confirmed by a careful medical examination, a urinalysis and, often, a color Doppler ultrasound that verifies that adequate blood flow to the testicle is present. Epididymitis is treated with pain relief and appropriate antibiotics.

There are some other conditions that produce pain in the scrotum. Orchitis is an infection or inflammation of the testis. It is usually seen as a part of epididymitis although it can also be acquired by viral infections, such as mumps, adenovirus and infectious mononucleosis, or by bacteria in the bloodstream. A rare cause of **acute** scrotum pain is an inflammatory disease called Henoch-Schonlein purpura, which is usually associated with bruises, abdominal pain, sore joints and kidney problems.

- A suddenly swollen, tender scrotum may indicate that there is torsion of the testicle. It's an emergency!
- A painful swelling in the groin that extends toward the scrotum may be an incarcerated hernia in which the bowel has become trapped.
- All scrotal swellings need a medical evaluation.

Finally, almost all male athletes can attest to the fact that scrotal trauma can produce pain. Although quite severe, pain resulting from trauma is usually transient and subsides in a few minutes. If the discomfort persists or significant swelling occurs, a medical evaluation is indicated. Surgically removing a blood clot may save an otherwise doomed testicle.

What can cause painless scrotal swelling? Understandably, discovering a scrotal mass or swelling can be alarming. Fortunately, the cause is most often both benign and treatable. The most common scrotal masses in childhood are hydroceles, inguinal hernias or **varicoceles**. A hydrocele is a collection of fluid surrounding the testicle. They are quite common in early infancy. Usually, these bluish, cystic swellings disappear in the first year of life but if they persist or develop after birth, they should be treated by a simple surgical procedure. An inguinal hernia is a bulge in the groin or a scrotal swelling that is created when a loop of bowel enters the remnants of a canal in the groin area. Both inguinal hernias and hydroceles can appear to be getting larger (but are still painless) when the baby is crying, coughing, straining to pass stool or even as the day goes on. Inguinal hernias are usually painless swellings but if the bowel gets stuck (or incarcerated), they can become hard, tender, painful and discolored. Varicoceles are common scrotal lesions in adolescence. In fact, 15 percent to 20 percent of boys will have one, almost exclusively on their left side. A varicocele is essentially a collection of varicose, or dilated, veins. Often varicoceles go unnoticed but, when he stands up, an adolescent may notice a mass near the left testicle that feels like a "bag of worms." Varicoceles will need surgical repair if they produce pain or if they interfere with the blood supply to the testis, impairing testicular growth. In this situation, failure to treat the varicocele may impair future fertility. Although many adolescents are understandably uncomfortable with a genital examination, it is partly for this reason that they should consent to being thoroughly checked at their annual health maintenance visit.

Finally, although rare, testicular masses might be the result of a tumor. Both benign and malignant scrotal tumors occur. They tend to be solid, firm and painless. It is important to remember that, once diagnosed, they can often be successfully treated.

Teething

What is teething? Teething refers to the normal appearance of new teeth erupting through the gums. Of a child's milestones, few are more variable and generally less important for a

ERUPTION PATTERN

	TOOTH	ERUPTION	FALLS OUT
UPPER JAW	central incisor	7–12 months	6–8 years
	lateral incisor	9–13 months	7–8 years
	canine	16–22 months	10–12 years
	first molar	13–19 months	9–11 years
	second molar	25–33 months	10–12 years
LOWER JAW	central incisor	6–10 months	6–8 years
	lateral incisor	7–16 months	7–8 years
	canine	16–23 months	9–12 years
	first molar	12–18 months	9–11 years
	second molar	20–31 months	10–12 years

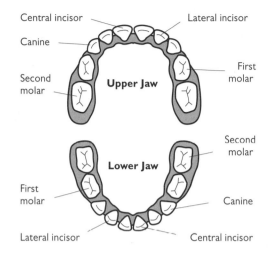

TEETH DEVELOPMENT
Deciduous, or primary, teeth erupt between the ages of 6 months and 3 years in a specific order. The pattern is the same in upper and lower jaws.

child's health or development than teething. Sometime between a few months of age and 1 year, the first teeth erupt. Most commonly, teething starts at 6 or 7 months when the lower incisors appear. Thereafter, more baby teeth erupt every month or two, starting with the incisors, then the first molars followed by the canines and, finally, the second molars.

What does teething look like? Usually, teeth simply appear without any symptoms at all. The baby may drool more and you will notice an increased desire to gum objects. The gums may appear a little swollen where the tooth will soon break through. Sometimes, particularly where the molars erupt, there may be some reddish or blue discoloration due to a little trapped blood. But discomfort is typically minimal. Crying, diarrhea and diaper rashes are also not a part of the teething experience, only common myths.

A lot of parents tend to blame a child's fever on teething. Actually, it's doubtful that teething really does produce a fever, and definitely not one of any significance. Rather, the age of teething coincides with the stage that infants start to contract the common childhood viruses. It is far more likely that any elevation in temperature in an infant is due to one of these. In any case, the parent who attributes a child's fever solely to teething is unwise. You should always seek the true cause of any unexplained fever in a young child.

How is teething treated? Most of the time, no treatment is needed. If the gums are swollen and the baby seems fussy, try massaging the gum with a clean finger for a minute or two. If this brings relief, you can repeat the massage

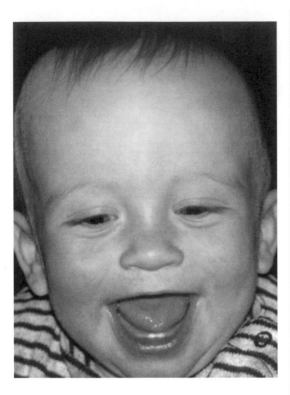

as needed. Babies can massage their own gums when they are provided with a teething ring or some safe object to gum. A wet washcloth or teething biscuit will do, but foods that may cause choking, such as carrot sticks, should be avoided.

If your child seems unsettled because of teething, you can try some oral pain relief. You can give your baby a dose or two of acetaminophen or ibuprofen, but persistent irritability is probably caused by something else. Find out what. A lot of parents choose to use teething gels to comfort their baby. The value of this is questionable and, like all medications, side effects although rare, can occur. It's probably best not to bother using them.

Urine and Stool Abnormalities

URINE

What does it mean if the color has changed? You might occasionally notice that your child's urine looks dark yellow or orange and that it smells stronger than normal. This usually means the urine is more concentrated and reflects on the degree of the child's hydration. This concentrated, dark yellow appearance is acceptable if the urine is the first passed in the morning as the child has not had anything to drink overnight. At other times, for example if the child has a fever or is vomiting, it may be a sign of dehydration. Very dark urine, particularly if it seems greenish, might be a sign of liver disease. In this situation, **bilirubin**, which is usually taken care of by the liver, is excreted in the urine producing a dark color. The stools are often quite pale.

The urine could contain blood or its breakdown products. In this case, the urine may change to a shade of red: it will look pink, reddish or tea- or cola-colored. Parents sometimes notice an orange or pink urine stain in the diaper of newborn babies and are concerned about blood in the urine. This is called the "pink diaper syndrome" and is caused by the precipitation of some crystals in the urine. There is no blood and no cause for concern, apart from ensuring that the baby receives enough to drink. Apart from this scenario, when urinary blood is suspected, a urine sample should be tested for the presence of blood.

There are many different causes of blood in the urine including urinary tract infections and inflammation of the kidneys (**glomerulonephritis**). In the case of infections, the child may have a fever, frequent urination and pain. Children with glomerulonephritis often have had a sore throat or a skin infection a couple of weeks earlier. They may also pass smaller amounts of urine and may have a slightly puffy or swollen appearance, particularly around the eyes. More rarely an injury to the lower back over the kidney area or a kidney stone could also result in blood in the urine.

If the urine dipstick test used by your doctor is negative for blood, the abnormal reddish color may be the result of a dye that is being excreted in the urine. This is usually seen after eating beets or while taking certain medications. Very rarely you may see green or blue urine caused by artificial coloring in foods or medications.

What about the urine's smell? The odor of urine can also be a clue to certain diseases. Foul-smelling urine might be the first sign of a urinary tract infection in babies. In this case, the urine can also appear cloudy or hazy. The child should see his doctor who will take a sample and check it for the presence of pus cells and bacteria. Maple syrup urine disease is a very rare inherited condition where the baby's urine smells like maple syrup, although it doesn't taste like it!

What if a child seems to void too often? Frequent urination may be a clue to an underlying problem. If the child seems to be passing increased amounts of urine (polyuria) and drinking a lot (polydipsia), your doctor should test the urine for the presence of sugar, caused by diabetes mellitus. These children also might have lost weight and be more tired than usual. If there is no increase in the amount of urine passed (just frequent, small amounts) then one should suspect a urinary tract infection, especially if the child is otherwise unwell with fever and pain on urination. Yet, as often as not, there is no real problem. Many younger children just get into the habit of drinking a lot of fluid and they must pee out the excess.

STOOL

What about the color of stools? Parents seem quite focused on the color of their child's stools and often expect others to be equally interested. The truth is that the color is usually of little significance. The bowel's job is to digest food, not produce a constant stool. Many changes in the color, consistency and smell of stool are caused by dietary change. Nevertheless, there are certain changes that may be considered normal and others that should alert you to consider specific problems.

Breast-fed babies will usually produce a mustard-colored, seedy stool but this can sometimes be green and runny as well. In older infants and children, green, watery and foul smelling stools are a sign of stomach flu (gastroenteritis). In this case, the child will often have vomiting, loss of appetite and even a **low-grade fever.** Stools that are very pale can be a sign of a blockage of the bile ducts, particularly in young babies during the first few months of life. In older children, hepatitis is a possibility, particularly if the urine is darker than usual and the whites of the eyes and the skin seem a yellowish color. Stools that are very pale, floating and foul-smelling can be a sign of malabsorption (see Diarrhea, pages 34–37).

What if there is blood in the stool? If the bloody stool is slimy or mucuslike, it usually is a sign of infection or inflammation of the large intestine or rectum. It is not unusual to see small amounts of fresh blood on the tissue in children who are constipated and strain when passing stools. A red-currant-jellylike appearance of the stool is typical for a rare condition called **intussusception** that occurs predominantly in children younger than 2 years of age. This condition occurs when a piece of the intestine telescopes into the next part of the intestine. The child usually suffers spasms of severe abdominal pain and is pale.

The sudden passage of a large amount of fresh red blood can classically be seen in young children with a condition called Meckel's diverticulum. Here, a remnant of a duct causes bleeding in the intestines.

Bloody diarrhea can be seen with bacterial gastrointestinal infections and should be suspected in children who have high fevers and abdominal cramps and appear unwell. You or your doctor should suspect this particularly if the child is a returning traveler or has been exposed to contaminated food or water. Teenagers with a longer history of bloody stools and abdominal pain need to be checked out for possible inflammatory bowel disease.

If the problem is higher up in the gastrointestinal tract, for example, involving the esophagus (gullet), stomach or small intestine, the blood will already be "digested" and the stool will look very dark or black and tarry in color. Peptic ulcers are unusual in young children but become more common in adolescence, especially if there is a family history of ulcers.

What about the consistency? Sometimes children between the ages of 1 and 3 years will pass watery stools with undigested recognizable pieces of food such as peas or carrots. This is typical of "toddler's diarrhea." The child usually doesn't have stools overnight. These children are generally healthy with good appetites and weight gain. One theory is that they drink too much fluid, especially fruit juices.

Vomiting

What is vomiting? Vomiting is the forceful expulsion of the contents of the stomach. It differs from regurgitation, which is effortless, typically more of a wet burp and usually seen in young babies. Vomiting can be described in different ways: the description can help determine the cause of the problem. For example, vomiting is called projectile if the stomach's contents, called vomitus, come out of the mouth at such speed that it seems they could hit a wall a few feet away. Your doctor will often enquire as to whether the vomitus is dark green, indicating the presence of bile, or blood-stained. Blood looks bright red if it is fresh but if it has been in the stomach for some time it can resemble coffee grounds in appearance. Often the vomited material appears to be simply partially digested food but, if the vomiting continues and the stomach gets emptier, the vomitus takes on a yellow color, caused by stomach juices, or even a watery appearance. Usually, vomiting occurs through the mouth but sometimes vomitus can come through the nose as well. Although this can alarm parents, it does not imply a more serious cause for the vomiting.

What could be causing vomiting? There are many different reasons why a child might vomit. Some are not particularly worrisome while others are potentially life-threatening and require urgent medical attention. The age of the child, the general behavior, the presence of other sick people nearby, the frequency and amount of vomiting, the presence of diarrhea and the presence of bile and blood in the vomitus are some of the factors in helping make this distinction.

WHEN SHOULD I WORRY IF MY CHILD IS VOMITING?

SEEK IMMEDIATE MEDICAL ATTENTION	CONCERNED ABOUT
Not keeping anything down for more than 6 hours and decreased urine output	dehydration
Unexplained drowsiness or dry tongue with sunken eyes	dehydration
Severe headache, irritability, neck stiffness with the vomiting	meningitis
Flat red or purple spots that do not disappear when pressing on the skin	meningitis, sepsis
Low back pain, urinary symptoms or foul smelling urine	urinary tract infection
Severe abdominal pain	appendicitis in older children intussusception if under 2 years of age
Presence of dark green bile in the vomitus	intestinal obstruction
Presence of an early morning headache and no nausea	raised pressure in the brain
Presence of blood in the vomitus (bright red or brown)	peptic ulcer, esophageal tear

Infection. Overall, infections make up the most common cause of vomiting. Many infections tend to be associated with a fever, so its presence suggests some type of infection as the cause of the vomiting.

Infections of the bowel (gastroenteritis) are very common in young children and usually start with a fever and vomiting, followed shortly thereafter by diarrhea. This is usually caused by a highly contagious virus, so other family members and friends may be affected as well. The vomiting usually settles down within 24 to 48 hours and seldom requires any specific treatment as long as the child does not become dehydrated (see above).

The most serious infection causing vomiting is **meningitis**. Although it is rare, meningitis is extremely dangerous and can be fatal if not recognized and treated urgently. Children with meningitis will often complain of high fevers, headache, irritability, neck stiffness and are either extremely lethargic or very difficult to settle. However, in young infants, these additional features may be absent or harder to pick up.

Urinary tract infections can often be a cause of vomiting. Affected children may complain of more frequent or painful urination or loss of bladder control. They may also have high fevers and back pain over the kidney areas. Once again, younger infants are unlikely to have much more than fever and vomiting, although parents may detect a foul odor to the urine when changing diapers.

Ear, throat or chest infections—such as pneumonia, **pertussis** and **bronchiolitis**—can cause vomiting, but this is usually part of a forceful cough that tends to empty the stomach at the same time and is often very mucuslike.

Bowel obstruction. Any problem that results in obstruction of the bowel will usually produce vomiting. If the blockage occurs after the first part of the small intestine where bile empties into the gut, the vomitus will be bile stained, or bilious. For example, on rare occasion, children will be born with intestines that have not gone through their normal developmental placement during the early fetal stage: the gut will be malrotated. This means that the many loops of the bowel are not properly anchored or folded in the embryo's gut and can potentially twist, causing an obstruction. Then, as a result of not being properly secured in the abdomen, the intestines can twist on themselves (**volvulus**), causing obstruction and bilious vomiting.

Intussusception is another obstructive cause of vomiting, usually occurring in children under the age of 2 years. This happens when one part of the intestine "telescopes" into the section in front, causing obstruction and affecting the supply of blood and nutrients to the piece of intestine being squeezed. Intussusception is uncommon but it is very important that a doctor recognize it because your child needs treatment early on. The baby usually becomes pale and limp while experiencing recurring bouts of severe abdominal spasms with drawing up of the legs. The pain is often associated with vomit-

ing, and may eventually be accompanied by the presence of blood in the stool that resembles red current jelly.

Any child who has had previous abdominal surgery can have obstruction due to the formation of scar tissue. Therefore, bilious vomiting after such surgery should alert you to the possibility of intestinal obstruction. Not all vomiting due to bowel obstruction is bilious. If the blockage is higher in the gut, such as the outlet of the stomach, the **pylorus**, there is usually no bile staining, but the vomiting is increasingly projectile. This condition classically occurs in first-born male infants from 2 weeks to 2 months of age.

Appendicitis tends to occur in older children and adolescents and occurs when the appendix becomes obstructed and inflamed. This usually results in pain in the abdomen, initially around the belly button and then moving to the right groin. Appendicitis is often accompanied by fever and vomiting, and the child tends to remain still because moving or coughing makes the pain worse.

Gastroesophageal reflux. In babies during the first months of life, by far the commonest cause of vomiting is gastroesophageal reflux (GER). This is a normal developmental process for many babies caused by a somewhat inefficient valve between the esophagus and stomach. Babies' lax muscle tone and the tendency for most infants to lie flat after a feed also contribute to the problem. GER is really just the regurgitation of stomach contents and, provided that your baby continues to gain weight appropriately, appears comfortable and has no fever, it would be appropriate to wait for this to gradually resolve. It usually does so by 9 to 12 months, much to parents' relief.

HOW SHOULD I TREAT THE VOMITING?

TIME FRAME	ACTION	
During the first 12 hours	If breast-feeding	continue with shorter feeds more frequently (every 2 hours) offer small amounts* of ORS** with each breast-feed
	If not breast-feeding	stop formula and solids and give ORS (2 tbsp./30 mL every 15–30 min), as the child improves, increase the amount of liquids
After the first 12 hours	If breast-feeding	continue to breast-feed
	If not breast-feeding	give small amounts of formula*** and milk and ORS (as above), and slowly start age-appropriate solids

Do not give your child medicines (for example, Gravol) unless recommended by your doctor. They can disguise the underlying problem and can also result in side effects.

*   Offer 2 tbsp. (30 mL); if your child keeps vomiting or refuses to drink, you can try using a teaspoon, medicine dropper or syringe to give the liquids.

**   ORS = oral rehydration solution, also called oral electrolyte solution, available from the drugstore as Pedialyte, Oralyte and Rehydralite. These liquids contain a mixture of water and salts required to replace your child's fluid loss and should be mixed carefully according to the instructions (some are available as ready-to-drink solutions).

*** You must feed your child more than just clear fluids after 24 hours.

Neurological causes of vomiting. Children with conditions leading to a rise in the pressure inside the skull will often vomit. In fact, vomiting can be the first sign of such a problem. Vomiting, for example, can indicate the presence of a brain tumor. These, fortunately, are very uncommon and the child will usually also have severe headaches, particularly in the early morning. Vomiting, when it occurs, is seldom accompanied by nausea or fever. Bleeding inside the skull, intracranial hemorrhage, usually occurs after trauma. It can be indicated by vomiting but, more frequently the vomiting that follows head injury is caused by a concussion.

Migraine headaches are often accompanied by nausea and vomiting. Cyclic vomiting is an unusual condition that is similar in some ways to migraine headaches. With cyclic vomiting, children vomit very frequently for a couple of days and then settle down usually for weeks or even months before the next bout of vomiting begins. These children may on occasion require intravenous fluids to treat dehydration. If your child only vomits during travel, the likely diagnosis is motion sickness.

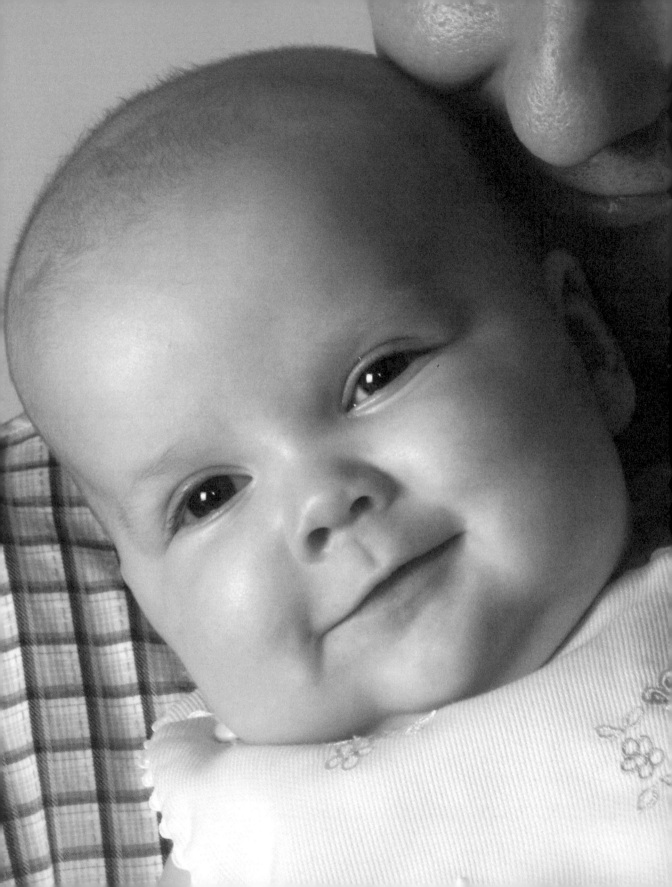

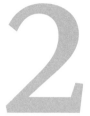

The Newborn

The Shape of Your Baby's Head

Many new parents express concerns regarding the shape of their new baby's head, and the swellings or lumps they may often feel along the surface of the skull. Here are some answers to questions you might have.

The skull of the fetus and newborn differs from the adult skull in several ways. The mature skull can be thought of as a single, fused bone whose primary purpose is to provide rigid protection for the brain within. A newborn's skull is formed from seven bones that are separated by openings called sutures. This serves two important functions. First, a skull comprised of several bony plates is flexible enough to allow the head to pass through the birth canal during delivery. Secondly, it allows for easy skull expansion during the first two years of life when the brain growth is most rapid. After two years, the brain has reached 75 percent of its full volume!

There are two areas, one at the top of the head and the other near the back of it, where three of the sutures intersect in such a way that larger openings, called **fontanelles** or "soft spots," are created. The smaller of these, the one near the back of the head, called the posterior fontanelle, usually closes when the bones fuse together between birth and 3 months of age.

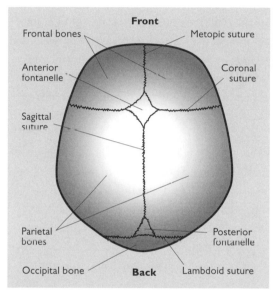

NORMAL SKULL OF THE NEWBORN
The newborn skull is made up of seven different bones separated by sutures. There are two soft spots (fontanelles).

The larger, anterior fontanelle normally closes between 6 months and 2 years of age.

What's wrong with the shape of my newborn's head? Many babies are born with what appears to be a dramatic and unusual head shape, usually an elongated skull, commonly referred to as a "cone head." This distortion of the head is called molding. It is a process whereby the bones within the skull have shifted and molded to allow the baby's head to descend through the birth canal. Don't worry about it. Within days, the bones reshape themselves back to the more rounded skull shape that most parents imagined for their unborn baby.

There is another swelling usually seen over the top part of the newborn's head that came out of the birth canal first. This is known as caput and is a soft and squishy swelling caused by the tight pressure on the scalp, often more prominent if a vacuum instrument has been used to help deliver the head. It can cross the midline and go over suture lines. It, too, is no cause for concern and will usually disappear within the first few days of life.

What is the bump on the side of my baby's head? Some babies are born with soft, mushy swellings, usually over the sides of the skull. These are caused by bruising from the pressure of the birth canal against the skull. They are called cephalohematomas, ("cephalo" for head, "hematoma" for bruise). They feel like small, and, occasionally, even large, sacs filled with fluid. In this case, the fluid is blood, and poses no danger or risk to the baby because it is outside the skull, just under the scalp. The swelling often disappears within weeks after birth. Sometimes, it can take months to clear up and can become quite hard, but there is no cause for concern as eventually it flattens completely. If it is very big, it will increase the risk of jaundice in the first week of life as the blood in the clot is reabsorbed and metabolized.

Why is my baby's head flat on one side? Since 1992, the recommendation has been to lay babies to

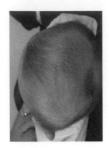

POSITIONAL PLAGIOCEPHALY
In positional plagiocephaly the head shape is a parallelogram.

sleep on their back or side. Fortunately this has led to a decrease in the incidence of **sudden infant death syndrome** (SIDS). However, it has led to a significant increase in a condition called positional plagiocephaly (also called deformational plagiocephaly). This horrendous-sounding medical term refers to the asymmetric flattening of the skull that occurs when an infant displays a preference for keeping her head turned one way or the other. If a baby spends most of the time on her back, and prefers to keep her head turned looking to the right, it is possible that the skull at the back on the right side will be flatter compared to the left side due to the pressure from the bed below.

The diagnosis of positional plagiocephaly is made by the visible skull asymmetry (best seen by looking directly down at the top of the skull) that becomes apparent around 3 to 4 months of age. The skull asymmetry may be cause for concern from a cosmetic point of view; however, there is no evidence that there are any adverse effects on brain growth or development. It's worth having the problem reviewed by your baby's doctor because, rarely, an asymmetrical skull is due to premature closure of the sutures, not positioning.

Positional plagiocephaly is almost always

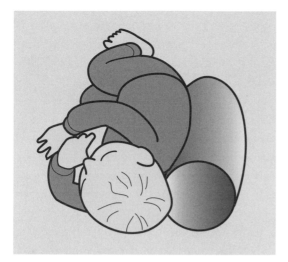

TREATING POSITIONAL PLAGIOCEPHALY
WITH COUNTER-POSITIONING
This infant is turned slightly on her left to reduce pressure on the flat right side of her head.

correctable with frequent head turning and ensuring that, during waking time, your baby spends time on her tummy several times a day. You can encourage her to turn her head by ensuring that the baby's sources of interest alternate from one side of the crib to the other. More severe cases of positional plagiocephaly are sometimes managed by temporarily having your baby wear a special type of helmet that helps mold the head to a more symmetrical shape.

Common Breast-feeding Problems

The benefits to babies and their families of breast-feeding are many. There are medical, developmental, emotional, economic and environmental advantages. Studies show that breast-fed babies develop fewer infections; have lower rates of **sudden infant death syndrome** (SIDS); and develop fewer chronic conditions such as asthma, diabetes and allergies. Despite continuing improvements in infant formulas, they do not equal human milk, which is the end product of millions of years of natural evolution. Human breast milk is the ultimate infant food.

Obviously, for first-time mothers breast-feeding is a completely new experience. Often, this supposed lack of expertise provokes anxiety. What if I can't do it? What if I don't have enough milk? It's important that you try to relax. First, breast-feeding is a natural process: while there is a learning curve, most women can successfully breast-feed and produce more than enough milk to feed and nurture their baby. Second, there is lots of help and support available for those who seek it from nurses, physicians and lactation specialists.

How do I get started? Many infants are ready to breast-feed immediately after birth. It is interesting to note that most infants are quite alert and will latch and suck well during the first few hours immediately after delivery. After the next 12 to 16 hours, infants often become less active and sleepier. This is a normal, common pattern.

The most important factor in establishing breast-feeding is obtaining a proper latch. A baby who latches well onto the breast will simply receive more milk. During the first several days, breast-fed babies receive a highly nutritious milk, called colostrum. This is the only source of fluid and nutrition that a newborn requires. In the first few days, there is usually no need to supplement with water or glucose water or formula. Typically, between the third to fifth days after delivery, your milk will come in and the amount available increases rapidly.

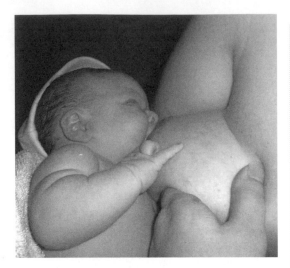

How can I tell if my baby is getting enough?
There are several ways to tell if she is receiving enough milk:

Weight gain. While all babies lose weight in the first few days after birth, a baby who is receiving ample amounts of milk will not lose more than 10 percent of her initial birth weight, and will usually be back up to birth weight between 1 and 2 weeks of age. A baby who is gaining weight is getting enough milk. In their first few months, on average, babies gain about an ounce (25 to 30 grams) per day.

Stooling. The pattern of stools often changes as babies get more milk. In the first one or two days, babies pass the newborn stool called meconium, which is black and tarlike. In the next two to three days, the stools become lighter in color and change from dark brown to dark, then light green: these are often called transitional stools. A baby with regular yellow, mustardlike stools is almost surely receiving adequate amounts of breast milk. These frequent "seedy" unformed, sometimes watery or pastelike stools should be a reassuring and welcome sight—even if they

appear two to three or even 10 times a day! A baby who is still passing meconium stools, or no stool at all, after the fourth or fifth day should be evaluated by a health care professional.

Urinating. A baby who is passing lots of urine is probably receiving enough milk. Babies should void at least three to four times per day. By the end of the first week, many babies are voiding six to ten times daily. With the ultra-absorbent diapers in use today, it can be difficult to tell if there is actually urine present in the diaper. If the diaper feels heavy compared with a new, unused diaper, there is urine present. Also, if there is stool in the diaper, there is likely also urine present. If the baby's fluid intake is marginal, the urine will appear more concentrated and a deeper yellow. Pink or orange crystals can even be seen on the diaper.

Sleep pattern. This is an *unreliable* way to tell if the baby is receiving enough milk. A baby who is receiving adequate amounts of milk will generally settle and sleep for a few hours after a feeding, then will spontaneously awaken to feed vigorously, then fall back to sleep. This must be differentiated from the constantly sleepy baby, who may be sleepy due to lack of milk intake.

Note that the duration of each feed; the feeling, or lack of, fullness in the breasts; as well as the inability to pump milk are not very reliable ways to determine the adequacy of milk supply.

How often should I feed my baby? Babies should be fed on demand, not by the clock: self-scheduling usually works best. No other mammal uses a watch to feed its young. Once your baby is latching well and beginning to gain weight, she should determine her own feeding and sleeping schedule. There is no need to awaken a thriving baby from sleep to feed. Besides, a very sleepy baby may not suck that well. And, if a thriving baby wants to be fed every hour or two, so be it!

Do breast-fed babies sleep less? No, there is no proof that breast-fed babies sleep more or less than formula-fed babies. Newborn sleep patterns vary widely. There is a commonly held misconception that babies who are formula-fed, or babies who receive an early introduction to infant cereal (before 4 or 5 months), sleep longer at night.

What about sore nipples? Some women experience a degree of soreness of the nipple or breast in the first few days. This is typically mild and transient. If there is a significant degree of pain, it is important to ensure that your baby's latch is optimal, as a poor latch is probably the commonest cause of soreness. This is best achieved with the help of someone with experience in this area. In some cases, a yeast infection (thrush) of the nipples, which is acquired from the baby's mouth, can cause nipple pain, burning, cracking and itching. This can be treated with topical antifungal creams.

Should I change my diet? This is a topic rife with mythology. There is no convincing evidence that proves that mothers need to alter their diets, or avoid certain foods, for the sake of their nursing babies. There is no proof that future food allergies in the baby can be prevented by altering the maternal diet, although the act of breast-feeding itself does confer some protection from future allergies. There is no proof that certain foods that the mother eats cause fussiness or "gas" in the baby. That said, if your baby clearly seems to react when you eat a specific type of food, perhaps you should stay away from it!

Does the baby need to eat or drink anything other than breast milk? No. Breast milk is the sole source of nutrition required in the first six months of a baby's life. There is no need for water, formula or any other nutrient until approximately 6 months of age. If you wish to supplement breast-feeding with infant formula or solids, for example when returning to work, it is a good idea to review things with your baby's health care provider.

Sunlight exposure on skin is an important source of vitamin D, which is important for the development of strong, healthy bones. In northern climates, where sunlight is limited, a vitamin D supplement is recommended. For most babies in northern states, the lack of year-round sunlight means that breast-fed babies require a single daily dose of vitamin D.

When should I start other foods? Most experts advise starting solid foods by 6 months of age and not before 4 months for a baby born at term. The specific timing should be determined by the preference of you and your baby. Exclusive breast-feeding until 6 months of age will provide all the nutrients required during this important period of growth and development.

Hiccups

Why does my baby get hiccups all the time? Most newborn infants have episodes of hiccups, at least some of the time, usually after feeding. This normal phenomenon has no established cause. It results from frequent or rhythmic contractions of the diaphragm muscle. The episodes of hiccups generally start at birth or even earlier. Many mothers recall feeling the hiccups while their baby was still in the womb! Hiccups tend to lessen and disappear by 1 or 2 months of age. They are benign in the sense that they are not a sign of any problem, nor do they cause problems of any kind. Hiccups generally bother parents much more than they do their babies.

How are hiccups treated? Most of the time, doing nothing is the best treatment: hiccups stop on their own. If they interfere with feeding, causing your baby to spit up, cough or cry, stop feeding for a few minutes. Try burping the baby and, when things settle down, resume the feeding.

Weight Loss and Dehydration in Newborns

"What does the baby weigh?" is usually one of the first questions asked by excited friends and relatives. It is a milestone that parents always remember. Many people are not aware that normal babies actually lose some weight before returning to their initial birth weight one or two weeks later.

Why do babies initially lose weight? It is important to understand weight loss after birth is a *normal* phenomenon. In the transition from life inside the womb to life outside, there are profound changes that occur in the baby's internal physiology. These changes encompass every organ system in the body, including the cardiovascular system and kidneys, which regulate the body's internal fluids. These changes lead to internal shifts in the body's fluid stores, which explain most of the weight loss in the first few days.

Feeding and fluid intake also play a role in the early weight changes. While both breast-fed and formula-fed infants lose weight early on, breast-

fed infants lose slightly more weight, on average, likely due to a lower volume of milk intake in the first several days. A third factor that contributes to the initial measured weight loss is the copious evacuation of meconium from the baby's bowel that frequently occurs in the first few days.

How much weight do newborns lose? The normal degree of weight loss in the first several days is typically 3 percent to 6 percent of the initial birth weight, but a loss up to 8 percent to 10 percent is acceptable. A loss of greater than 10 percent of birth weight is cause for concern that the intake is insufficient and your baby may be dehydrated.

The most accurate assessment of hydration or dehydration at any age is an accurate weight. In fact, dehydration is defined by these weight changes. While this may seem simple in today's highly technical world, there are many factors that often interfere with the accuracy of weight measurements. First of all, there is variability from scale to scale, which becomes important in comparing birth and discharge weights from the hospital to those from offices or clinics. Also, there can be a large discrepancy when comparing the baby's weight when dressed and diapered to how much she weighs naked.

How can I tell if my baby is dehydrated? Apart from the weight changes, there are some clues to a baby's state of hydration. A baby who is active, feeds vigorously and awakens spontaneously to feed is not likely to be dehydrated. A baby who passes urine frequently (every three to four hours) and has frequent stools is probably receiving an adequate amount of milk.

Some of the features of dehydration in older children, such as the presence or absence of tears and degree of moisture within the mouth, are inaccurate or subtle in newborns. The clinical assessment of hydration in newborns is a challenge and an art; even experienced clinicians rely on weight changes. The importance of the degree of weight loss is further underscored by the recommendation that parents of newborns discharged from hospital are advised to see their health care provider within 48 hours of discharge. This is mainly to assess weight and hydration, as well as jaundice.

When will my baby regain her birth weight? Most newborns regain birth weight between one and two weeks after birth; in some instances it occurs more quickly. As long as your baby feeds well she should gain an average of 2/3 to 1 ounce (20 to 30 g) per day from this point until about 3 months of age. Babies who fail to gain weight within the expected time need to be carefully evaluated to determine if the problem is related to lack of adequate intake—which accounts for the vast majority—or if there is an underlying medical problem.

How are excess weight loss and dehydration treated? A healthy baby is everyone's goal. The dehydrated and hungry baby needs extra fluid and nourishment. How that is achieved becomes a matter of choice and, often, it becomes an emotional experience for all if you are breast-feeding. Too often, this situation creates a sense of failure. Lactation counseling, emotional support and supplementation, with either expressed breast milk (if available) or formula, is advised. Supplementation can be achieved by feeding from a cup or a lactation device (a tube extending from the bottle taped to the nipple or fingertip); some mothers will choose to supplement with a bottle.

Jaundice in the Newborn

What is jaundice? The term neonatal jaundice refers to the yellow color seen in the skin and eyes of many newborn babies. It is caused by a naturally occurring body chemical called **bilirubin**, which circulates in the bloodstream until it is eventually eliminated via the liver. Bilirubin is a breakdown product of hemoglobin, which is responsible for carrying oxygen in the red blood cells. All people have some bilirubin circulating in their bloodstream from the hemoglobin that is constantly being broken down. The level is much higher in newborns, especially if they are premature, because the newborn's liver is slightly immature and is slower at processing, or eliminating, bilirubin from the bloodstream. In addition, babies are born with relatively high hemoglobin levels that provide a proportionately bigger supply of bilirubin for the liver to manage than older children and adults.

The majority (50 percent to 70 percent) of babies will develop jaundice to some degree. It typically becomes visible on the baby's face, including the whites of the eyes, around the second or third day of life. In most instances, jaundice is completely harmless. In fact, some experts feel that mild jaundice may be beneficial to babies because bilirubin has antioxidant properties. If bilirubin levels increase, the jaundice moves from the face downward, and becomes more apparent on the baby's trunk and extremities. Visual estimation of the degree of jaundice, even by experienced professionals, provides a rough guide of the level of bilirubin but is generally not accurate enough to be relied upon alone, especially in babies with darker skin. For this reason, the health care provider may choose to do a blood test to measure the bilirubin.

JAUNDICED NEWBORNS: INDICATIONS FOR CLOSE MONITORING

- Prematurity (babies born three or more weeks before their due date).
- Significant bruising (including a **cephalohematoma** under the scalp).
- History of significant newborn jaundice in immediate family members.
- Jaundice that becomes noticeable in the first 24 hours of life.
- "Incompatibility" between the mother's and newborn's blood groups (occurs more commonly in mothers with type o or Rh-negative blood, if the baby inherits her blood type from a type A or B, or Rh-positive father).
- Breast-feeding that is not going well.
- Weight loss greater than 10 percent of baby's birth weight.

It is only when bilirubin levels are excessively high that there is the potential for harm to the baby. In a rare condition called kernicterus, damage to parts of the brain occur due to bilirubin precipitation and toxicity. This can result in a range of permanent neurological problems including deafness, movement problems and mental retardation. Fortunately, this outcome is extremely rare and is preventable.

Neonatal jaundice is very different from jaundice that first appears in children outside of the first few weeks of life. A host of other problems, many serious, can be responsible.

When should I be concerned? It is important to remember that jaundice in the great majority of newborns is benign. In some newborns, there are identifiable risk factors that should lead to careful monitoring of the jaundice. Some of these factors are listed in the table at left.

In some newborns, especially those who are breast-fed, the jaundice can last for several weeks after birth and is called breast milk jaundice. As long as the degree of jaundice consistently decreases and your baby is well and gaining weight, there is no need for you to be concerned and no need to interrupt or discontinue breast-feeding.

How is jaundice treated? While most newborns do develop jaundice to some degree, the majority require no treatment. For most newborns, adequate feeding leading to good weight gain is sufficient to keep bilirubin levels low.

When the bilirubin levels reach certain thresholds that vary depending on your baby's age, your health care provider might determine that treatment is necessary. Your baby will then be placed under a special set of fluorescent lights and receive "phototherapy." These lights have been proven to be safe and effective for treating jaundice. Usually within one to two days the bilirubin levels decline so that no further treatment is needed.

In very rare cases, when the bilirubin level is dangerously high, or rising quickly despite phototherapy, a more complicated medical procedure, called an exchange transfusion, is performed. This requires that some of the jaundiced blood is removed and replaced or exchanged for new blood. In the more serious cases of neonatal jaundice, tests are performed to detect any potential diseases that may be producing the marked jaundice.

Many new parents are told that they should place their babies in sunlight, either direct or indirect through a window, to help eliminate the jaundice. While there is some data that shows that sunlight, like phototherapy, has the ability to lower bilirubin levels, there is not enough data to support its safe and practical use in newborns. You could partially undress the baby in order provide greater skin exposure to the light and end up with a cold infant who is still yellow.

Blocked Tear Ducts

Tears are constantly produced in small glands under the upper outer portion of each eyelid. After lubricating the eye, tears track down and drain into small holes that are located on the nasal side of the eyelid. These holes serve as the entry point for a complex drainage system whereby the tears drain into the back of the nose. (This explains why the nose sometimes becomes congested after you cry.) In some infants, the nasolacrimal duct (see illustration at the top right), is partly or completely obstructed. The result is excessive tearing or discharge. The symptoms often appear several weeks after birth when your baby produces more tears than before.

What are blocked tear ducts? During the first several months of life, many newborns and young infants have noticeable tearing and thetears seem to "overflow" down one or both cheeks. In some instances, there may also be a white or yellowish discharge that leads to persistent crusting in the corner of the eye, mostly after sleep. The commonest cause of these symptoms is a blocked tear duct otherwise

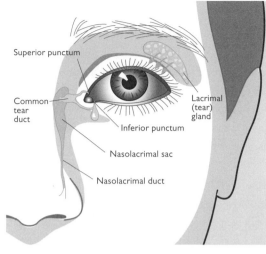

THE NORMAL TEAR DUCT
The frontal view of the eye highlights the lacrimal (tear) gland and nasolacrimal drainage system.

known as nasolacrimal duct obstruction. This occurs in approximately 5 percent of normal newborns.

Fortunately, in the vast majority of cases, this blockage resolves spontaneously. The problem disappears in more than 90 percent of children by 18 months of age without any medical treatment.

When should I be concerned? While blocked tear ducts are common, and generally benign, there are instances where you might have to take your baby to her doctor. Occasionally, the surface of the eye can become infected. In this instance, the eye whites will appear red and the tearing becomes a thick and green discharge. This infection is called **conjunctivitis** and antibiotic drops or ointments might be needed to treat it. A less common infection can occur in the lacrimal sac, a part of the tear duct itself. This results in localized redness and swelling over the nasal portion of the lower eyelid, called dacryocystitis. This usually requires oral and occasionally intravenous antibiotics.

While most blocked tear ducts unblock spontaneously, there are some children whose symptoms do not improve. If your child's symptoms have not improved toward 1 year of age, referral to an eye doctor (ophthalmologist) is often necessary.

How do I treat blocked tear ducts? While most blocked ducts improve with no treatment at all, some experts recommend a technique called tear duct massage. The idea is to gently press down with a clean finger over your baby's lower eyelid, against the bridge of the nose, and gently "milk" downward, to try to move the tears through the duct. Your doctor can demonstrate the technique. In those children whose ducts have failed to spontaneously open by 1 year of age, ophthalmologists may recommend a brief surgical procedure called tear duct probing, whereby a thin wire probe is used to open the duct.

Newborn Screening

What is newborn screening? The process of screening involves applying a test to an entire population in order to detect conditions before they cause problems. This is a key concept in preventative care and public health. Newborn screening tests typically involves taking a small blood sample, usually from the baby's heel, on the second or third day of life.

Newborn screening began in the United States in the early 1960s, when a blood test was performed on all newborns shortly after birth to detect **phenylketonuria** (PKU). This is a genetically inherited condition where affected individuals lack the ability to metabolize, or break

down, a common dietary component. Undetected and untreated, individuals with PKU would develop irreversible brain damage leading to mental retardation and seizures. If PKU is detected early, prior to any damage occurring, individuals can lead normal, healthy lives simply by following a specific diet and avoiding certain foods. This is a dramatic example where a screening test has led to early detection of a condition and its complications can be avoided.

Another condition that can be detected by screening a newborn's drops of blood is medium-chain acyl-CoA dehydrogenase (MCAD) deficiency. A baby with MCAD deficiency lacks or has insufficient enzyme to break down simple fats to make energy. Once detected the treatment is simple—a low-fat, high-carbohydrate diet. If undetected, the child can die or suffer severe mental retardation if she goes without eating for even a short period. More jurisdictions are testing for MCAD deficiency, but it is still not universally monitored for. If you have one child with MCAD deficiency you have a higher risk of having another.

While the concepts of early detection and prevention seem obvious, not all conditions are amenable to screening. A program should satisfy the following criteria:

1. The condition being screened for is an important health problem that occurs often enough to justify testing an entire population;
2. The treatment for the condition is acceptable and more effective when started early; and
3. The test is simple, safe and reliable.

Today, there are dozens of conditions for which screening tests are available. Every state and country has a different list of conditions for which they screen. Most places screen for PKU as well as hypothyroidism; there is a long record of success in screening for these two conditions. In some places, there are also screening tests for cystic fibrosis, sickle-cell disease and a host of other conditions. And, in many places, newborns are screened to detect hearing loss as early as possible.

When should I worry? Screening tests are really just preliminary investigations. Even the best of them will have a few false positive results. This means that the test has falsely identified someone with a condition that they do not truly have. If you have been notified about an abnormal screening result, arrangements will be made to either repeat the test or proceed to more definitive testing. Although a positive screening result is bound to be upsetting, it may help to remember that, even if the disease is confirmed, effective treatment is available and it can start as early as possible.

Newborn Skin Conditions

MILIA

What are milia? Milia are small cysts containing material from the upper layer of the skin, called keratin. They are commonly seen in the newborn period in up to 50 percent of babies. Milia can appear spontaneously or secondary to some other skin condition.

What does milia look like? Milia lesions consist of pinpoint, pearly white, shiny raised bumps. They are typically found on the nose and forehead.

How do I treat milia? No treatment is necessary. Milia lesions disappear on their own after a few weeks or months.

MILIARIA

What is miliaria? Miliaria, also called "heat rash" or "prickly heat," is the result of blockage of sweat glands, trapping sweat under the skin. The appearance depends on the depth of the blockage. Overbundling, increased environmental temperature and/or fever are common contributors.

What does miliaria look like? Miliaria lesions are usually on parts of the body that sweat most, for example on the forehead, neck, armpits and trunk. When the obstruction in the sweat glands is superficial, they look like crystal clear, sweat-filled fluid sacs (**vesicles**) that resemble dew drops and are a few millimeters in diameter. When the obstruction is in the deeper levels of the skin, miliaria look like clear vesicles on a red base.

How do I treat miliaria? No specific treatment is required for miliaria. Cooling the skin by decreasing the number of clothing layers and/or a lukewarm bath is usually sufficient. The temperature in your baby's room should be comfortable for you wearing light clothing.

CRADLE CAP

What is cradle cap? Cradle cap is a crusty, greasy scalp condition that commonly occurs in the newborn and infantile period. It is the result of accumulation of sebum, which is an oily substance produced by the sebaceous glands to lubricate the skin and hair. Cradle cap can occur on the scalp alone or in association with other areas, such as the diaper area and neck and underarm folds, and is then called seborrheic dermatitis.

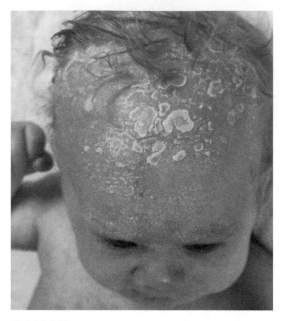

CRADLE CAP

This yellow, greasy crusting on the skalp is typical of cradle cap.

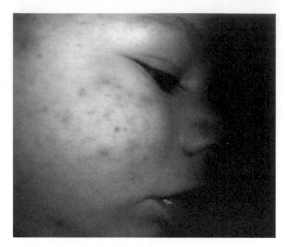

BABY ACNE

The papules and pustules of baby acne.

BABY ACNE

What is baby acne? Baby acne or infantile acne is essentially the same problem as adolescent acne. It is the result of interplay between hormones transferred from the mother and local organisms, such as bacteria and fungi. It is a self-limited condition that usually clears up by itself within a few months. Persistence of the acne lesions after the age of 6 months requires medical attention.

What does baby acne look like? Baby acne appears as raised red lesions (**papules**) and pus-filled pimples (**pustules**). Typically, blackheads (**comedones**) are rarely seen. The acne lesions are found on the cheeks, chin and forehead. Rarely, they can spread to the upper body.

How do I treat baby acne? Most of the acne lesions require no specific treatment and will clear up by themselves. In more involved cases, topical applications of antibiotics or benzoyl peroxide prescribed by a physician can be helpful in controlling the severity of the lesions.

What does it look like? Cradle cap is a thick crust of yellow, greasy material on a red background. Primarily found on the crown of the head, in the creases behind the ears and occasionally on the forehead and eyebrows, the crust adheres to the skin but can be removed if saturated in oil. It is generally not itchy. Most of the crusts will be eliminated in a few months to one or two years.

How do I treat cradle cap? Treatment of cradle cap involves lifting up the crust, which is usually accomplished by applying oil, such as mineral oil or baby oil, 30 minutes prior to bathing. This allows you to remove the crust painlessly with a narrow-toothed comb and is followed by regular shampooing. You have to repeat the process several times. For thick, resistant crusts or the ones with underlying redness, topical application of a mild to moderate corticosteroid prescribed by a physician is beneficial.

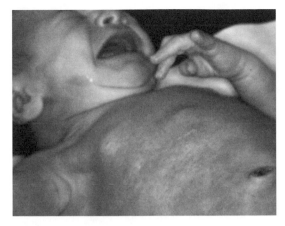

TOXIC ERYTHEMA
The blotchy red rash with tiny pimples seen in toxic erythema of the newborn.

TOXIC ERYTHEMA OF THE NEWBORN

What is it? First, in spite of its name, toxic erythema is not toxic. Affected newborns are completely healthy and the condition is not related to infection. It is one of the most common skin rashes, occurring in about 50 percent of full-term newborns. Toxic erythema usually shows up after 24 to 48 hours of life. The cause of this condition is not known.

What does toxic erythema look like? Toxic erythema appears as red blotches on the body and face. They are not found on the palms or soles. Often, tiny, pinpoint, water-filled pimples are found in the middle of the red patches. Each individual patch disappears within hours to a few days, while other areas are becoming affected.

How do I treat toxic erythema? In most cases, the rash disappears without intervention within the first two to three weeks of life. Rarely, the eruption can persist until your baby is 6 weeks of age. A persistent rash or a sick-appearing newborn requires medical attention.

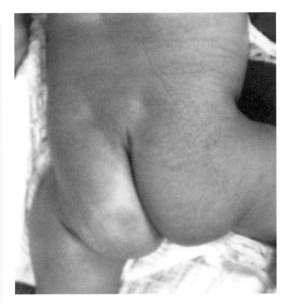

MONGOLIAN SPOTS
A Mongolian spot over the buttocks of a newborn baby.

MONGOLIAN SPOTS

What are Mongolian spots? Mongolian spots, whose more formal name is dermal melanocytosis, are noticeable patches commonly seen in darker skinned babies and represent a temporary pigmentation of the skin.

What does a Mongolian spot look like? Mongolian spots are usually found in the middle of the lower back or over the buttocks. Less commonly, other areas of the body can also be affected. The spots can be single or multiple. They appear as a large, flat, poorly circumscribed blue-gray discoloration. Bruising is sometimes confused with Mongolian spots, but bruises tend to change color after a few days.

How are Mongolian spots treated? The spots fade slowly in most children during childhood. No intervention is necessary.

Thrush

What is thrush? Thrush is a common, benign infection in a baby's mouth caused by a yeastlike fungus called *Candida albicans*. It can appear as early as the first week of life and is common in the first months of life. A small amount of candida occurs naturally in the mouth, skin and bowel in harmony with a range of natural bacteria. It rarely causes mouth disease in healthy adults, but does cause infections in about 5 percent of healthy infants due to a relative immaturity of their immune system. Toddlers and older children can develop thrush following a course of antibiotics. This is caused by a temporary disruption of the balance between candida and normal bacteria in the mouth that keep it under control. The fungus that causes thrush thrives in a warm, moist environment, which explains the typical locations—the mouth and diaper area.

What does thrush look like? Thrush appears as white patches on the gums, inner cheeks, tongue and palate. These might resemble milk curds but do not wipe off easily. In some cases, the yeast infection spreads to the diaper area and causes a red, irritated diaper rash that will last for days to weeks unless treated. Many infants with thrush have no symptoms; some develop fussiness and feeding difficulties. A significant impact of a baby's oral thrush is that the infection can spread to the mother's nipples. Many lactation consultants feel that this can lead to nipple pain, unusual sensitivity, itching and irritation, as well as a stabbing pain deep within the breast.

How is thrush treated? Given that thrush is usually benign, and often produces no symptoms, mild cases can be left to resolve on their own. Most authorities recommend treating a breast-fed infant, or any infant with symptoms, with an oral antifungal medication, such as nystatin. You should simultaneously treat your breasts with antifungal creams to prevent the infection from spreading back and forth from your baby to you. Diaper rash caused by yeast is usually treated with an antifungal cream.

Umbilical Cord Problems

What is the umbilical cord? The umbilical cord was the lifeline that provided precious nutrients to the fetus during the pregnancy. At delivery, it was clamped and cut. Initially, the cord is thick, rubbery and translucent, but after a few days it dries, shrivels and appears as an unsightly stump protruding from the abdomen of an otherwise beautiful baby. Fear not. The stump typically falls off between 1 and 3 weeks of age and the area becomes a belly button.

What do I do with the umbilical cord? Most parents are relieved to hear that the care of the cord is simple. Ignore the thing, as it needs no special attention. In the past, parents were advised to clean the area around the cord with antiseptics, for example alcohol; but now many authorities advise no special cleaning apart from normal hygiene. The cord falls off more quickly if left alone, and there is no proof that topical antiseptics prevent infections, which are rare to begin with.

Keep in mind that the cord is useless, dead tissue. It may smell strongly and look awful, but this decay is normal and ultimately leads to the cord falling off. A small amount of bleeding may occur just before or after the cord detaches. It usually stops with gentle pressure, and alone, it is not a cause for concern.

What happens after the stump falls off? The umbilical stump normally falls off one to three weeks after birth. In most cases, the story of the cord thankfully ends here. In some cases, there may be a small, pink piece of leftover tissue called a cord **granuloma**. This is not symptomatic, but can continue to create a small amount of discharge from where the cord was attached to the baby's abdomen. The granuloma will disappear over several months if left alone; in some cases, treatment by your health care provider with silver nitrate will help the granuloma to disappear more quickly.

When should I worry? Rarely, the tissue around the cord does become infected and requires treatment. Omphalitis refers to an infection of the umbilical stump and surrounding skin. In this case, the skin on the abdomen around the stump becomes reddened, and there may be pus coming from the umbilical stump. There may be an increased smell. In some cases, your baby may show signs of illness including fever, poor feeding and lethargy. Any of these symptoms

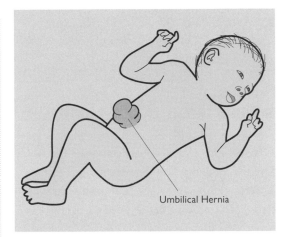

UMBILICAL HERNIA
An umbilical hernia is a protruding lump from the belly button that is more prominent when the baby cries or strains.

should lead to immediate medical assessment.

Some parents will notice a lump protruding from the baby's belly button long after the cord falls off. The lump, which usually protrudes more when the baby is crying or straining, is an umbilical hernia. This hernia is caused by the protrusion of abdominal contents covered with normal skin, through a temporary hole in the wall of the abdomen under the belly button. It does not cause any discomfort for the baby, and the hole usually closes in the first few years and, for the great majority, by 4 to 5 years of age. It is much more common in infants of African ancestry and premature babies. While some types of hernias require surgery to repair, an umbilical hernia rarely requires surgical treatment. Do not worry about it!

Much more rarely the abdominal contents protrude into the base of the umbilical cord covered only in a transparent membrane with no layer of skin. This is always quite obvious at the time of delivery and is known as an omphalocele. This condition will need specialized surgical repair.

Sudden Infant Death Syndrome

What is sudden infant death syndrome? The whole topic of sudden infant death syndrome (SIDS) is a frightening and emotional one for new parents. After all, what is more horrifying than the unexpected death of a seemingly healthy infant? SIDS is defined as the sudden and unexpected death of an apparently healthy baby in the first year of life, which remains unexplained after a comprehensive investigation. Most cases occur between 2 and 4 months of age and 95 percent of all cases happen before 6 months. While there has been a decrease of over 50 percent in the number of deaths due to SIDS in the United States since 1990, SIDS is still the third leading cause of death in infants, and the first leading cause of death among infants aged 28 to 364 days. It is estimated that SIDS occurs in about 1 per 2,000 births in the United States. Our understanding of SIDS is increasing, but we still do not understand exactly why it occurs.

What can be done to prevent SIDS? Although the specific cause of SIDS remains unknown, studies have revealed some risk factors:

- Babies who sleep on their tummies have an increased incidence of SIDS compared with babies who sleep on their back or side. Therefore, babies should be placed to sleep on their backs. When babies are awake they will need to spend some time on their tum-

mies to help their development and avoid flattening of the back of their head. Once babies are old enough to roll over from the back to the tummy, it is not necessary to force them back onto their backs for sleeping.
- The risk of SIDS is increased by bed sharing, especially if the parent who shares the bed with the infant is a smoker or has been drinking alcohol or taking drugs that may impair responsiveness.
- Maternal smoking during pregnancy and exposure to second-hand tobacco smoke are both important risk factors for SIDS.
- Babies who become too hot have an increased risk of SIDS. As a guide you should assume that if the room temperature is comfortable for you then it is fine for the baby. Don't dress the baby any warmer than you find comfortable.
- Breast-feeding may help protect against SIDS.
- Anything that could potentially suffocate the baby, for example, soft mattresses or soft bedding such as pillows, comforters and bumper pads, should be avoided. This also applies to stuffed toys and plastic wrapped products of any kind.

What happens afterward? As traumatic and horrifying as the reality of the death of an infant may be, there is still a grueling process to follow. Medical staff and quite possibly police officers usually will ask specific questions surrounding the circumstances of death. In many jurisdictions, the decision to perform an autopsy is made not by the parents, but by a coroner. These are some of the many steps that are required in order to make a diagnosis of SIDS.

You need to understand that in the vast majority of instances, you were not in any way responsible for your child's death. Remember, the cause of SIDS is unknown. Even though the child's health care provider may have examined her a few days previously, there are no clinical findings to predict which child will die from SIDS. Numerous studies have shown that vaccination does not increase the risk of SIDS.

There are grief specialists and support groups to help to find ways of dealing with the painful feelings.

If you have suffered such a loss, you should be aware that there is a slightly higher risk of SIDS for future infants; fortunately, this risk is less than 1 percent. Most experts do not feel that SIDS is hereditary.

RECOMMENDATIONS TO MINIMIZE RISK OF SIDS

- Place normal healthy infants to sleep on their back.
- Care for infants in a smoke- and drug-free environment.
- Dress/cover infants in a manner to avoid overheating.
- Breast-feed your baby if at all possible.
- Use firm, flat bedding with sheets and light blankets as needed.

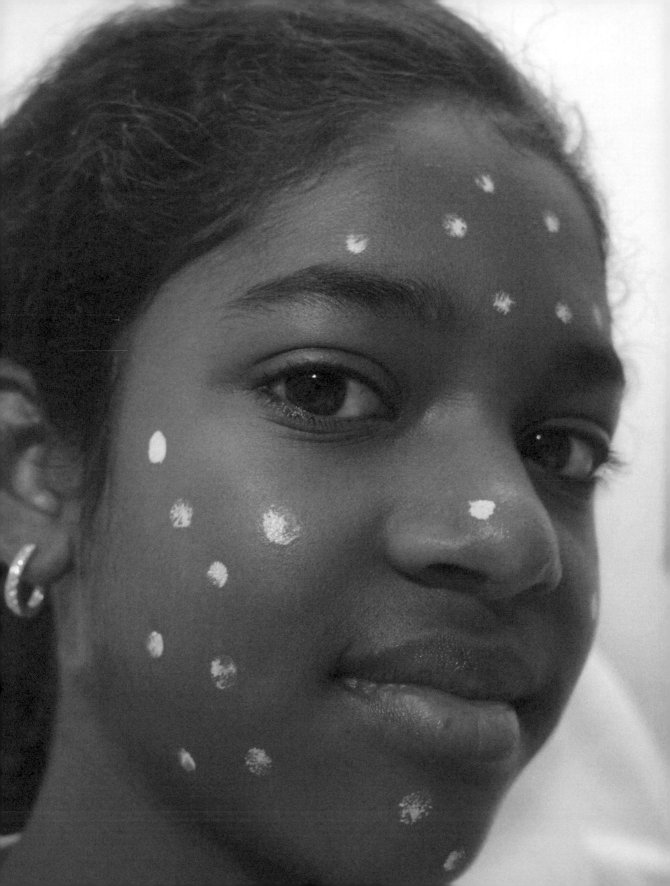

Childhood Infections

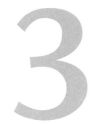

Botulism

What is botulism? Botulism is caused by an infection with bacteria called *Clostridium botulinum*. This bacterium produces a chemical, or "toxin," that interferes with the transmission of signals from the nerve to the muscle, thereby impairing muscle movement and causing paralysis. Botulism is a very rare infection. It can occur in infants, usually younger than 6 months of age, where it is called "infantile botulism." This happens after eating food contaminated with spores of *Clostridium botulinum*, usually when food is preserved or stored improperly. Botulism is not transmitted from person to person. In infantile botulism, the source of the spores is often not known. However, honey is a known source, and therefore you should not give it to your baby.

What does botulism look like? In infantile botulism, the symptoms usually evolve over days to weeks. The typical symptoms are constipation, followed by lethargy, poor feeding, a weak cry and weakness in the muscles of the eye. The weakness can go on to affect many other muscle groups and cause generalized weakness and a floppy body.

In older children, the symptoms typically occur more quickly. The weakness starts at the

head and then moves downward, with both left and right sides being affected equally. The initial symptoms may include double vision, blurred vision, dry mouth and difficulty swallowing and talking. This usually progresses to generalized weakness.

How do I treat botulism? Children who develop botulism need urgent medical care and hospitalization. Antibiotics are not routinely recommended. A special medication that fights against the toxin produced by *Clostridium botulinum* has been developed, but is only recommended in certain situations because of its potential side effects.

Bronchiolitis

The lung is made up of a branching network of airways, shaped like a tree. The main trunk is called the trachea, with major branches coming off called bronchi. The bronchi then branch into smaller airways, the smallest of which are called bronchioles.

What is bronchiolitis? Bronchiolitis is a viral infection in the lungs that tends to occur in young children under 2 years of age. An infection by a

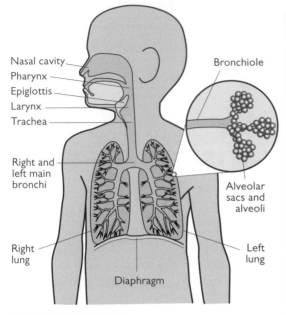

Nasal cavity
Pharynx
Epiglottis
Larynx
Trachea
Right and left main bronchi
Right lung
Diaphragm

Bronchiole
Alveolar sacs and alveoli
Left lung

THE RESPIRATORY SYSTEM

In bronchiolitis, a viral infection causes swelling and increased mucus in the small airways, especially the bronchioles.

virus causes swelling and increased mucus in the small airways, especially the bronchioles. The peak period for bronchiolitis is in the colder months, usually from November through April in the United States.

There are several viruses that can cause bronchiolitis. The most common one is called respiratory syncytial virus (RSV). The other viruses that cause it include parainfluenza, influenza, adenovirus and rhinovirus. These viruses are usually transmitted by unwashed hands infected with nasal secretions and, less frequently, through the air. Infection with RSV is common in childhood, with more than 80 percent of children being infected by the age of 2. Most frequently an older brother, sister or adult with a cold passes the virus on to the baby. The incubation period, that is, the time from when the virus is picked up until symptoms appear, varies from two to eight days.

What does bronchiolitis look like? Initially, the symptoms are similar to the common cold. Often your baby has a runny nose, cough and a **low-grade fever**. Then symptoms and signs of infection spread to the lungs or lower respiratory tract. His breathing rate increases, as does the apparent work of breathing. His chest appears to be moving in and out faster, the spaces between the ribs seem to be more sucked in, his nostrils may be flaring and he might make a grunting noise with every breath. There may be general symptoms such as restlessness, lethargy, a low-grade fever and decreased feeding. When listening to the lungs with a stethoscope a doctor or nurse will most likely hear wheezing, crackles or both.

In babies who are very young or have underlying medical conditions (such as prematurity, chronic lung disease, congenital heart disease or immunodeficiency), bronchiolitis can result in severe complications. These include apnea, where the baby doesn't take a breath for more than 10 to 15 seconds, or respiratory failure, where the lungs can no longer perform their vital function—taking oxygen into the body and getting rid of carbon dioxide—effectively.

How do I treat bronchiolitis? The vast majority of infants who have bronchiolitis do not require hospitalization and get better without any special treatment or medications. The disease lasts one to two weeks, which is similar to what happens when a child has a bad cold. Unfortunately, as in the common cold, there is no specific medication or treatment that makes a big difference in treating babies with bronchiolitis.

If you notice that your child is breathing faster and working hard to breathe, it is urgent that a medical professional examine him. The health care professional will then decide with you whether your infant can be safely looked after at home, or requires specific treatment or observation in the emergency room or hospital.

Several tests can be performed on babies who are suspected of having more severe bronchiolitis. An oxygen saturation level is measured by a monitor attached to the baby's finger or toe. This test indicates whether the lungs are doing their job of getting oxygen into the bloodstream. A chest x-ray can be done to look for pneumonia caused by a bacteria or to exclude other disorders. A swab from the nose can be sent to the laboratory to identify the virus causing the infection. This is typically done only in children with bronchiolitis who are seen in hospital.

Supplemental oxygen is required for babies with low oxygen levels—generally a saturation level less than 90 percent to 92 percent. This can be given by a mask applied to the face, through small prongs in the nostrils or, in very young infants, through a clear plastic box placed over their head, a bit like an astronaut.

It is important that your child receive adequate fluids to prevent dehydration. Often young infants may have difficulty coordinating their breathing with swallowing when they are working so hard to breathe, as is the case in bronchiolitis. They may also be exhausted from the effort and the infection, and therefore show minimal interest in feeding. Feeding smaller amounts more frequently may be helpful. However, if feeding is significantly reduced, your child may require intravenous supplementation to provide fluids. Another option would be a nasogastric tube passed through the nostril into the stomach, which can be used to provide formula and fluids.

Chest physiotherapy refers to various ways of tapping on the chest to help remove mucus

from the lungs. There is no evidence that this helps in bronchiolitis, and thus it is generally not recommended.

There are a number of medications that have been tried with varying amounts of success. Albuterol (generally called salbutamol outside the United States) is an inhaled medication that works by relaxing the muscular wall of the airways, thereby opening them up. It is very effective in children with asthma. However, in bronchiolitis, although it does seem to be helpful in some babies, there is no convincing evidence that it works particularly well. Many doctors will try albuterol, see if it helps and if there is no benefit, stop it. Epinephrine is another inhaled medication. It also works by decreasing the swelling in the airways. Like albuterol, the studies of its use have produced conflicting results. Some doctors like to use it, while others do not. Both albuterol and epinephrine are usually given through a compressor in the hospital setting, although albuterol can also be given at home with a compressor, for very young babies, or a puffer with a spacing device. Inhaled epinephrine is not given at home.

Steroids work by decreasing the inflammation in the airways. There is no strong evidence that inhaled steroids work in bronchiolitis but some doctors believe that one dose by mouth can help those babies sick enough to come to hospital. Further studies into the use of steroids for bronchiolitis are underway. Ribavarin is a medication that works against the most common virus that causes RSV bronchiolitis. For children with RSV bronchiolitis who have serious underlying medical conditions and, therefore, are considered at high risk for serious complications, ribavarin is a consideration. However, its benefit is also controversial. Remember that bronchiolitis is caused by a virus, and antibiotics will therefore be of no benefit. However, they will be required if the baby develops a bacterial infection on top of the bronchiolitis.

Can I prevent my child from getting bronchiolitis? Preventing healthy infants from getting bronchiolitis by avoiding contact with other people infected with a virus is difficult, if not impossible: it's like the common cold. Remember, most children will be exposed to RSV before their second birthday and the majority of them will sail through with a nasty cold or no illness at all.

There is no immunization currently available to protect against RSV infection. However, infants who have serious underlying medical problems and are at high risk for getting seriously ill from bronchiolitis might gain some protection against RSV infection and bronchiolitis from a monthly injection during the winter season of pooled antibodies to RSV.

Can my child get bronchiolitis more than once? It is possible to get bronchiolitis more than once. That is because the RSV virus changes from season to season and even within the same season. Also, there are different strains of the RSV virus, each of which can cause bronchiolitis. Furthermore, several different viruses can cause bronchiolitis. For example, RSV may cause bronchiolitis the first time and influenza may cause it the second. Thus, bronchiolitis is different from the chicken pox virus, which you typically "get" only once.

Cellulitis

What is cellulitis? Cellulitis is an infection of the skin and underlying soft tissues that can occur anywhere in the body. These infections are caused by bacteria; most commonly group A streptococcus and *Staphylococcus aureus*. In cer-

tain circumstances, such as dog or cat bites, or in children with a problem in their immune system, other types of bacteria can also cause cellulitis.

Cellulitis occurs most commonly following some sort of break in the skin that allows the bacteria to invade and infect the area. This can happen after a fall, scrape or insect bite. Cellulitis may also occur as a complication of chicken pox. The skin around the "pox" gets secondarily infected with bacteria, commonly group A streptococcus, leading to cellulitis and, rarely, to the very severe flesh-eating disease, called **necrotizing fasciitis**. Children who have a problem with their immune system, such as an immunodeficiency or diabetes, are more prone to cellulitis.

What does cellulitis look like? The skin becomes red, warm and swollen, and may be tender. The child might have a fever and chills and feel unwell but this is not always the case. Swollen glands, which are really enlarged lymph nodes, can be found near the area of cellulitis. For example, cellulitis of the leg or foot produces swollen nodes in the groin, and cellulitis of the arm or hand leads to enlarged lymph nodes in the armpit (axilla). The doctor might decide to do a blood test to look for the bacteria causing the cellulitis, particularly if your child has fever or chills or an immune problem. But, in most cases, the bacteria will not be found in the blood.

Cellulitis around the eye, or **periorbital** cellulitis, is of particular concern. It is important that urgent assessment and treatment occur so that the infection does not spread inward to the vital structures of the eye. Worrisome signs that the infection has indeed spread to the eye producing orbital cellulitis include pain when your child moves his eye, decreased vision and a protruding eye.

How do I treat cellulitis? Cellulitis is treated with antibiotics. Depending on your child's age, underlying health and the extent of the cellulitis, the antibiotics will be given either by mouth or by intravenous infusion. If the infected area involves the hand or foot, elevation of the limb will help to decrease the swelling. Most cases of cellulitis will begin to improve within 48 hours of your child receiving antibiotics. It is important that your child take the entire course of antibiotics, usually for 7 to 10 days, to ensure that the bacteria are completely eradicated.

If your child is treated with antibiotics at home and the cellulitis is spreading or your child is experiencing a lot of pain or becomes very unwell, consult your doctor or return to the emergency room immediately.

Chicken Pox (Varicella)

What is chicken pox? Chicken pox, or varicella, is an infection caused by the varicella-zoster virus. It is extremely contagious. The virus is spread from person to person by direct contact or through the air by breathing in droplets containing varicella-zoster virus. You can also get it by being near someone with chicken pox who is coughing or sneezing. Because of this infectious nature, chicken pox is very common: before the introduction of the varicella vaccine in 1995, there were about four million cases of the disease in the United States each year. Children are usually contagious from one to two days prior to the onset of the rash and for about five days afterward. The virus infects the cells lining the nose and throat. After an incubation period of about two weeks the virus causes illness as it spreads to lymph glands and into the blood and the skin.

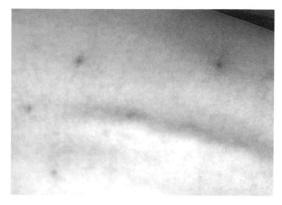

CHICKEN POX

The vesicles of chicken pox seen on the back early in the course of the disease.

What does chicken pox look like? Children with chicken pox often begin their illness with a fever, headache, muscular aches and a typical rash. This rash is made up of spots that look like small water blisters (**vesicles**) a few millimeters in diameter on top of a reddish base. Some children have only a few blisters and others have as many as 500. Usually after four or five days, the blisters dry up and form scabs. The rash can be quite itchy, especially during the healing phase when the scabs are forming.

The complications of chicken pox are rare but can be life-threatening. If the blisters get infected with streptococcus, a secondary bacterial skin infection, **impetigo**, can result. Rarely, the streptococcus produces a deeper soft tissue infection, the so-called flesh-eating disease (see Necrotizing Fasciitis, pages 96–97), which can even be fatal. In developing countries, secondary infection with **tetanus** can also produce tragic results. Chicken pox can be very severe or even life-threatening in newborn infants and anyone who has a weak immune system. Children with chicken pox occasionally develop involvement of the lungs (pneumonia) or brain (**encephalitis**). The signs of brain involvement are clumsiness and difficulty with balance as a result of the cerebellum being affected. Babies who get chicken pox from their mothers before birth can be born with birth defects including skin scars, eye problems or deformities of the arms and legs.

How is chicken pox treated? There are specific antiviral medications for chicken pox, such as acyclovir, but these are generally not recommended for routine use in otherwise healthy children. The decision to use antiviral therapy, how to give it and for how long should be based on the age of your child (usually only to those older than 12 years of age), the extent of infection and whether or not he has a weakened immune system.

Healthy children should be treated for their symptoms. If they are feverish and achy, they can take acetaminophen or ibuprofen. Never use aspirin for chicken pox: it can result in a serious condition called Reye's syndrome. If there is significant itching, trim his fingernails to prevent secondary bacterial infection. He can take soothing oatmeal (Aveeno) baths and oral antihistamines, such as diphenhydramine, reduce the itch and promote better sleep.

The best protection against chicken pox is prevention, using varicella vaccine. One dose is recommended for children over 12 months but younger or equal to 12 years of age. Two doses separated by an interval of at least four to eight weeks are recommended for individuals older than 12. Varicella vaccine does not guarantee that your child will never develop chicken pox, but it does significantly reduce the probability. Furthermore, vaccination seems to prevent most of the serious complications that can occur.

Cytomegalovirus (CMV) Infections

What is CMV? Cytomegalovirus is a common virus that can show up in a variety of situations. It is generally spread by contact with a person's secretions; and infection requires close, intimate contact with someone who is shedding the virus in his saliva, urine or other bodily fluids. The virus can be passed from a pregnant mother to her fetus through the placenta (congenital infection) or at delivery as the newborn passes through the birth canal. Transmission can even occur through breast milk during feeding or through transfusion of blood or blood products and has occurred with transplantation of organs. Even after the symptoms have disappeared, CMV remains dormant in the body for life.

CMV is common throughout all parts of the world. In developing countries, most children are infected in early infancy. In the United States up to 85 percent of adults have had CMV infection. Some studies have shown that as many as 70 percent of children 1 to 3 years of age in child care centers excrete the virus. The **incubation period** for developing disease when CMV is passed between people is unknown.

What does CMV look like? CMV causes different types of illnesses depending on the child's age and his immune system. Most children develop no symptoms after CMV infection. They remain entirely well, and there are no long-term health consequences. Adolescents and adults can develop infectious mononucleosis-like symptoms with a prolonged fever and a mild hepatitis. (See Infectious Mononucleosis, pages 105–106.)

Infections acquired by the developing fetus during pregnancy are called congenital infections. Congenital CMV infection affects 1 percent of all live births in the United States. Most congenital CMV infections have no symptoms. Of infants who have had congenital CMV infection, about 10 percent to 15 percent might have problems with hearing or learning later in life. Congenital CMV is a common infectious cause of hearing loss in children. Around 10 percent of newborns with congenital CMV will be very sick. They can be born very small and jaundiced, with skin rashes, an enlarged liver and spleen, a smaller than expected head and brain that may contain calcium deposits, and disease in the back of the eye called retinitis. Blood tests can reveal a low platelet (the blood cells that help with clotting) count. These children can have severe neurological problems affecting their learning and intellect. It can also lead to cerebral palsy. The risk of severe neurological problems is greatest when fetal infection occurs in the first half of pregnancy. Infection at the time of birth or through breast milk is not linked with any disease.

To diagnose congenital CMV infection several blood and urine tests may be required. For the older child or adolescent, blood tests are required.

How is CMV treated? Specific antiviral medications are available for treatment of CMV infection in children with immune system problems. However, the benefit of using these medications for healthy children is still uncertain. Treatment should be considered in newborns with congenital CMV. One study found that treating newborns with congenital CMV decreased their chance of developing hearing loss.

Pregnant women who are not immune to CMV are advised either to avoid close contact with young children who are likely to be releasing the virus, if practical, or at least practice meticulous hygiene, especially hand washing.

Coxsackie Virus Infections

What are coxsackie virus infections? Infections caused by coxsackie viruses are very common in childhood. These viruses belong to a group known as **enteroviruses**. Spread of the virus in childhood can occur through saliva and secretions from the nose and mouth or by the fecal-oral route in which there is ingestion of a virus that is shed in feces. These viruses can survive outside the body on surfaces for periods long enough to allow transmission. Coxsackie virus infections are common in the summer and early fall in temperate climates. The usual **incubation period** is three to six days, except when coxsackie causes pink eye (**conjunctivitis**) in which case the incubation period is just one to three days. People who have had coxsackie virus infection can continue to shed the virus for several weeks after the infection through their stools, and for about a week from secretions from the nose and mouth.

What does coxsackie look like? Coxsackie virus shows up in several ways. Most commonly, children have a fever and feel unwell. They can have a "cold," sore throat or herpangina. In herpangina, the virus causes small fluid-filled blisters and ulcers in the back portion of the mouth. Children with herpangina will have a pain in their mouth, and may drool and have difficulty swallowing liquids and food because of the pain. Coxsackie virus can also cause pneumonia.

Children infected with coxsackie virus might have a rash. For example, hand, foot and mouth disease is caused by coxsackie virus (see Hand, Foot and Mouth Disease on pages 99–100). The virus can also cause diarrhea and vomiting with abdominal pain. Coxsackie virus can cause conjunctivitis. More uncommonly, it can also cause an infection in the heart, **myocarditis**, or the space around the heart, **pericarditis**. Children with this type of coxsackie infection will be very sick with trouble breathing, a fast heart rate and may have low blood pressure due to heart failure. Coxsackie virus can also cause a form of **meningitis** or **encephalitis**.

Newborns can become very sick with coxsackie virus infection. They can eat poorly, have fever, a distended belly, and look very ill.

For common coxsackie virus infection, where the child is not severely ill, the diagnosis can be made by your doctor without any specific tests.

How is coxsackie treated? Antibiotics are not helpful for coxsackie virus infections. For rare but life-threatening infections, a specific antiviral medication for enteroviruses (which include coxsackie viruses) has been used with some success. However, this is still being studied. Most children with typical coxsackie virus infections can be treated at home. It is important to ensure that your child drinks adequate amounts of fluids to prevent dehydration. In the case of severe infections, hospitalization may be required, but this is very uncommon.

Croup

What is croup? Croup is a distinctive respiratory condition caused by inflammation mainly in the windpipe, or trachea—hence, its other name, tracheitis. Most often croup is due to an infection caused by a virus called parainfluenza, which is spread from person to person by direct contact with infected saliva or nasal mucus. Infection usually occurs in preschool children

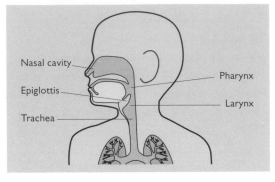

CROUP

In croup, the inflammation is mainly in the upper part of the airways (i.e., the larynx and trachea).

and is most dangerous in young infants because they have narrower airways.

What does croup look like? Croup begins suddenly, often at night, in a previously healthy child who wakes up coughing. The cough is typically very sharp, dry and brassy-sounding, commonly described as being like the noise made by a seal or like a dog's bark. Usually, the child has a very hoarse voice. Infants and children who have more severe croup will also make a distinctive gasping noise when they breathe in, called stridor, as the air tries to pass through their windpipe, narrowed by swelling. Sometimes, after a day or two, the infection will settle in the chest where it can cause wheezing.

How is croup treated? You will probably find your croupy child frightening. Generally, most children with croup get better by themselves and require no treatment. For years, parents have been told to use humidity to manage croup. Usually, this involves sitting in the bathroom with the shower running. Although parents and physicians alike have long felt humidity helps loosen secretions in croupy children, there is little scientific evidence that it actually works. The same applies for the suggestion that taking a child outside into cold air is useful. Both treatments are pretty harmless and may be worth a try, but they aren't proven therapy.

Specific antiviral therapy is not available. Antibiotics are ineffective and should be reserved for those children who develop a complication, such as bacterial ear infections or pneumonia.

What does work? If the trachea is narrowed enough to produce stridor, anti-inflammatory medication (steroids) are given orally to reduce swelling. For those children with significant respiratory distress, inhaled epinephrine given with a **nebulizer** and mask is used to open the airway rapidly. In severe cases, the child may require hospitalization to get oxygen and other supportive treatment until the croup gets better.

Cat Scratch Disease

What is cat scratch disease? For those who love cats, they are the perfect pet. But sometimes, even the perfect pet can present problems. Cat scratch disease is one of them. It is an infection caused by the bacteria *Bartonella henselae*. The germ is passed to humans by contact with infected cats. Fleas can also transmit the bacteria between cats, but it cannot be passed between people. More than 90 percent of people with cat scratch disease have had recent contact with apparently healthy cats, often kittens.

What does cat scratch disease look like? Children with cat scratch disease are generally not very sick. They may have fever. It usually takes about 7 to 12 days from the time of the scratch to the appearance of a skin lesion and about 5 to 50 days before enlarged and tender lymph nodes (swollen glands) become prominent. The skin lesion is usually a small raised spot, or **papule**, that is often found at the site where the cat scratched the skin and where the bacteria entered the body. The lymph nodes that drain the area where the body has been scratched become enlarged, tender, warm and red. For example, if your child was scratched and infected in the lower arm, the lymph nodes around the elbow, underarm and neck become affected. In some children, the nodes may start to drain pus.

Rarely, cat scratch disease can also cause more serious problems, such as **encephalitis**, **meningitis**, persistent fevers, hepatitis, pneumonia, infection in the liver, spleen or bone, and other types of rashes.

Cat scratch disease can be diagnosed by performing special blood tests. Sometimes, your child's doctor might order a biopsy of the enlarged glands to help the diagnosis.

How is cat scratch disease treated? Cat scratch disease usually gets better by itself, without treatment, in two to four months. A needle may be used to remove the fluid and relieve the pain of enlarged lymph nodes that are filled with pus. Antibiotics are recommended only for children who are very sick, have uncommon forms of cat scratch disease, for example in the liver or spleen, or who have an immune system problem.

In general, children should be instructed to avoid playing roughly with cats and kittens to prevent scratches and bites. If a child is scratched or bitten by a cat, the site should be cleaned right away. If you have a cat, it's important to control its fleas.

The Common Cold

What is the common cold? Although the common cold is a minor and self-limiting viral infection, it still can make kids miserable. The cumulative burden of upper respiratory tract infections on society is truly immense, costing billions of dollars annually and resulting in countless hours of lost work. It is important that you know a little bit about the common cold so you can understand the natural course of the disease, what should concern you, what treatments work and which ones don't.

The common cold is caused by a number of respiratory viruses, the most common of which is the rhinovirus. On average, young children get about four colds a year but often there are years when a child seems to get more than his fair share of colds.

What does the common cold look like? Typical symptoms are a stuffed or runny nose, poor appetite, headache and mild tiredness. The nasal discharge is usually watery and clear at the onset but often becomes yellow or green and thicker after a few days. This thickening of the mucus is expected and does not necessarily

imply a secondary bacterial infection. Children might complain of sore eyes, sore throat, hoarseness or neck gland swelling.

Unlike the "flu," fever is infrequent and seldom high with a cold. The common cold usually remains confined to the nose and throat and does not affect the chest. Parents often underestimate the usual duration of a cold. Although symptoms may last only a few days, particularly in older children, it is common for a child to remain unwell for at least a week. In about 10 percent of preschoolers, the symptoms will persist for two weeks.

How is the common cold treated? The shelves of pharmacies are filled with cough and cold remedies, both traditional and naturopathic. Would that they actually worked! Oral decongestants are not very effective and can cause rapid heartbeat and sleeping difficulties in children. Antihistamines don't work for colds. Cough medicines may appear to be useful for hacking coughs but they too have been proven to work no better than a placebo. Furthermore, remember viruses cause colds; antibiotics are ineffective for the common cold.

What does help? Time, mainly. Children cure themselves. You can use acetaminophen or ibuprofen for relief of pain, aches or fever. Avoid aspirin (acetylsalicylic acid), or any cold medicine containing it, for children and teenagers because it can lead to brain and liver damage (Reye's syndrome). Encourage your child to drink plenty of fluids and to rest where possible. Nose drops or sprays are difficult for children to use, but can provide brief relief for the runny nose.

You have two basic jobs when your children have the symptoms of the common cold. First, comfort them as best you can and, second,

REASONS TO SEE YOUR DOCTOR

- wheezing
- rapid breathing
- increased work of breathing
- earache
- increasing drowsiness
- new fever, days after the cold first appeared

observe them for any signs that suggest the cold is turning into something more serious. These include wheezing, rapid or labored breathing, earache, increasing drowsiness or the development of a new fever days after the cold first appeared.

Diphtheria, Polio, Tetanus, Pertussis and *Haemophilus influenzae* Type B Infections

It is important that you know about these infections. Not because they are common, but, ironically, because they no longer are. In the past, thousands upon thousands of young children died every year because of these diseases. Now they don't. A simple series of vaccines has virtually eliminated mortality from diphtheria, tetanus, pertussis, polio and *Haemophilus influenzae* type b in the developed world. It has been one of modern medicine's greatest achievements.

A vaccine called DTaP is a three-in-one needle that protects against diphtheria (D), tetanus (T) and acellular pertussis (aP). Kids get three shots of DTaP vaccine at 2, 4 and 6 months of age. This is called the primary (initial) immunization series. A booster is given between 15 and 18 months, and another between 4 and 6 years. Later, between the ages of 11 and 12 years, a shot for tetanus and diphtheria only (Td) is given. Separate shots are given for polio (IPV) and *Haemophilus influenzae* type b (Hib) infections. Primary immunization is at 2 and 4 months, with an additional Hib shot at 6 months. Boosters for IPV and Hib are given between 12 and 15 months, with another for IPV between 4 and 6 years. There is a combination DTaP/Hib shot,

and while it should not be used for primary immunization it can be used as a booster for any Hib vaccine. These vaccines are highly effective and extremely safe. Serious reactions are rare.

DIPHTHERIA

What is diphtheria? Diphtheria is a serious infection caused by the bacteria *Corynebacterium diphtheriae*. It is spread by direct contact from one person to another by coughing or sneezing. Healthy people can be carriers of diphtheria bacteria and may also spread the bacteria without being visibly sick. In those who have not been vaccinated against diphtheria, the bacteria can enter the body and inflame the upper airway by releasing a toxin that injures the body.

What does diphtheria look like? Diphtheria causes a sore throat, fever and chills, and serious problems with breathing. The tonsils and upper airways can become so inflamed that a crustlike membrane forms and actually blocks airflow. The affected child will drool and struggle to get air. Diphtheria can also affect the heart causing an inflammation called **myocarditis**. Heart failure can result. Nerve damage can result from the toxin, causing muscle weakness and paralysis of the vocal cords. Diphtheria kills 1 out of every 10 people who get the infection. Infants who become infected are even more likely to die from it.

How is diphtheria treated? Treatment must be started immediately at the time of diagnosis using an intravenous injection of antitoxin, a substance that blocks the effect of the toxin. Antibiotics do not affect the duration or severity of the illness but they do shorten the contagious period.

TETANUS

What is tetanus? Tetanus is a serious infection caused by bacteria that live in soil, dust and manure. It is also known as lockjaw. Tetanus is not contagious and does not spread from person to person. This makes it different from the other infections that can be prevented by vaccination. Tetanus bacteria enter the body through a break in the skin as a result of a puncture, cut or bite. These bacteria then grow in the body and release a nerve toxin that enters the spinal cord and brain. The infection of the nervous system causes a loss of spinal reflexes that in turn leads to an excess stimulation of muscles, causing spasms throughout the body.

What does tetanus look like? Symptoms begin within one to seven days of the skin injury. The child's muscles may go into paralyzing spasms. The first muscles affected are the ones in the jaw, hence the term "lockjaw." This is very painful and the child may not be able to swallow or open his mouth. Tetanus also causes cramping of the muscles of the arms, legs and stomach and can cause painful convulsions. If tetanus affects the breathing muscles, the child can die very quickly from respiratory failure. Children who survive tetanus can have long-lasting problems with speech, memory and thinking.

How is tetanus treated? Even with early treatment, tetanus kills 2 out of every 10 children who get the disease. Tetanus **immunoglobulin**, a preparation extracted from donated blood, should be given by injection into a muscle. Treatment also requires surgical cleaning of wounds and relieving and preventing muscle spasms with drugs. Prevention is the best treatment. Immunization in infancy and periodic boosters with tetanus toxoid has essentially eliminated tetanus in North America. If a child's immunization status is uncertain, a booster dose of tetanus toxoid can be administered in the emergency department when a wound is treated.

PERTUSSIS (WHOOPING COUGH)

What is pertussis? Pertussis is more commonly known as whooping cough. It is caused by a bacteria called *Bordetella pertussis* that can infect the lining of the air tubes and lungs. Pertussis spreads very easily from an infected person to others through coughing and sneezing, often by an adult with milder symptoms. A toxin on the surface of the bacteria damages the child's air tubes.

What does it look like? Pertussis usually begins with mild cold symptoms. However, instead of getting better with time, the cough typically gets worse and eventually turns into violent coughing spasms. These coughing spasms can produce vomiting or cause the child to stop breathing for a short period of time. The cough may last for weeks making it hard for infected children to eat, drink or even breathe. Pneumonia will occur in 2 out of every 10 children with pertussis. Infants are in particular danger if they develop whooping cough. One out of 400 babies under a year old who get pertussis will end up with brain damage and some may die. Young infants with whooping cough may stop breathing or have convulsions and go into a coma. In older children and adults, whooping cough is a milder disease, but infected individuals may still have severe coughing that can last from 6 to 12 weeks.

How is pertussis treated? Children who are presumed to have pertussis and their close contacts are prescribed an antibiotic, such as erythromycin. This is done to prevent spread of the disease to others: it doesn't significantly reduce symptoms once the coughing spasms have begun. Temporary quarantine is also required. The treatment for whooping cough is largely supportive. Young infants whose coughing produces blue spells or who experience breathing stoppage (**apnea**) are admitted to hospital for care. This includes suctioning the excess mucus and saliva, maintaining hydration and nutrition, and providing oxygen when needed.

POLIO

What is polio? Polio is a viral infection caused by one of three strains of the poliovirus. Poliovirus is found in the throat and stool and is spread by coughing, sneezing or by touching other people with hands that are not washed. Transmission can also occur by swallowing contaminated water or food. Once in the body the virus spreads through the blood into the brain and spinal cord along the nerve fibers.

What does polio look like? Some people with polio don't feel sick at all. Often, however, polio causes fever, headache, vomiting and severe muscle pain. It can also make children very tired and cause stiffness in the neck and back. About 1 child out of every 100 infected with the virus will get the severe form resulting in paralysis with an inability to move the arms or legs for the rest of their lives. Some children who contract polio die.

How is polio treated? There is no specific treatment for polio, only supportive measures. But, it is totally preventable by immunization.

Hib (*HAEMOPHILUS INFLUENZAE* TYPE B) INFECTION

What is Hib? "Hib" stands for *Haemophilus influenzae* type b and is a kind of bacteria. Even though *influenzae* is part of its name, the bacterium has nothing to do with the influenza virus that produces the flu. Hib is most dangerous when it infects the fluid around the brain and spinal cord causing a very serious disease called **meningitis**. Hib can also cause pneumonia, bacteremia (infection in the blood, often called blood poisoning), and even infections in the bones and joints. In addition, Hib can produce a serious infection of the throat near the larynx. This is called epiglottitis and makes it so difficult for the child to swallow and breathe that death can result.

What does Hib meningitis look like? In young infants the symptoms of meningitis include fever, irritability, feeding difficulties, drowsiness, coma, vomiting, stiff neck and a bulging **fontanelle** (the soft spot on top of the skull). Older children with meningitis usually have a fever and a major change in behavior such as drowsiness, reduced consciousness, fussiness or agitation. Other symptoms include severe headache, pain when moving the head or neck, general aches and pains, joint pain and convulsions. For the first few hours, meningitis can initially mimic a simple viral infection.

How is Hib meningitis treated? Without treatment, almost all children who get Hib meningitis will die or suffer brain damage that lasts for the rest of their lives. Even with appropriate management, about 5 percent of children with Hib meningitis die and approximately a third of the survivors will have brain damage or deafness. The other serious Hib infections of the blood, lungs, bones and joints can also kill. Fortunately, since the development of the Hib vaccine in the 1980s, the incidence of serious disease due to *Haemophilus influenzae* has declined dramatically. Before 1990, Hib was the most common cause of bacterial meningitis in the United States. The incidence of Hib from 1980 to 1990 was 40–100 for every 100,000 children, but since 1990 the incidence has decreased to 1.3 per 100,000 children.

Encephalitis

What is encephalitis? Encephalitis is an uncommon infection of the brain usually caused by viruses or, less often, by bacteria. This infection in the brain causes swelling of the brain cells and potentially permanent damage. Normal brain functions, such as thinking, speaking, feeling, moving and even breathing can be disrupted. Encephalitis is different from meningitis where the infection affects primarily the fluid and space around the brain.

The common causes of encephalitis in childhood are viral infections. Viruses can reach the brain and infect it through the bloodstream. For example, following an insect bite, the virus enters the blood and can spread to various parts of the body including the brain. Viruses can also reach the brain by infecting a nerve in another part of the body, and then spreading through the connection of nerves that leads to the brain.

Of the viruses that cause encephalitis, herpes simplex accounts for about 10 percent of all cases of encephalitis in the United States. The herpes simplex virus can be transmitted through contact with infected mouth secretions or from an infected skin lesion. Other viruses that can cause encephalitis include **enteroviruses**, influenza, Epstein-Barr virus (mononucleosis) and adenovirus. Some viruses are transmitted by mosquitoes and ticks and are more common in certain parts

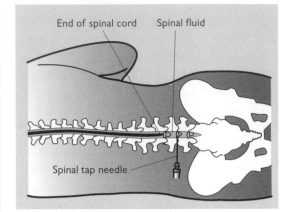

LUMBAR PUNCTURE
Meningitis is diagnosed by performing a lumbar puncture (spinal tap). A sample of fluid is taken from the space below the end of the spinal cord so that the needle will not touch the spinal cord.

of the world where these insects live (for example, West Nile virus, Japanese encephalitis). *Mycoplasma pneumoniae* is the most common bacterium that can cause encephalitis in childhood. Despite many tests, a specific infecting organism is not identified as the cause of the encephalitis in some patients.

What does encephalitis look like? Children with encephalitis usually have fever, headache and an altered level of consciousness. They might be disoriented, which means that they may not know where they are, and not recognize the people around them. They can have behavioral and speech disturbances. Some children with encephalitis will have seizures. They can also have difficulty moving parts of their body. This might include difficulty swallowing and eating.

The diagnosis of encephalitis is confirmed by performing several tests. One important procedure is the **lumbar puncture**, or spinal tap. In this test, a needle is placed in the lower back into a fluid-filled space below where the spinal cord ends. A small amount of **cerebrospinal fluid** (CSF) is removed. The fluid is then sent to the laboratory where the number of white blood (pus) cells is counted, and tests for bacteria and viruses are also performed. Imaging of the brain by means of a CT or MRI scan is usually necessary. An **electroencephalogram** (EEG), which looks at the pattern of electrical brain waves, is sometimes helpful to detect evidence of abnormal brain activity or seizures.

How is encephalitis treated? Children with encephalitis need to be hospitalized. Fluids and nutrition may need to be provided by an intravenous or **nasogastric tube** if the child is unable to swallow. Seizures need to be treated with anticonvulsant medication. In cases of herpes simplex virus encephalitis a specific antiviral medication, called acyclovir, is given intravenously. An antibiotic will be used if the encephalitis is caused by the bacterium *Mycoplasma pneumoniae*. The prognosis for children who have had encephalitis is variable. Some children will make a full recovery while others are left with significant neurological impairment or they can even die. Children handicapped by encephalitis can have difficulties moving parts of their body, difficulties in the way they think or speak, difficulties with seeing or hearing, or have problems with seizures. They often require a rehabilitation program with the help of physiotherapists and occupational therapists.

Fifth Disease (Erythema Infectiosum or Slapped Cheek Disease)

What is fifth disease? Fifth disease is a very common childhood infection caused by a virus called parvovirus B19. Half of all teenagers have evidence in their blood that they have been previously infected by parvovirus B19, but about a quarter of people who become infected show no symptoms at all. Parvovirus B19 is transmitted between people by droplets in the air that we inhale.

What does fifth disease look like? The two major features of fifth disease in children are flulike symptoms and a characteristic rash. The flulike symptoms start between four to 14 days after the virus enters the body, but can take up to three weeks to develop. These flulike symptoms typically include chills, headaches and muscle aches. About a third of children with fifth disease have a fever.

The classical rash of fifth disease usually begins about two to three weeks after the virus enters the body. Children develop a distinctive rash with red cheeks, sometimes referred to as the "slapped cheek rash." The rash can also occur on the body, starting on the chest and moving to the arms, buttocks and thighs. It starts as small red dots and goes on to a blotchy or lacy appearance. This rash may be more pronounced after a warm bath and can be itchy. It may come and go for a few weeks during the illness, and can come back during emotional episodes, exercise or exposure to sunlight or heat for weeks or months after the illness. This rash is not harmful or dangerous.

Children with fifth disease are most infectious before the rash appears, and, in fact, they are unlikely to be infectious after the rash appears. Thus, children with fifth disease and a rash can attend school because they are no longer contagious.

Parvovirus B19 can make the anemia of children with certain types of anemia like sickle cell or thalassemia much worse. This is called an **aplastic crisis** (see page 262).

How do I treat fifth disease? Because fifth disease is an infection caused by a virus, antibiotics will not work. There is no specific lotion or medication that is required for the rash. Children who are otherwise healthy will get better by themselves. As with other viral illnesses, you should make sure that your child is drinking adequate amounts of fluid, and you may give him medications such as acetaminophen or ibuprofen to treat the fever if it appears to be causing discomfort. If anyone in contact with your child is pregnant, she should talk to her doctor, as parvovirus infection early in pregnancy can occasionally lead to miscarriage.

Necrotizing Fasciitis, or "Flesh-Eating Disease"

What is necrotizing fasciitis? Flesh-eating disease, or necrotizing fasciitis, is an uncommon but life-threatening bacterial infection. It affects the skin, the fat just below the skin and a layer below the fat called the fascia. As the bacteria spread through the soft tissue, the blood vessels are damaged and the result is impaired blood flow to the skin and fat layers. Necrotizing fasciitis spreads rapidly and causes swelling and cell death, or "necrosis," in the skin, subcutaneous fat and fascia. Damage to these soft tissues is very extensive, hence the name "flesh-eating disease." The flesh is not actually eaten by bacteria!

This is a rare condition. It can occur after some sort of "break" in the skin that allows bacteria to invade and infect the area. This can happen after a fall, scrape, insect bite or burn. Many cases seen in American children are the result of infected chicken pox lesions. Certain underlying diseases predispose patients to

developing the disease, including conditions that affect the immune system (diabetes mellitus, HIV/AIDS and cancer) or patients with preexisting skin conditions. Although necrotizing fasciitis is rare, the bacteria that produce the condition are themselves quite common: group A streptococcus or *Staphylococcus aureus*.

What does necrotizing fasciitis look like? Necrotizing fasciitis can affect any area of the body, but most commonly it affects the legs or arms. Early on, patients have symptoms similar to **cellulitis**, a more superficial infection (see Cellulitis, pages 84–85). The skin appears red, swollen, shiny and tense. However, unlike in cellulitis, pain is severe the infection progresses very rapidly in a matter of hours, and the redness of the skin turns purple or purple-black as the tissue dies. Numbness may occur in the affected areas as the nerves that supply the skin are damaged and die. The infection spreads into the deeper layers as well. Children who develop necrotizing fasciitis are very unwell. They have high fever and chills and are very weak. The infection can result in failure of the other organs in the body.

CT and MRI scans have been used to help confirm the diagnosis. Samples of discharge from the infected skin and blood samples are taken to culture in order to identify the responsible bacteria.

How is necrotizing fasciitis treated? Probably the best form of treatment is prevention by vaccinating your child against chicken pox. If a child does develop necrotizing fasciitis he will require emergency specialized care in hospital. Often close monitoring in an intensive care unit is required. The treatment includes antibiotics given through an intravenous catheter. Sometimes surgery is required to control the infection by removing the infected areas of skin and soft tissue (**debridement**). A special blood product, intravenous **immunoglobulin** (also called immune globulin intravenous, or IVIG), has been shown to be effective against certain types of bacteria.

Gastroenteritis

What is gastroenteritis? Gastroenteritis ("gastro" or "stomach flu") is an infection of the bowel, including the small and large intestines. It is extremely common in young children. The major symptoms of gastroenteritis are diarrhea and, frequently, vomiting. Diarrhea exists when the stools are looser, more watery and, usually, more numerous than normal (see pages 34–37).

By far the commonest cause of gastroenteritis in North America is viral but it can also be brought on by bacteria or parasites. Rotavirus, **enteroviruses**, adenovirus and astroviruses are the most common viral causes, while shigella, E. coli, campylobacter and staphylococcus are the major bacterial culprits.

Transmission of these viruses and bacteria can occur between people or through contaminated water or food. It is important that everyone wash their hands with soap after going to the toilet and that you do the same after changing diapers and before preparing food.

What does gastroenteritis look like? The illness, particularly if viral, will often start with vomiting and a **low-grade fever**. Diarrhea occurs as an initial symptom or follows very shortly. If there is blood in the diarrhea, the illness is more likely to be caused by a bacterium. Abdominal cramps and loss of appetite and energy are also commonly seen.

Dehydration is a major concern with gastroenteritis, particularly in young children. It occurs when the body's total water content decreases as a result of loss of water and salt through diarrhea and vomiting. Signs of dehydration include loss of tears when crying, eyes that appear "sunken," dry lips, decreased amount of urination (fewer wet diapers), lethargy, cold hands and feet, and a fast heart rate. Low blood pressure is a sign of severe dehydration. When a child gets dehydrated his body weight drops.

How is gastroenteritis treated? The most important aspect of dealing with gastroenteritis is to ensure that your child is taking the right type and amount of fluids to prevent dehydration. In the vast majority of children, gastroenteritis does not require any medication and gets better on its own.

If your child becomes dehydrated, it is important not to give plain water or soft drinks as the sole replacement for the stool losses, particularly for infants and small children. These fluids contain the incorrect amounts of salt and sugar, and can be harmful if given alone during a diarrhea illness. There are many different types of oral rehydration solutions (ORS), which are made up of water, sugar in the form of glucose, salt and bicarbonate. In the stores they are sold under various different names, for example Pedialyte, Oralyte and Rehydralyte. They have been formulated in the right mixture so the body can absorb salt and glucose readily, and are specifically made for use in gastroenteritis. Oral rehydration solution, often called oral electrolyte solution, has been used extensively around the world for many years and, when used properly, works very well in preventing and treating dehydration from gastroenteritis. Oral rehydration solution does not treat the diarrhea. The diarrhea will get better in time. Diarrhea in older children who aren't that sick can often be managed with clear fluids, such as a combination of broth and diluted juices.

Children who weigh less than 22 pounds (10 kg) can take 2–4 ounces (60–120 mL) of ORS for each episode of vomiting or diarrhea. Children weighing more than 22 pounds, can take 4–8 ounces (120–240 mL) of ORS for each episode of vomiting or diarrhea.

Children with mild-to-moderate dehydration should be taken to their doctor or health care provider, who will instruct you on how to rehydrate your child. Children who are vomiting can successfully take oral rehydration fluids by being given small sips very frequently; for example, every two minutes with a spoon or syringe. This takes a lot of time and patience for success.

A minority of children with gastroenteritis will become severely dehydrated. These children need urgent attention by a doctor and will require an intravenous for fluids. When they are no longer dehydrated, they are ready for oral rehydration solution.

What types of food can I give? It's probably best to let your child's appetite dictate how much solid food he eats. Offer him something: withholding food for more than a day is not appropriate. The types of foods that are best tolerated during gastroenteritis are based on general experience rather than scientific studies. It is advisable to avoid foods high in simple sugars, such as sweetened tea, juices and soft drinks. Foods consisting of complex carbohydrates (such as rice, wheat, potatoes, bread and cereals), yogurt, fruits, vegetables and lean meats are usually tolerated. The BRAT diet (bananas, rice, applesauce and toast) is usually tolerated but does not supply adequate nutrition.

Infants and children who have mild diarrhea and are not dehydrated should continue to breast-feed and/or eat their regular diet. It is reasonable to give children who are not dehydrated oral rehydration solution in addition to their regular diet to keep up with fluid loss through diarrhea. Most children with gastroenteritis will be fine with milk or formula. A lactose-free milk is only necessary if the child has explosive stools and cramping when ingesting milk, or the diarrhea persists for more than a week.

Are medications necessary to treat gastroenteritis? In general, medications should not be used to treat gastroenteritis. Antibiotics are not necessary for gastroenteritis caused by viruses, although they may be indicated for some of the bacterial causes. Antidiarrheals and antiemetics (for vomiting), while useful in adults, are not recommended in children.

Should my child go to school or day care? Young children with diarrhea should stay at home. They should return to school or day care when the diarrhea is resolved, they are drinking and eating properly, and they can participate in activities comfortably without extra care. Repeat stool tests need to be done in the cases of some types of bacterial diarrhea before a child can return to school or day care. Your doctor and/or public health department will guide you in this situation.

Giardiasis

What is giardiasis? Giardia lamblia is a parasite that is found in all parts of the world. Giardia infection, or giardiasis, can affect two parts of the body: the small intestine and a part of the liver called the biliary tract, which drains bile produced in the liver into the upper portion of the gastrointestinal tract, the duodenum.

Children can become infected with giardia by hand-to-mouth transfer of the parasite from the feces of an infected person, or by drinking water or food that is contaminated by infected feces. Animals, such as dogs and cats, can also become infected with giardia and then contaminate water with their feces.

After infection with giardia, symptoms develop one to four weeks later (this is the **incubation period**). A person who has giardiasis can excrete the organism in his feces for months.

What does giardiasis look like? Some children can have a giardia infection and have no symptoms at all. Those with symptoms can have a sudden onset of watery diarrhea with abdominal pain. Others might have foul-smelling stools and a distended belly, pass lots of gas and lose their appetite. The bowels may not be able to absorb normal nutrients, leading to weight loss and anemia. Children with anemia may be pale and tired. There is usually no blood seen in the stools. Children with giardiasis can become dehydrated because of diarrhea and reduced appetite.

Giardia can be diagnosed by sending the stool for testing. It is also possible to diagnose giardia by taking a sample of fluid or a biopsy from the duodenum and testing this.

How is giardiasis treated? If a child with giardia infection is dehydrated due to diarrhea, he may require oral rehydration solution (ORS) or even intravenous fluids for rehydration. Several medications are available but metronidazole is the antibiotic that is most commonly used to treat giardia. It is given for five to seven days. In general, children who have giardia in their stools but are very well without symptoms, should not be treated. The illness will clear up on its own.

If an outbreak of giardia occurs, public health officials should be notified to ensure that everyone with symptoms is treated and also to determine where the infection came from.

Campers and backpackers should avoid drinking directly from streams that may be contaminated with giardia. Boiling water will kill the giardia parasite and other organisms that can cause infection.

Hand, Foot and Mouth Disease

What is hand, foot and mouth disease? Hand, foot and mouth disease is an infection caused by a virus called **coxsackie**, in particular, type A16. This viral infection can occur at any age but is most likely to affect young children during the summer and fall seasons. The virus that causes the infection is found in saliva and spreads from one child to another through the air or by touch, the same as cold viruses. Coxsackie viruses can also survive on the surface of toys for periods long enough to allow spread from these surfaces to children. The incubation period, the amount of time it takes for the virus to grow in the body until symptoms start, is about four to six days. A child is usually contagious for one to two weeks after developing symptoms.

What does hand, foot and mouth disease look like? As the name implies, the disease is most noticeable on the hands, feet and mouth. The most common signs are small, painful ulcers in the mouth and a skin rash, which consists of small blisters on the hands and feet, although they do occur on the palms and soles as well. The rash

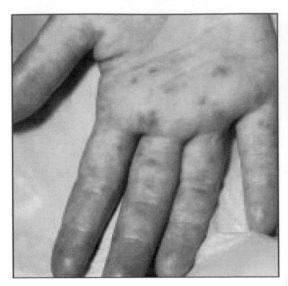
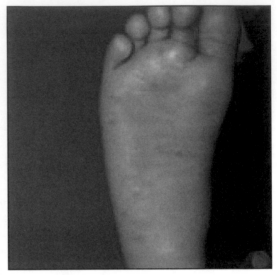

HAND, FOOT AND MOUTH DISEASE
The rash on the palms and soles of a child with hand, foot and mouth disease.

can affect other parts of the body as well such as the buttocks. Accompanying symptoms include fever, loss of appetite and irritability. Older children might complain of headache, sore throat and lack of energy.

How is hand, foot and mouth disease treated? There is no specific treatment for hand, foot and mouth disease. You should make the child comfortable and continue to offer food and liquids. You need to wash your hands after wiping the child's nose, changing a diaper or using the toilet, and before preparing food. If the child has a more severe infection and doesn't drink enough to prevent dehydration, it is important that a doctor examine the child and give additional advice regarding treatment. Antibiotics will not help because they don't work for viral infections. The infection gets better on its own and the symptoms usually last for 7 to 10 days. Infected children can keep going to day care or school if they feel well enough to take part in these activities.

Hepatitis

What is hepatitis? Hepatitis occurs when there is an inflammation of the liver. This is most commonly caused by a viral infection. There are five main viruses that directly infect the liver causing hepatitis and these have been labeled hepatitis A, B, C, D and E. Only two of them can be prevented by vaccination: hepatitis A and hepatitis B. Many other conditions can produce hepatitis, including drug side effects and complications of other common viral infections, such as infectious mononucleosis.

Hepatitis A can affect anyone and can occur as isolated cases or in epidemics. The hepatitis A virus is found in the stool of infected people and can spread directly from person to person or in food or water that has been contaminated with stool containing the virus. It is especially likely to spread if people do not wash their hands after changing diapers or going to the washroom.

Hepatitis B is different from hepatitis A in that it spreads when body fluids are directly passed from person to person; for example, from a woman to her baby during birth, or through sexual intercourse without condom. Hepatitis B can also be spread by sharing infected needles, such as in drug abuse or in a tattoo shop. It is *not* spread by sneezing, coughing, hugging or using the same dishes or cutlery. In the United States, about 70,000 new people are infected with the hepatitis B virus each year. The number of babies born with hepatitis B is lower now than it used to be, and this is largely because pregnant women are tested for the disease and, if found to be a carrier, their babies are vaccinated as soon as they are born.

Hepatitis A is usually quite mild and rarely results in any permanent liver damage unlike hepatitis B, which can cause serious damage to the liver and long-lasting adult liver disease, particularly if the infection is acquired as an infant or child. Persistent infection occasionally occurs: chronic hepatitis B is one of the main reasons adults get liver cancer. Hepatitis C, D and E are rare and are uncommon in North America. All forms of hepatitis can only be diagnosed by a blood test.

What does hepatitis look like? People with hepatitis often have fever, loss of appetite, nausea and "feel sick all over." Many infected individuals have no symptoms at all. Hepatitis affects the functioning of the liver. As a result, it often causes the skin and whites of the eyes to take on a yellow color, a condition called jaundice.

How is hepatitis treated? Prevention is best. A vaccine is now available to prevent hepatitis A infection and may be used for people traveling to areas where there is a high occurrence of hepatitis A virus or in situations of overcrowding, such as in military barracks and student dormitories. After a person has been exposed to the hepatitis A virus, an injection of immunoglobulin can

prevent infection. Immunoglobulin contains protective substances, called antibodies, against hepatitis A virus. There is no specific medication to treat hepatitis A once it occurs. Treatment is supportive and includes proper rest, fluid and nutrition.

There is no cure for hepatitis B, just supportive treatment. Still, its spread can be prevented in several ways, the most effective of which is by vaccination. Two or three shots are needed to provide complete protection against hepatitis B infection and these shots are usually given over a six-month period. Hepatitis B vaccine is one of the safest vaccines used today. Other ways to prevent the spread of hepatitis B:

- Avoid illicit drugs. If used, needles should not be shared between individuals.
- Use a condom when having sex with multiple partners or a new partner.
- Pregnant women must have a blood test to see if they have hepatitis B. If so, they are carriers. If the mother is a carrier, the baby should be vaccinated against hepatitis B as soon as he is born.

Herpes Simplex Infections

What is herpes simplex? Herpes simplex virus, or HSV, is a common virus that can cause disease in newborns, children, adolescents and adults. There are two types of herpes simplex viruses, type 1 (HSV-1) and type 2 (HSV-2).

What does HSV look like? The many ways that the herpes simplex viruses can show up depend on the age of the child, the strain of virus and whether or not the disease is an initial infection or a recurrence. After the initial infection, the herpes simplex virus persists in the body for life in a latent or dormant form.

Newborns can get infected with HSV, usually HSV-2, during their path down the birth canal. The infection risk for the newborn is highest if the mother is first infected during pregnancy. It is much less of a risk if the infection is a reactivation of an old herpes infection. The majority of mothers of newborns who develop infection have no signs or symptoms of HSV infection before or during pregnancy. Infection in the newborn usually takes one of three typical forms: disseminated disease, localized disease or localized central nervous system disease, involving the brain. In disseminated HSV, the newborn is very sick with evidence of infection in many organs including the lungs, liver and maybe the brain. In localized HSV disease, symptoms are confined to a particular area, for example, the skin, eyes and mouth. In localized central nervous system disease, the brain is infected. Newborns with disseminated HSV usually get sick in the first week of life, whereas newborns with disease of the brain usually get sick between the second and third weeks after birth. These newborns may not have any skin lesions.

Infected children might have no symptoms at all. The typical symptoms of HSV infection in children involve the skin and the mucous membranes of the mouth and genitals. Infection with HSV-1 usually results from direct contact with infected mouth secretions or a lesion, such as a cold sore. Infection with HSV-2 usually results from direct contact with infected genital secretions or lesions through sexual contact.

Cold sores, which look like single or grouped fluid-filled blisters (**vesicles**) around the mouth, usually on the border of the lips, are a very com-mon form of HSV infection. Cold sores can come and go over time, and often occur in association with stress (see page 385.)

Gingivostomatitis is caused by HSV-1 infection and involves the gums and mucous membranes of the mouth. It is usually quite painful, and can make eating and drinking unpleasant. Fever can accompany this infection.

Herpetic whitlow is an infection of the end of the finger with single or multiple vesicles. This can occur at the time of a primary HSV infection of the mouth or genitalia.

HSV can also cause **encephalitis**, a serious and life-threatening infection of the brain. This is usually caused by HSV-1. Children will have a fever, and altered level of consciousness, seizures, weakness and/or personality changes. (See Encephalitis, pages 94–95.)

How do you treat HSV? Pregnant women who have HSV infection that is visible at term should deliver their babies via an elective cesarean section. This reduces the risk of newborns getting the infection if surgery is performed before the waters break or very early thereafter. Newborns who develop HSV infection will need to be hospitalized and started on an antiviral medication called acyclovir.

Children with herpes gingivostomatitis need to be treated early on with acyclovir by mouth. It is important to ensure that the child take adequate fluids so that he does not become dehydrated. Oral acyclovir can be useful to reduce the number of sores and symptoms in cold sores, or herpes labialis, if given early, when symptoms are just beginning. Acyclovir also comes in a cream. However, studies have shown that it is not particularly effective for cold sores.

HIV/AIDS

What is HIV/AIDS? Human immunodeficiency virus (HIV) is the virus that causes acquired immunodeficiency syndrome (AIDS) in children and adults. Full-blown AIDS is the most severe end of the HIV disease spectrum. At the other end are children who have HIV without obvious symptoms. HIV causes disease in children by weakening their immune system. Because of their impaired immune systems, children with HIV have difficulty fighting off everyday germs or they develop infections caused by unusual germs that wouldn't cause disease in healthy children. This immune deficiency also places them at risk of developing specific types of cancers. HIV infection can also impair a child's growth and development.

The HIV virus can be spread from person to person by,

1. sexual contact: vaginal, anal or oral;
2. exposure to contaminated blood or other body fluids containing a high concentration of HIV, either through the skin (from needles or sharp objects) or mucous membranes, like the mouth;
3. transmission from mother to infant before or around the time of birth; or
4. breast-feeding.

In countries where strict precautions and screening of donated blood exists, transmission of HIV through transfusion of blood or blood products is very rare.

In North America, more than 90 percent of HIV-infected children under 13 acquire the infection from their mothers at birth. Over this age, the virus is spread primarily through sexual exposure. Once a person has been infected with HIV, it stays in his body for life.

In developed countries, where health care and medications are readily available, HIV infection in children has dropped dramatically over the past 15 years. This is largely due to the availability of medications that can prevent transmission of infection from an infected mother to her newborn. Unfortunately, in developing countries, where HIV infection tends to be common, these medications are not available or affordable. With today's medical knowledge and medications, HIV infection in children should be considered a preventable disease. Sadly, for millions of children it is not.

What does HIV *look like?* HIV infection can cause disease involving many parts of the body. By damaging the immune system, HIV can result in infection and cancer. Prior to immune system damage, some children with HIV infection can be very well but once the immune system is severely affected, they will become very sick.

Children with HIV develop a wide range of problems, many of which are seen in other common conditions. These include enlarged lymph nodes throughout the body, enlarged liver or spleen, failure to gain weight, severe thrush in the mouth, diarrhea that lasts for weeks, swollen parotid glands (glands in the cheeks that produce saliva), heart failure, hepatitis, kidney problems and neurological disease including delayed development. HIV infection can result in anemia and low **platelet** counts.

Infants with HIV infection can have severe lung infections. This often occurs in the first six months of life and is commonly due to pneumocystis carinii pneumonia (PCP), a fungus that does not cause disease in patients with a normal immune system. It can be a life-threatening illness. Infants and children appear very sick with breathing difficulties. The lungs' ability to maintain normal body oxygen levels is often impaired. Children of all ages can develop this. Infants can also have serious problems gaining weight. This might be due to repeated intestinal infections (gastroenteritis) or absorbing the nutrients in food. Infants who are diagnosed with HIV infection usually have a large liver and spleen and enlarged lymph glands throughout the body. Their development can be delayed and they have neurologic signs similar to cerebral palsy.

Older children diagnosed with HIV infection often have had mild symptoms for many years. They go to the doctor for reasons similar to other children with immune system problems; for example, with frequent milder infections, particularly ear infections, **sinusitis** and frequent colds; or one or two serious infections, such as **meningitis**, pneumonia and bone infections. They can also have more severe bouts of common childhood infections such as chicken pox. Their liver and spleen might be enlarged. Older children can have problems with concentration, language and school performance related to neurological involvement. Children with HIV can get a specific lung disease, called lymphocytic interstitial pneumonitis (LIP).

When infection with the HIV virus occurs for the first time (primary infection) during adolescence, it can result in an illness with fever, sore throat, muscle aches, enlarged lymph glands, rash and fatigue. This type of illness with primary infection does not occur in younger children. Infection during adolescence might not result in symptoms of HIV until adulthood.

HIV is diagnosed by blood tests. In children and adolescents, tests look for the presence

of an **antibody** to the HIV virus. Infants under 18 months need special tests to diagnose HIV infection. The presence of antibodies in their blood does not automatically indicate infection in these infants but may only be due to the presence of maternal antibodies passed through the placenta from their mother's blood.

How is HIV/AIDS treated? There is currently no cure for HIV infection. In order to prevent transmission of HIV from a pregnant woman to her baby, it is imperative that pregnant women are tested for HIV and given medications if they have HIV infection. These medications are excellent at reducing the risk of transmission of infection from the mother to the baby. The mother begins taking them at 14 to 34 weeks into the pregnancy, as well as an intravenous dose during labor, and then the newborn is treated for six weeks.

Mothers with HIV infection should not breast-feed. This will prevent transmission of the virus from the mother to the newborn through breast milk.

Infectious disease specialists are involved in the medical care of children with HIV infection. Medications, called antiretrovirals, are given in combination to control the HIV infection. They do not cure the disease, but help minimalize the effect of HIV infection on the immune system. HIV viral load is a blood test done to see whether the infection is under control. It measures the number of copies of the virus in the plasma (the portion of the blood without red blood cells). This test helps to see how well the medications are working. When the immune system of a person with HIV is not working well, he is often placed on additional medications taken daily to prevent certain types of infections. This is called **prophylactic therapy**.

Children who are taken care of by an HIV team of doctors and health care workers and take medications can remain healthy. Many aspects of the care are directed toward providing support for the child and family, and helping them deal with this long-term illness.

Infectious Mononucleosis

What is infectious mononucleosis? Infectious mononucleosis is a well-known infection caused by the Epstein-Barr virus (EBV). EBV is transmitted primarily in the saliva, hence the term "kissing disease." EBV infection is common, and in some developing countries 80 percent to 100 percent of children are infected by the age of 3 to 6 years. In more developed countries, infection tends to occur mainly in adolescents or young adults.

What does mononucleosis infection look like? Young children with EBV usually have no obvious illness or else a mild disease consisting mainly of cold symptoms, sore throat and, perhaps, fever.

Older children develop a characteristic illness known as infectious mononucleosis, or mono. The initial symptoms can include generally feeling unwell, a reduced appetite and chills. After that, the child usually develops a fever, sore throat and lack of energy with swollen glands (lymph nodes) in the neck and elsewhere. A headache is common. The fever can be prolonged and even last for one to two weeks. It can be a few weeks more before the child starts to feel well again. A few patients, less than 5 percent, may have fatigue for as long as three to four months.

The throat of those with infectious mononucleosis appears red and inflamed. Typically, the tonsils are covered with an ugly white coating. Often this is thought to be due to a bacterial infection like strep throat and, consequently, the doctor might prescribe antibiotics. But, if

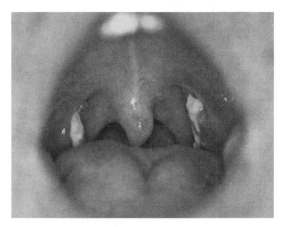

INFECTIOUS MONONUCLEOSIS
With infectious mononucleosis, the throat is red and inflamed and the tonsils are covered with an ugly white coating.

children with EBV infection are given the antibiotic amoxicillin, they will develop an itchy, red rash 7 to 10 days after the first dose. Also, in mononucleosis, the spleen, an organ that sits under the ribs on the left side of the abdomen, commonly becomes enlarged. The liver, under the ribs on the right side, can become swollen and tender as well. In addition there may be swelling around the eyes.

Common laboratory tests will confirm the diagnosis. A simple blood count and film often suggest that an infection is due to "infectious mono." Increased numbers of a particular type of blood cells, called atypical lymphocytes, can be seen on the blood film. The numbers of other blood cells, such as **platelets** and **neutrophils**, decrease. The child might have anemia, indicated by a low hemoglobin level. These blood abnormalities are usually temporary and insignificant. EBV infection can be diagnosed with a blood test that detects antibodies produced by the body against the virus. There are rapid but less specific **antibody** tests, such as looking for heterophile antibodies (monospot), as well as slower more involved antibody tests that can accurately identify EBV infection. There can be evidence of hepatitis (inflammation of the liver), which is usually mild and resolves without treatment. Very rarely, some children can develop an infection of the brain, known as **encephalitis**.

How is mono treated? There is no specific treatment. It is important to ensure that your child takes adequate fluids and avoids overexertion. If his spleen is enlarged, he has to avoid contact sports to prevent the rare chance of the spleen rupturing. He can take acetaminophen or ibuprofen for fever or sore throat, if they are causing discomfort. However, antibiotics are not helpful in treating infectious mononucleosis, as it is a viral infection. Some children develop severe swelling of their tonsils that interferes with the ability to breathe. Prednisone, which is a powerful anti-inflammatory drug, can help decrease swelling if this happens.

Influenza

What is influenza? Influenza, commonly known as "the flu," is a generalized infection caused by the influenza virus, of which there are two main types: A and B. Influenza is transmitted from person to person by droplets containing the virus. The droplets are spread by coughing or sneezing, or by direct contact with articles such as toys recently contaminated by an infected child's coughing or sneezing. During community outbreaks of influenza, the highest rates of illness occur among school-aged children who then spread the infection to adults and other children within families. Influenza is

highly contagious and is most infectious during the 24 hours before the onset of symptoms. It can continue to be infectious for up to 10 days from the onset of the illness. Each winter season 10 to 40 percent of healthy children get the flu. Approximately one out of 100 require hospitalization because of a complication such as pneumonia. Those hospitalized are often under 2 or have chronic heart or chest diseases.

What does the flu look like? True flu, meaning infection caused by the influenza virus, is different from the common cold and is characterized by the sudden onset of high fever, often with chills, headache, sore throat, runny nose, muscle pains, a feeling of weakness and a dry cough. Red eyes, stomach ache, nausea and vomiting can also occur. In young infants, influenza can look like a very serious illness and be mistaken for **meningitis**. Complications of influenza include pneumonia and encephalitis (infection of the brain).

How is the flu treated? Generally, treatment is aimed at making your child comfortable. You should control the fever with acetaminophen or ibuprofen. These are useful and should be used liberally. However children with influenza should not take salicylates such as aspirin because of the resulting increased risk of developing a condition known as Reye's syndrome, which produces headache, vomiting, liver inflammation and low blood sugar.

There are antiviral medications available to treat influenza but these are generally only used in special situations and not for otherwise healthy children. These medications should be considered for children with a severe or life-threatening illness, or preventively in those children in whom shortening the course of the illness would be beneficial, such as in children with severe heart or lung disease or cancer and in children with special environmental, family or social situations for which ongoing illness would be harmful. There are new medications that have recently been approved for treatment of uncomplicated influenza A and B. These are somewhat effective if used within two days of onset of symptoms. These medications, however, may only shorten the influenza illness by 1 to 1 ½ days.

Prevention of influenza infection is now partially possible by an annual influenza vaccination. Immunization is recommended for all healthy children from 6 months to 2 years of age and for children over 6 months of age who have chronic illnesses, such as heart disease, cystic fibrosis, chronic kidney disease and cancer. Any individual, child or adult, who wishes to be vaccinated against the flu should have a shot.

Lyme Disease

What is Lyme disease? Lyme disease is the most common tick-borne infection in the United States, where 12,000 cases are reported annually. Most cases occur in the northeastern, mid-Atlantic and upper north-central states, and in a part of northwest California. Lyme disease is caused by a bacterium, *Borrelia burgdorferi*, and it is transmitted to humans by a deer tick. It is spread primarily through bites from the tick, which feed predominantly in the late spring and early summer.

What does Lyme disease look like? The disease is characterized by a rash, called "erythema migrans." The rash begins with a single red spot that expands over days to weeks to form a large red area that is 2 inches (5 cm) or more in size, sometimes with a partial clearing in the center creating a ringlike appearance; or it may be made up of many such spots all over the body. Fever, drowsiness, headache and mild neck stiffness can accompany the rash. More importantly, Lyme disease can affect various body parts including the nervous system, where it sometimes causes facial weakness, the heart and the joints. Joint involvement can occur as a late symptom and often affects the knees, so that the condition mimics juvenile rheumatoid arthritis.

How is Lyme disease treated? Antibiotics are recommended. The choice of antibiotic is based on the age of the child and the severity of the infection. There is a vaccine to prevent Lyme disease in susceptible individuals. Checking children for tick bites if they play in tick-infested areas during the warmer months can reduce the chance of infection.

Malaria

Malaria is a curse for millions of people, causing great suffering and death. The disease is very common throughout the tropical parts of the world. It is most prevalent in sub-Saharan Africa, parts of Central and South America, and parts of Oceania and Southeast Asia. Everyone needs to be aware of malaria because, in this age of international travel, visitors can get the disease. When going to areas of infection, it's important to take preventative measures.

What is malaria? It is an infection caused by the parasite plasmodium. There are actually four types of *Plasmodium* species that can infect humans: *P. vivax*, *P. malariae*, *P. ovale* and *P. falciparum*. Human infection occurs when a female anopheles mosquito, itself infected with the parasite, bites a person.

The malarial parasites first go to the liver (the liver stage) where they grow and divide within the liver cells. Then they enter the bloodstream and invade the red blood cells (the blood phase). In all malarial infections, the symptoms and signs of illness occur during the blood phase. The liver phase of the malaria infection varies in duration depending on the type of malaria species. For *P. falciparum* the liver stage is completed in one week whereas *P. vivax* and *P. ovale* can remain dormant in the liver for months to years, and only cause infection and symptoms once they enter the blood phase.

What does malaria look like? Malaria symptoms will occur at least seven to nine days after infection by the parasite. These symptoms can start months later if the child was using some antimalarial medication because even if the child was taking antimalarial medication, he can still contract the disease.

The typical symptoms of a malaria infection are high fever with chills, sweats and headaches. This can occur every day or in cycles that occur every second or third day. Children can also develop nausea, vomiting, diarrhea and coughing. Pain around the joints, in the abdomen or back may also be seen. The spleen, an organ in the left side of the abdomen, can become enlarged. Some children look pale, or have jaundice. Infection with *Plasmodium falciparum* can result in a severe illness with involvement of different organs, for example the lungs and kidneys, as well as the brain, and can even be life-threatening.

If your child has a fever and has recently been to an area of the world where malaria is common, take him to his doctor to be tested for malaria.

Malaria is diagnosed by a blood test. The blood is examined under a microscope to see if the parasites are present and, if so, which species it is. Sometimes, the blood test might not initially identify any malaria parasites even though infection is in fact present. In these circumstances where malaria is a possibility and the test is negative, the blood test should be repeated every 12 to 24 hours over a 72-hour period.

How is malaria treated? Depending on the child's condition, treatment for malaria can occur in hospital or at home. Medications are available for treating malaria. The type and number of medications required will depend both on the species of malaria, and where the child acquired it. In some countries, the parasites are resistant to some of the regular antimalarial drugs.

How do I prevent my child from getting malaria? If you are traveling to an area where malaria is common, you can take several measures to prevent being bitten by mosquitoes. The anopheles mosquito prefers to bite at night, so prevention is even more important from dusk to dawn. Remain indoors in well-screened areas, if possible, and wear protective clothing while outside. You should sleep under bed nets impregnated with insecticide and use mosquito repellents containing DEET. Ask your doctor about what type of DEET is safest and most effective, and how best to use it (see West Nile Virus, pages 130–31). Prophylactic antimalarial medications to prevent developing malaria are recommended for travelers to areas where malaria is common. There are different types of medication depending on where you are visiting but most have to be taken one week before travel, so that the medication has time to start working, and also needs to be continued for some time after returning in order to work effectively. Depending on where you are traveling, your doctor will give you specific instructions about which medication to take and when to start and stop it. It is extremely important to follow these instructions, because if the medication is stopped early after returning, it is still possible to get sick.

Measles, Mumps and Rubella

Worldwide, measles, mumps and rubella infections are quite common. A combined vaccine containing all three viruses (MMR) has significantly diminished the frequency and suffering caused by these infections. Children should get the MMR vaccine twice. They should get the first shot when they are 12 to 15 months old. The second shot can be given as early as one month after the first MMR shot or, more commonly, before they start elementary school, between the ages of 4 to 6. The vaccine should not be given before 12 months of age.

MEASLES

What is measles? Measles is a virus that can cause serious illness. It spreads quickly by sneezing and coughing and is very easy to catch. Over 90 percent of those who have not already had measles, or are not protected against measles by vaccination, will get it after exposure to an infected person. When you breathe in the droplets containing the virus, it infects cells lining the nose and throat. After a few days the virus spreads into the blood and throughout the body. Eventually, the virus is present in the eyes, skin, respiratory tract and lymph glands and will produce symptoms in these areas. It can also spread to the brain. The **incubation period** is about 10 to 12 days.

What does measles look like? Measles begins with a high fever, runny nose, severe brassy cough, red eyes and photophobia (eyes that hurt in bright light). After a few days a bright red rash begins to appear around the face, chest, arms and legs. Measles virus can also cause ear infections and pneumonia. In 1 out of every 1,000 children who get measles, inflammation and swelling of the brain develops. This **encephalitis** can lead to seizures, deafness, mental retardation or death. Complications of measles are common because the virus impairs the functioning of the white blood cells that fight infection.

How is measles treated? Treatment is supportive, aimed at making the child as comfortable as possible. Fever and discomfort can be alleviated with ibuprofen or acetaminophen. Antibiotics are ineffective and should not be given just to prevent bacterial complications of measles. An antiviral drug is available to treat measles but is only used to treat severely ill, hospitalized children. Large doses of vitamin A have been shown to decrease the death rate of infants in developing countries. **Immunoglobulin**, which is concentrated antibodies made from blood donations, has also been used for severely ill children.

MUMPS

What is mumps? Mumps is an infection caused by the mumps virus. It is most common in children; 90 percent of patients are under the age of 15.

The virus is spread by close contact between people and by sneezing and coughing. The incubation period is longer than that for measles; about 16 to 18 days.

What does mumps look like? About 20 percent of children infected with mumps have no symptoms at all. More often, however, mumps causes a fever, headache, aches and pains and loss of appetite. Characteristically, there is painful swelling of the parotid glands, which are the salivary glands in front of the ear and alongside the angle of the jaw. This swelling of the parotid glands makes the cheeks puff out. About 1 in 10 children with mumps will actually develop meningitis, an infection of the fluid around the brain and spinal cord. Mumps meningitis is usually mild and does not cause permanent damage. Mumps can also cause deafness, painful swelling of the testicles in teenage boys and men (and, rarely, sterility) and a painful infection of the ovaries in women.

How is mumps treated? The most effective treatment is prevention by immunization. There is no effective treatment for mumps. Antibiotics are ineffective. Any pain or significant fever can be treated with acetaminophen or ibuprofen.

RUBELLA

What is rubella? Rubella is also known as "German measles." Like real measles, it is caused by a virus and is spread by close contact between people and by sneezing and coughing. Rubella is a mild illness in children and many have no symptoms at all. It is usually more severe in teenagers and adults. The greatest danger comes from infection of the unborn child, when the virus produces the syndrome of congenital rubella. The incubation period for rubella is about 14 to 21 days.

What does rubella look like? Rubella typically causes a mild rash made up of small red spots that first appear on the face and scalp and that last for one to three days. There can also be a fever, sore throat, aches and pains, and **swollen glands**, especially behind the ears and at the back of the head.

The most serious complication of rubella occurs when a woman catches rubella during the first 20 weeks of pregnancy. The infected mother can pass the disease on to her fetus while it is in the womb where it may cause malformations of the baby's brain, eyes, ears, heart and other organs. It can even cause death of the fetus. The chances of this happening are very high; it occurs in 80 percent of cases. Other complications of rubella include painful joints, thrombocytopenia (a decrease in platelets, the particles in the blood responsible for blood clot formation) and encephalitis.

How is rubella treated? There is no specific treatment for rubella. Symptoms such as headache and aches and pains can be relieved with acetaminophen or ibuprofen. There is also no treatment for the infected fetus where the damage that happens is irreversible and permanent.

Once again, the best treatment is prevention by vaccination with the MMR vaccine. Before getting pregnant, you can get a simple blood test that will tell if you had rubella as a child. If you are still susceptible to infection, the complete MMR shot should be given right away. The vaccine cannot be given if you are pregnant.

Meningitis

What is meningitis? Meningitis refers to an infection of the fluid and membranes that cover the brain and spinal cord. The main types are viral and bacterial. Viral meningitis is the most common form and is much less serious than bacterial meningitis. Bacterial meningitis is a very serious disease at any age.

Each year about 2 out of every 100,000 people in the United States develop bacterial meningitis. Most cases are caused by one of two bacterial germs called meningococcus, or *Neisseria meningitidis*, and pneumococcus, also called *Streptococcus pneumoniae*. Other causes of bacterial meningitis include group B streptococcus, *Escherichia coli* (E. Coli) and *Haemophilus influenzae* type b (Hib), but these are much less frequent.

Both meningococcus and pneumococcus can also cause serious disease by infecting the blood. This is called bacteremia or "blood poisoning." Bacteremia can lead to a more dangerous condition, septicemia, which is essentially bacteremia with shock or low blood pressure. These bacteria can also infect the lungs (producing pneumonia), joints (septic arthritis), bones (osteomyelitis) or the heart tissues.

Which children are at greatest risk? For both meningococcal and pneumococcal infections, the risk is highest for children under 2 years of age. There is a second, smaller rise in the risk of meningococcal infection among those 15 to 24 years of age. Other risk factors include a compromised immune system or having sickle-cell disease or some other chronic illnesses. Overcrowding (such as in day care centers, dormitories, military barracks, etc.) also increases the risk that the germs will spread more easily.

How does a child get meningitis? The bacteria that cause meningitis are quite common. Many people, both children and adults, do not develop any symptoms of illness after being infected by them. These germs live harmlessly in the back of noses and throats. These people are called "healthy carriers" and account for most of the spread of infection, compared with those who are clearly sick with disease. It is estimated that 40 percent of children become carriers of pneumococcal bacteria in the first year of life. About 20 percent of teenagers and adults are healthy carriers of meningococcus. For the disease to spread, people must have close direct contact, such as kissing, coughing or sneezing. It can also be passed through saliva or when people share things like food, cups, water bottles, cigarettes, lipstick, straws, toothbrushes or even musical instruments with mouthpieces. The germs die quickly outside the body, which is fortunate, making these bacteria not very contagious.

What does meningitis look like? Infants under a year of age will usually develop a fever, become very irritable and may experience feeding difficulties or drowsiness. These babies might vomit, have a stiff neck or develop a bulging **fontanelle** (soft spot on the top of the skull). In older children, the early signs of meningitis are fever and a major change in behavior such as drowsiness, reduced consciousness, fussiness or agitation. Other symptoms include severe headache, pain when moving the head, neck stiffness, general aches and convulsions (seizures). About two-thirds of children with meningococcal meningitis get a skin rash of red spots that don't disappear or blanch when pressed. The spots can get quite large and spread very quickly.

Without treatment, especially antibiotics, all children who get meningitis will die or suffer permanent damage. Even with treatment, about 1 in 20 children can't be saved. Many of the survivors will have some form of brain damage.

How can you tell if your child has meningococcal septicemia? Children with this form of meningococcal disease get sick very quickly, typically in a few hours. Almost all will have a rash that starts as red or bluish spots that don't disappear when pressed. The spots increase in size and number quite rapidly. Infected children become drowsy, semiconscious, irritable or agitated. Low blood pressure (shock), coma, convulsions, bleeding problems and severe breathing difficulties can all be part of the disease. Blood clots can also form, cutting off the supply of oxygen to the outer parts of the limbs. Even with treatment, about half of the children with meningococcal septicemia will either die or have permanent damage.

Which vaccines protect against meningococcal and pneumococcal infections? There are two types of vaccine available that protect against meningoccal and pneumococcal infections: polysaccharide vaccines and conjugated vaccines.

The original polysaccharide vaccines are effective in older children and adults. They are ineffective in children under 2, which is the time that children are most vulnerable to these infections. The polysaccharide vaccines do, however, have broader coverage than the conjugated vaccines. The polysaccharide meningococcal vaccine protects against four groups of meningococcal infection and the pneumococcal vaccine protects against 23 strains of pneumococcal infection. Boosters may be necessary with these older vaccines.

The new conjugate vaccines are effective for children younger than 2 as well as older children. These new vaccines consist of purified polysaccharides ("complex sugars") linked (conjugated) to a purified protein. The current meningococcal conjugate vaccine protects only against meningococcal group C, the most common group that causes meningococcal meningitis in North America. The current pneumococcal conjugate vaccine protects against the seven most common strains of pneumococcus, which are the cause of over 80 percent of pneumococcal meningitis.

Infants should get three shots of conjugated pneumococcal vaccine at approximately 2, 4 and 6 months of age, with a booster between 12 and 15 months. Meningococcal conjugate vaccine should be given at the age of 11 or 12 years. The meningococcal polysaccharide vaccine may be recommended for children in high-risk groups; two doses are given three months apart between the ages of 3 months and 2 years.

Both meningococcal and pneumococcal vaccines are very safe and do not cause any serious reactions. Local reactions, such as redness, swelling or pain at the place where the needle is given, can occur in 15 percent to 20 percent of those vaccinated. Fever may occur in some children. You can give acetaminophen or ibuprofen for pain or to reduce any accompanying fever.

Osteomyelitis and Septic Arthritis

What are they? Osteomyelitis is defined as swelling or inflammation of bone. Children most commonly get osteomyelitis as a result of a bacterial infection that spreads from the original source through their bloodstream to the bone, causing infection. It can also occur after trauma or surgery, or spread from an infection in the soft tissues, such as skin, near the bone. The long bones of the arms and legs are most frequently involved, although any bone can become infected.

Septic arthritis is a bacterial infection in the joint, often the hip. Bacteria can get into a joint by first infecting the bloodstream, or by entering through the skin over the joint.

The most common bacteria that result in infection of the bone or joint in children include *Staphylococcus aureus*, group A streptococcus and *Streptococcus pneumoniae*.

What do these infections look like? Children with osteomyelitis or septic arthritis usually have fever. They might have pain and swelling over the affected bone or joint. The area might feel hot when touched. They often have limited movement of the infected limb. This can result in a child with a limp or who refuses to walk. When the infection is in the bloodstream, the child can look very unwell.

Several types of test are done to diagnose osteomyelitis or septic arthritis. A blood culture will look for the presence of bacteria in the bloodstream. Other blood tests look for indirect signs of infection, such as a high white blood cell count or an elevated level of the markers of inflammation, particularly the **erythrocyte sedimentation rate** (ESR) or **C-reactive protein** (CRP). An x-ray of the affected area helps diagnose osteomyelitis, but it can take up to two weeks from the time the infection began before changes are seen on an x-ray. Ultrasound, CT scan or MRI scan can also be helpful. A bone scan is another test that can help to diagnose bone infections. In this test, a substance is injected into the bloodstream through a catheter inserted into a vein. The substance will go to the infection or inflammation site and show up

on the scan. Often a sample of the bone or some fluid from the joint will be required to confirm the presence of infection and help the health care providers decide which antibiotics to use.

How are they treated? Osteomyelitis due to infection from bacteria needs to be treated with antibiotics. Often a child needs a course of intravenous antibiotics to get the infection under control. Once he is using the limb normally, the antibiotics can be taken by mouth. The treatment is longer than for other infections, and usually lasts for weeks.

Septic arthritis might need a combination of surgery and antibiotics. Because the infected fluid can destroy the inside of the joint and lead to long-term problems, it may be necessary for a surgeon to drain all of the fluid out and clean the joint. Similar to osteomyelitis, antibiotic treatment is usually continued for weeks.

Otitis Media (Middle Ear Infection)

What is otitis media? Anatomically, there are three main components to the ear: the external ear, which is the visible part of the ear plus the ear canal that leads to the eardrum; the middle ear that contains small bones to amplify sounds; and an inner ear containing the hearing and balance apparatus. Otitis media is an infection of the middle ear. Middle ear infections are caused by viruses or bacteria that get inside the middle ear, most commonly following a common cold, and cause an infection or inflammation. Ear infections are very common and most children will have had at least one or more ear infections by age 3. Most ear infections are not serious and heal completely.

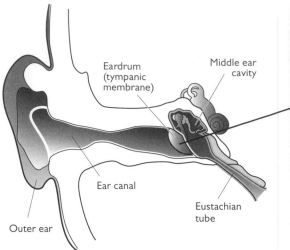

Eardrum (tympanic membrane)

Middle ear cavity

Ear canal

Eustachian tube

Outer ear

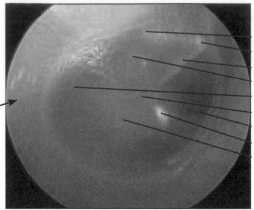

THE NORMAL EAR

The healthy tympanic membrane is translucent and pearly gray. The bone of the middle ear can be seen behind the eardrum.

What does otitis media look like? Earache is the main complaint of children who are able to speak. In addition, they might have the usual symptoms of a cold, including fever, sore throat, lack of energy and loss of appetite. Younger infants are usually fussy and irritable. They have trouble sleeping, tug or pull at their ears, and lack response to quiet sounds. When the doctor looks in the ear, the eardrum appears red and swollen and the middle ear behind the eardrum is filled with pus obscuring the bones of the middle ear.

How is otitis media treated? Almost all middle ear infections in children younger than 2 are treated with antibiotics. Most infants feel better within the first two or three days after starting medication. In the meantime, you can relieve their pain with analgesics such as ibuprofen or acetaminophen. But, to cure the infection, you must give them all the medication prescribed. We now know that 8 out of 10 middle ear infections in older children will get better on their own without antibiotics. So, if a child is older than 2 and the ear infection isn't causing too many problems, the doctor might suggest a painkiller alone, and reexamine the child two or three days later to see whether he needs antibiotics.

Although the **acute** problem generally subsides in a few days, fluid will remain in the middle ear for some time afterward. This condition is called **otitis media with effusion**. It differs from acute otitis media in that there is no associated pain or fever. This stage of healing can take weeks to get completely better and further antibiotic use doesn't really help.

Many young children have so many ear infections or the effusion lasts so long that something further needs to be done. A simple surgical procedure in which tiny tubes are placed in the eardrum to better ventilate the middle ear can be performed to reduce the recurrence of otitis media.

Pinworms

What are pinworms? Pinworms are tiny worms that live in the intestines and are really more of a nuisance than a disease. It sounds worse than

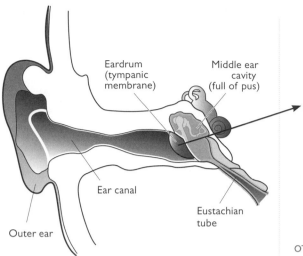

Eardrum (tympanic membrane)

Middle ear cavity (full of pus)

Ear canal

Eustachian tube

Outer ear

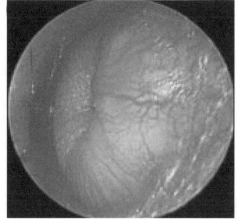

OTITIS MEDIA (MIDDLE EAR INFECTION)
In acute otitis media, the eardrum is red and bulging because the middle ear is filled with pus.

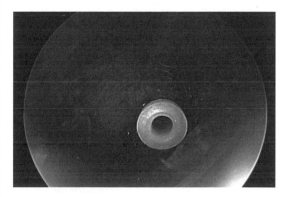

TYMPANOSTOMY TUBE
These are often inserted to treat chronic otitis media (otitis media with effusion) and prevent recurrence. They allow normal ventilation of the middle ear.

it really is! They are very common in children and spread easily among them and staff in child-care facilities. The worms crawl out of the anus at night and lay their eggs on nearby skin causing irritation. They are spread when an infected child scratches the itchy area and gets pinworm eggs on his fingers or under his fingernails and then touches another child or adult. The eggs can survive for several weeks outside the body on toys, bedding or clothing.

What do pinworms look like? Pinworms are tiny, white threadlike worms. Usually, children with pinworms have no symptoms. However, some children can get very itchy around the anus and vagina. The condition is usually diagnosed by observing the adult worms that are most likely to be seen around the anal area a few hours after the child is asleep. The doctor will sometimes suggest a "pinworm prep" to make the diagnosis. This merely involves applying a sticky transparent plastic slide to the anus and then having it examined under a microscope for eggs and worms.

How are pinworms treated? Pinworm infection can be treated with medicine (mebendazole or pyrantel) taken orally. Sometimes the whole family needs to be treated to prevent reinfection. Other preventive measures include making sure all household members and any others who come in contact with the child wash their hands thoroughly after going to the toilet, changing diapers and before preparing or eating food.

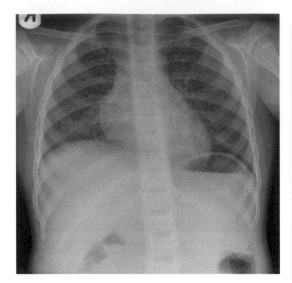

NORMAL CHEST X-RAY

In this normal x-ray, the two lungs appear as dark shadows on both sides of the heart (which appears white).

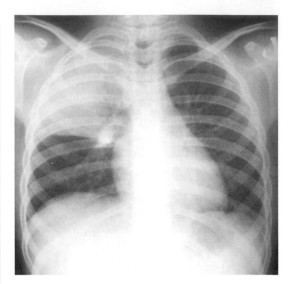

PNEUMONIA

The pneumonia is seen on this x-ray of the chest as the white area in the top half of the right lung (on the left-hand side).

Pneumonia

What is pneumonia? Pneumonia is a very broad term that describes inflammation of the lungs, usually caused by an infection. A child with pneumonia can be seriously ill or, more commonly, just mildly sick, depending on the cause and the extent of the inflammation. The old term "double pneumonia" refers to an infection in both lungs. Walking pneumonia refers to the mildly ill child who does not require hospitalization and remains active and fairly well.

In otherwise healthy children, most cases of pneumonia are caused by viral infections. Some of the more common viruses include respiratory syncytial virus (RSV), influenza, parainfluenza, adenovirus and rhinovirus. Children with bacterial pneumonia tend to be sicker. Usually, they are infected with *Streptococcus pneumoniae*, *Staphylococcus aureus*, *Haemophilus influenzae* or *Mycoplasma pneumoniae*. Rarely, a child can get

pneumonia by inhaling food or an object (for example a peanut or small toy part) into the lungs. This is known as aspiration pneumonia.

What does pneumonia look like? Pneumonia, especially if it is viral, might start with the symptoms of the common cold. Children with pneumonia commonly have fever and a cough. Young children will sometimes vomit as a result of their coughing. The most important sign of pneumonia is if your child is breathing fast and/or working hard to breathe. The skin between his ribs may be sucked in and he might make grunting noises with each breath. These are all referred to as the signs of "respiratory distress." Children normally breathe faster during or just after crying, so it is important to observe them for signs of respiratory distress while they are calm. Often, a child with pneumonia will be tired, not want to eat and generally feel unwell. If the infection is in the lower lobe of the lung, which sits on the diaphragm, your child can seem to have pain in his stomach. If his doctor suspects your child has pneumonia, a chest x-ray will confirm the diagnosis.

How is pneumonia treated? Viruses account for the majority of pneumonias in children, so antibiotics might not be essential. However, differentiating viral causes from bacterial causes of pneumonia can be difficult. If the chest x-ray shows pneumonia (which appears as a white area) or your child has a high fever and seems unwell, antibiotics are usually prescribed. You need to ensure that your child takes all the antibiotic as prescribed. Most children can be treated at home. But some children who are very young, look very sick or who require supplemental oxygen or intravenous fluids, might be hospitalized.

Your child may not feel like eating while he is sick. This is okay as long as he is drinking sufficient fluids to prevent dehydration. Medication for the fever (acetaminophen or ibuprofen) is recommended if he seems uncomfortable with the fever, or has other aches and pains. Over-the-counter cough medications do not help. Your child can go outside, although he should limit exercise until he does not have to work too hard to breathe. Pneumonia does not generally cause any permanent damage to the lungs. Therefore, as long as your child appears well, his doctor will usually not request a repeat chest x-ray after he is better.

Rabies

What is rabies? For centuries, the word "rabies" brought terror to people's minds. Now, in the developed world, the disease is fortunately very rare. Rabies is caused by the rabies virus that is passed from animals to humans, usually through a bite. Sometimes, it can be passed by saliva from an infected animal through an abrasion in the skin or the mucous membrane of the eyes, nose or mouth. Many types of animals can pass rabies to people. Wild mammals—raccoons, skunks, foxes, coyotes and bats—are the major sources of infection in North America. Dogs, cats and even cattle can pass rabies to people. Worldwide, most rabies cases in humans are actually from dog bites. Small rodents, such as hamsters, squirrels, guinea pigs and rabbits, almost never spread rabies.

What does rabies look like? In humans the time from infection to disease, the **incubation period**, is usually from four to six weeks, but can last from five days to a year. Children who are infected with rabies become sick with fever and headache. They can then develop neurological symptoms: for example, anxiety, confusion, sleepiness, difficulties with swallowing and eventually seizures. Some children develop weakness or paralysis. The illness almost always leads to death.

How is rabies treated? Once symptoms of rabies develop, there is no treatment that helps. Very few patients with rabies have survived. This is why prevention is so important. If your child is bitten by any animal, talk to your doctor or health care provider right away. Vaccination after exposure to rabies works very well in preventing disease.

After a bite, it is important for the area to be thoroughly cleaned with soap and water. A rabies vaccine and rabies immunoglobulin are available and should be given after a child has been bitten by a wild or potentially infected animal. The rabies immunoglobulin is made up of antibodies, which are proteins that help the body fight this infection. The decision to give either or both of these should be made by your doctor, often in communication with the local public health department. Any animal suspected of having rabies that has bitten a person should be reported to the local health department.

It is important to protect your household pets from rabies. They should have the appropriate rabies vaccination and be seen regularly by a veterinarian. Pets should be kept under supervision to prevent contact with possible stray animals. Spay or neuter your pets to keep the number of unwanted stray "visitors" to a minimum. If you see stray animals around, call public health or animal control.

Educate your children to avoid interaction or contact with wild animals or touching dead animals. When traveling to parts of the world where rabies in dogs is common, warn all family members to avoid contact with stray dogs. Talk to a health care provider or travel clinic about the risk of exposure to rabies in that area, whether you should receive a vaccination before going and what to do if you get bitten.

Roseola

What is roseola? Roseola is a common viral infection that is also known as "exanthem subitum" or "sixth disease." It affects mainly younger children: roseola is rare in those younger than 4 months of age or those older than 4 years. The disease is caused by a virus called human herpesvirus 6 (HHV-6). This virus is not very infectious and it is not known how it spreads from person to person.

What does roseola look like? Infected infants and children usually develop a fever that is charac-

teristically high (over 103°F/39.5°C). Usually the fever persists for about three days, but can sometimes last up to seven. Infants are often cranky and very irritable while the fever is elevated but settle down nicely once the fever is brought down with medication. Classically, the fever subsides after three or four days, and then is followed by the development of a red spotty rash lasting hours to days. It is difficult to diagnose roseola until the rash appears, in its distinctive sequence, after the fever subsides. Up to 10 percent or 15 percent of children can have febrile seizures.

How is roseola treated? Children with roseola get better without any treatment and complications are very rare. The use of medication to lower fever, such as acetaminophen or ibuprofen, can be helpful but may not necessarily prevent seizures associated with fever.

Salmonella Infections

What are salmonella infections? Salmonella are a group of bacteria that can cause a variety of diseases in children. This section deals with the types of salmonella that cause diarrhea and not typhoid fever, which is specifically covered in the section on typhoid fever.

The bacteria are transmitted by eating food of animal origin, including chicken, beef, eggs, dairy products and fish. Fruits and vegetables have also been reported to be a source of infection if they have been in contact with an infected animal or human. Infection can also occur when a person drinks contaminated water. People can get salmonella if they are in contact with the feces of an animal and don't wash their hands. Pet reptiles (turtles, lizards and snakes), ducklings and baby chicks are particularly known to pass salmonella to people. Other animals including dogs, cats and farm animals can pass it on as well.

What does salmonella infection look like? Some children with salmonella infection will have no symptoms at all. They are called "asymptomatic carriers" who, although well, can transmit the disease to others. The most common symptoms in children who have the disease are diarrhea, fever, abdominal cramps and tenderness. The **incubation period** is short, ranging from 6 to 48 hours.

Children can sometimes develop an infection in their bloodstream. As a result, they can be feverish and quite sick, or "septic." The bacteria can spread to other areas of the body and cause infection there, such as bone infections or even **meningitis**.

When a child has diarrhea, salmonella infection can be diagnosed by testing a stool sample to see if it grows the bacteria in the laboratory (stool culture). Depending on your child's symptoms, a sample of urine, blood or other tissue might also be necessary.

How is salmonella treated? Children with diarrhea alone do not require treatment with an antibiotic, merely supportive care with adequate fluids and fever control (see pages 97–98). This is because antibiotics do not shorten the number of days of illness, and can prolong the time that the bacteria remain in the stools after the illness has cleared up. Most children will be better within seven days. Treatment with an antibiotic is recommended for very young infants, younger than 3 months of age, or other children with underlying chronic disease and immune system problems. Children with more complicated or serious disease from salmonella, such as blood infections, need treatment with antibiotics. They will likely need hospitalization and initial treatment with an antibiotic given intravenously.

To prevent infection with salmonella, cook eggs and other food of animal origin properly. Do not eat food containing raw eggs. Practice good hand hygiene. Wash your hands with soap and running water after contact with animal feces, after touching reptiles or any objects and surfaces that a reptile has touched. Also, when a child or person has salmonella, notify the public health department to help identify the source of infection in outbreaks. This protects other people from getting infected. In general, for nontyphoid salmonella, a child or staff member in a day care who has the disease should stay away until completely well.

Severe Acute Respiratory Syndrome (SARS)

What is SARS? SARS is a new infection that burst onto the world stage in 2003. Much is still unknown about this life-threatening disease. It is caused by a virus that primarily leads to disease in the upper respiratory tract, producing coldlike symptoms, or the lower respiratory tract, where it can cause pneumonia. The name of the virus that is suspected to cause SARS is the coronavirus.

What does SARS look like? In adults, SARS can be very serious and life-threatening. Adults usually have fever and mild symptoms during the first week, and then develop disease in their lungs in the second week, which can result in a need for supplemental oxygen. About 25 percent of adults will develop severe disease in their lungs, requiring admission to an intensive care unit.

SARS in children seems very different. It is much less severe. The incubation period is 5 to

10 days. Children develop a fever, dry cough and a runny nose. These symptoms are similar to children who develop the "common cold." Children do not usually develop muscle aches, dizziness or chills as adults do. Examination of the lungs with a stethoscope is usually normal. The fever is usually gone within seven days, and there is rarely any increased work of breathing. Some children will have evidence of infection on chest x-ray. No children died of SARS during the 2003 outbreaks. Some children who were infected with the coronavirus during the SARS outbreaks did not even develop any symptoms. Adolescents may have more serious disease than younger children.

How is SARS treated? Treatment for SARS is still being studied. Because children do not develop severe disease, treatment is supportive. This means that supplemental oxygen is given if required, as are intravenous fluids and nutrition. Isolation of cases is an important part of preventing SARS from spreading, and your local public health agency can provide updated information regarding this.

Scarlet Fever

What is scarlet fever? Scarlet fever is caused by an infection with a bacterium known as group A streptococcus. Strep is also responsible for infections in the throat (strep throat) and the skin (**impetigo, cellulitis**). This bacterium can produce a specific protein, or toxin, that results in a characteristic rash that is very red—hence the name "scarlet." This happens in about 10 percent of children who develop strep throat. Scarlet fever most commonly occurs between the ages of 4 to 8, and is uncommon in children

younger than 2. Generally, it is a fairly mild disease but is quite contagious.

What does scarlet fever look like? Within two to four days of being exposed to strep, children usually develop a fever, headache, nausea, vomiting, abdominal pain and muscle aches, and feel generally unwell. If it occurs as part of a strep throat, they will have a sore throat as well.

The characteristic rash develops 12 to 48 hours after the fever starts. It appears as red patches on the skin first on the neck, chest and in the armpits. The rash then spreads over the course of the next day to the arms and legs, giving the child the appearance of a "boiled lobster." Typically, there are small bumps, or "goose pimples," that give the skin a rough sandpaperlike texture. The redness in the skin folds, particularly in the neck, underarms, elbows and groin area, is accentuated. Around the mouth, the skin is characteristically pale. The tongue initially may have a white coating that peels after a few days to reveal a bright red "strawberry" tongue. The rash gradually disappears in about a week. The skin then starts peeling about 7 to 10 days after the rash, and this can continue for weeks. This peeling is most prominent in the underarms, groin and tips of the fingers and toes. Fortunately, the rash does not leave any scars.

How do I treat scarlet fever? Children who develop scarlet fever should be treated with penicillin for 10 days. Your doctor will swab your child's throat before antibiotics are started to help confirm the diagnosis. Antibiotics can help shorten the duration of fever, treat the sore throat and reduce the spread of infection. They also prevent some of the complications of strep infections, such as rheumatic fever. Children should not return to school or child care until at least 24 hours after beginning treatment with antibiotics, providing the fever has settled and they are feeling better.

Other family members or children who have been in contact with children with scarlet fever do not need specific treatment. If they develop a rash or are unwell they should see their doctor.

Shingles (Herpes Zoster)

What is shingles? Shingles, also known as herpes zoster, is an infection caused by the varicella-zoster virus. This is the very same virus that causes chicken pox. Shingles is more common in adults but can occur any time after a child has been infected with the chicken pox virus. After causing chicken pox, the varicella-zoster virus then attaches to sensory nerves in the dorsal ganglia next to the spinal cord. There, the virus can remain inactive indefinitely. However, reactivation of the virus in the nerve can occur and, when it does, the result is shingles. The average interval between chicken pox and childhood shingles is about four years if chicken pox occurred in the first year of life and about six years if chicken pox occurred after the first year.

Very rarely, shingles occurs after vaccination for chicken pox. It is much less likely for a child to develop shingles after the chicken pox vaccination than after getting chicken pox. Unlike chicken pox, shingles is much less contagious. Shingles is spread by contact with the skin rash. Children are not considered contagious if the rash is covered by a bandage or clothing.

What does shingles look like? Shingles begins with localized tingling or pain in the skin and a red raised rash. This develops into a patch of small, bumpy, fluid-filled blisters. The clue to the diagnosis is that the rash is distributed along a

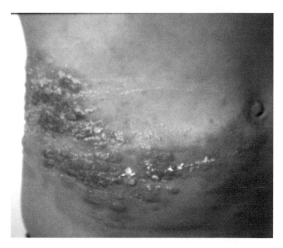

SHINGLES

The blisters of shingles rash affecting the patch of skin supplied by the infected nerve.

specific, more or less straight patch of skin on one side of the body only, which is the part supplied by the nerve infected with the virus. The most common area for the rash to occur is on the chest. Typically your child will not have a fever and is otherwise well. Later during the first week, the rash starts to scab and "crusts" up. Healing occurs within weeks and only rarely will the rash cause some scarring.

When the virus infects a nerve supplying the face, shingles can sometimes affect the eye. This can be expected if the rash involves the side or tip of the nose. Clues that your child's eye is involved include a painful red eye.

In adults, pain can persist after the rash has disappeared. Fortunately, this is very uncommon in children and, even when pain does persist after the rash, it usually clears up in fewer than eight days.

How do I treat shingles? Because shingles is an infection caused by a virus, antibiotics will not work in fighting the infection. Antiviral medications are available for treatment in adults but antiviral therapy has little effect on reducing the rash or symptoms. The main reason to treat shingles is to reduce the pain after the rash has gone. Because this occurs very rarely in children, routine treatment of shingles with antiviral medications is not usually recommended. Treatment with antivirals is recommended when shingles affects the eye or if there is a severe rash with pain in otherwise healthy children. The pain in shingles can be treated with ibuprofen, acetaminophen or codeine, but never aspirin as this has been associated with Reye's syndrome.

Sinusitis

What is sinusitis? The sinuses are the air-filled cavities on both sides of the face, located beside the nose and around the eye. These facial sinuses are connected with the nasal passages. Sinusitis occurs when the lining of these cavities becomes inflamed or swollen because of bacterial infection. This can happen whenever the drainage of secretions from the sinuses into the nasal passage is impaired, usually as a result of nasal congestion due to colds or allergies. When the secretions remain trapped in the sinuses, bacteria can then multiply causing an infection. Sinusitis is more common in a child over 10 but can occur in younger children as well.

What does sinusitis look like? There are two characteristic ways sinusitis shows up in children. The most common one consists of persistent cold symptoms with little or no improvement after 10 days. These symptoms include a runny nose and cough that is worse when your child lies down. The second, less common presentation is a severe upper respiratory tract infection,

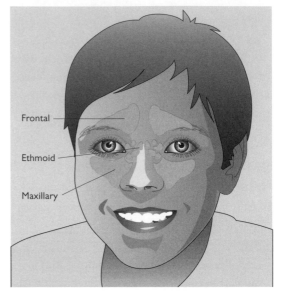

THE SINUS CAVITIES
The sinuses are air-filled cavities on both sides of the face. They are connected to the nasal passages.

including high fevers and thick greenish-yellow (pussy) mucus coming out of the nose for at least three days. There may also be some swelling around the eye, or facial pain.

Your doctor can diagnose sinusitis from the above symptoms and signs without any tests. Sinus x-rays are often not very helpful in diagnosing childhood sinusitis. CT scans may be useful for selected patients but are not considered routine for the diagnosis of sinusitis.

How do I treat sinusitis? Sinusitis is treated with antibiotics. With the correct antibiotics an improvement should be expected within 48 to 72 hours. Initially, medication for pain relief, such as acetaminophen or ibuprofen, may be required as well. While some doctors may recommend decongestants that are sprayed into the nose, their use is controversial. If there is an underlying condition, for example seasonal allergies, they will need to be treated as well.

Tonsillitis and Strep Throat

What is tonsillitis? Tonsillitis is an infection of the back of the throat involving the tonsils. The tonsils are the two lymph glands at the sides of the throat, which help fight off infections as part of the immune system.

Bacteria or viruses can cause tonsillitis, although viral causes are more common in children. Streptococcus, specifically group A hemolytic streptococcus, is the most common bacterium that causes tonsillitis and is known as "strep throat" or, more formally, as streptococcal pharyngitis. In tonsillitis the rest of the back of the throat, called the pharynx, is frequently also infected. This is known as pharyngitis. Often, the words tonsillitis and pharyngitis are used interchangeably.

Streptococcal pharyngitis occurs at all ages but is more common among school-aged children and adolescents. It is much rarer in children under 3. Pharyngitis from streptococcus usually happens after contact with another person's infected secretions from the mouth or nose. The incubation period is between two to five days.

What does tonsillitis look like? Children with tonsillitis have a sore throat, particularly when swallowing, and may have a fever. They may also have a headache, abdominal pain, nausea and vomiting. However, cough, runny nose and diarrhea are not usual features of strep throat; they suggest a viral infection. The tonsils might appear enlarged, red, with some white patches of pus. It can be very difficult to tell the difference between viral and streptococcal pharyngitis based purely on appearance.

There are some rare complications with strep throat. Some children develop a collection of pus in or around the tonsils called a peritonsillar abscess. This is associated with pain, difficulty opening the mouth, prolonged fever and difficulties with swallowing. Children can develop a rash with strep throat called scarlet fever (see pages 120–21). Some children with a strep throat, who have had no treatment or only incomplete treatment, can develop a heart problem, swelling of the joints and, days later, rashes. This is called rheumatic fever. In rheumatic fever, the body's immune system responds inappropriately to the streptococcal infection and starts attacking different parts of the body, including the heart. A similar reaction to streptococcal infection can cause kidney problems (post-streptococcal **glomerulonephritis**). Unfortunately, treatment of strep throat with antibiotics does not prevent this rare occurrence.

If your child's tonsillitis is caused by a virus, he can have a cough, pink eye (**conjunctivitis**), hoarseness, sneezing, ulcers in the throat, redness and swelling of the front part of the mouth or diarrhea. These features are usually not common with strep throat. Children infected with Epstein-Barr virus (EBV) have fever, enlarged lymph glands, a tired feeling and may have an enlarged spleen. (See pages 105–106.)

Your doctor will confirm the diagnosis of strep throat by a throat swab test. These results come back in one to two days. There are rapid swab tests for streptococcus that doctors can do in their offices and get results almost immediately. If the throat swab is negative for strep then it is usually assumed that the cause of the pharyngitis is viral. There is a blood test that can diagnose Epstein-Barr virus.

How is tonsillitis treated? Some children with tonsillitis may find it difficult to eat solids. In order that they do not get dehydrated, get them to drink adequate fluids. Acetaminophen or

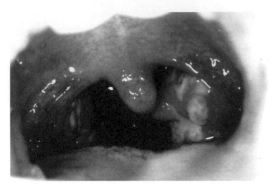

TONSILLITIS

When infected, the tonsils can become red, swollen and covered in pus.

ibuprofen can provide comfort from the fever and sore throat.

Because strep throat is caused by a bacterium, it is treated with an antibiotic. Penicillin is used, unless your child has an allergy, and it is taken for 10 days. Children with streptococcal pharyngitis should not return to school or child care until at least 24 hours after beginning antibiotic treatment. This is to prevent spread to other children. No specific treatment is generally required for other members of the family who are well. If they develop symptoms or have just had symptoms they should be tested for streptococcal pharyngitis. There is no specific treatment for viral causes of pharyngitis, which gets better by itself.

Children with tonsillitis rarely require surgery, or tonsillectomy. This may be necessary only when there are significant problems with breathing or many episodes of infection in a year.

Toxoplasmosis

What is toxoplasmosis? Toxoplasmosis is an infection caused by a parasite called *Toxoplasma gondii*. The disease occurs throughout the world and in different species. Cats generally acquire the infection by feeding on infected animals, such as mice, or on uncooked household meats. They can spread the disease to their owners. Humans usually become infected after eating undercooked meat or food containing the parasite. A large outbreak linked to contamination of a municipal water supply also has been reported. In babies born with toxoplasmosis, the mother became infected during pregnancy and passed the infection on to her newborn.

What does toxoplasmosis look like? At birth, 80 percent of newborn infants with congenital toxoplasmosis infection have no symptoms. However, problems with vision, learning disabilities or mental retardation can become obvious in a number of these children several months to years later. Those who do have evidence of congenital toxoplasmosis at birth can have a red, bumpy and spotty rash, enlarged lymph nodes, enlarged liver and spleen and jaundice. Some may have **thrombocytopenia**, in which case the blood particles that help form clots are reduced. Brain abnormalities, seizures and deafness can also develop. Some of the severely affected infants die in their mother's womb or within a few days of birth. Infection of the heart muscle and lung are rare complications. Sometimes only the eye is affected by toxoplasmosis.

Toxoplasma gondii infection acquired after birth is usually not associated with any symptoms. If symptoms develop, they are nonspecific and include tiredness, fever, sore throat, muscle aches and swollen neck glands. The illness is usually quite minor and gets better on its own.

How is toxoplasmosis treated? Although there are specific drugs available to treat toxoplasmosis, a previously healthy child who acquires the infection does not require treatment. Infants born with congenital toxoplasmosis, however, will require a special combination of antibiotic treatment for a period of one year. Breast-feeding by an infected mother provides no risk to her infant. Infected children are *not* contagious.

If you are pregnant or contemplating becoming pregnant, prevention of congenital toxoplasmosis is possible by following basic hygiene principles. Eat meat only if it is properly cooked, or if it is smoked or cured. Wash your hands thoroughly and clean kitchen surfaces after handling raw meat. Keep your hands away from the mouth and eyes while handling uncooked meat, and unwashed raw fruits and vegetables. Avoid contact with cat feces or litter boxes or wear gloves. Also avoid children's sandboxes, which cats think of as large litter boxes.

Tuberculosis

What is tuberculosis? Tuberculosis (TB) is an infection caused by the bacterium *Mycobacterium tuberculosis*. The worldwide incidence of tuberculosis has been increasing. Children in developed countries account for less than 5 percent of all cases worldwide. However, because of increased travel and immigration, tuberculosis is increasingly being seen in developed countries.

M. tuberculosis is usually transmitted through the air from one person to another. Transmission or infection can occur when a child inhales droplets from an adult or adolescent with infectious tuberculosis of the lung, who is coughing or sneezing. The bacteria can settle in the child's lungs and begin to multiply. From there they can move through the blood to other parts of the body.

What is the tuberculin skin test? A TB skin test is used to help diagnose infection in children who have no symptoms. It contains a protein that is injected through a needle just under the skin. The area is then examined and measured between 48 to 72 hours later to see how big the bump on the skin is. A positive skin test implies that the child has tuberculosis infection or disease. It can take up to three months after becoming infected for the skin test to turn positive. Based on several factors, such as the presence of any symptoms, x-ray findings, underlying immune problems and travel to places where TB is common, the skin test is read as positive or negative. Routine tuberculosis skin testing of all children is not recommended. Rather, certain groups who are at risk for TB infection should be tested, which is why immigrants from countries with a high incidence of TB are always tested. The problem with testing everyone is that the test can be falsely positive in otherwise well children.

What can happen if my child comes into close contact with M. tuberculosis? Tuberculosis "exposure" means that a child has had a recent contact with someone with suspected or confirmed contagious pulmonary TB, but he is well and has a normal chest x-ray and a negative tuberculin skin test.

Tuberculosis "infection" refers to a person who has a positive tuberculin skin test but has no evidence of disease and the chest x-ray is normal or only shows some **granulomas** or calcifications in the lung or lymph glands in the chest. Granulomas or calcifications are the body's response to the infection and can be seen on chest x-ray or CT scans. Tuberculosis infection might also be referred to as "latent TB infection," because people with this don't feel sick but can develop TB disease later in life if they do not receive appropriate treatment.

Tuberculous "disease" refers to a person who has signs and symptoms of infection, and/or lung disease evident on a chest x-ray. Tuberculosis can cause disease when the child is first infected (primary infection) or later on in life (reactivation, or post-primary disease).

What does TB look like? Children can be infected with *M. tuberculosis* and have no symptoms at all. The bacteria can attack any part of the body, but they usually attack the lungs.

The initial infection can cause inflammation or swelling in the lymph glands of the chest (lymphadenitis). This can show up on a chest x-ray. In most cases this clears up by itself, and might leave some scarring or calcium deposition in the lymph gland, which, by itself, is not a problem.

Children who have symptoms of disease can have disease in the lungs and/or outside of the lungs. Regardless of where the disease is, children with TB can have fever, chills, sweating at night, weight loss and no appetite.

TB in the lung can look similar to regular pneumonia, with cough and fever. On a chest x-ray this will show up as a white area. The body reacts to the infection in a special way, forming what is called a "granuloma" in the lung. The infection can also affect the lining of the lung, called the pleura. This can result in fluid collecting around the lung, a pleural effusion, which can cause chest pain. The infection can invade the blood vessels of the lung, resulting in it spreading around the lung and to other parts of the body. Some older children and adolescents might cough up blood or sputum. Miliary tuberculosis describes the special form of tuberculosis where the infection has spread to other parts of the body through the bloodstream.

Tuberculosis outside the lungs is less common than in the lungs. It occurs in about one-quarter of infants and children under 4 who get TB. It can affect almost any part of the body. The most common form of disease outside of the lungs is lymphadenitis. This can occur in the lymph glands in the neck. Tuberculosis can also infect the space around the brain and cause **meningitis**. It occurs in about 4 percent of children with tuberculosis. The bacteria can infect the bone or joints (osteomyelitis or septic arthritis), causing swelling and pain. Rarely, it can cause disease in the bowels or kidneys.

How is TB diagnosed? In order to diagnose tuberculosis, your child's doctor will take a careful history of symptoms and possible exposure to an infected adult, complete a detailed physical exam, perform a tuberculin skin test and order a chest x-ray. Further blood tests and other investigations, such as a CT scan of the lungs, might be done based on your child's specific symptoms. If TB is present, it is necessary to try to isolate the bacteria from the body. This will help determine which medications will provide effective treatment. Adults can easily cough up phlegm from the lungs but this is very difficult for children. A common way of finding the germs in children is to do a "gastric aspirate." Overnight, the body pushes mucus from the lungs, which contain the *M. tuberculosis* bacteria, up the windpipe and this is swallowed into the stomach. In this test, a tube, called a nasogastric tube, is placed through the child's nose into his stomach and used to obtain an early morning sample of the stomach contents for testing before the child eats or drinks. If there is evidence of TB in other parts of the body, there might be special samples required from lymph nodes, spinal fluid, bone or joint fluid.

How is TB treated? The first step is to determine whether a child has tuberculosis exposure, infection or disease. If a child has tuberculosis exposure and no infection or disease, he might have a repeat skin test in three months and no medications. Children with tuberculosis infection require medications for six to 12 months to prevent getting sick from tuberculosis disease. Tuberculosis disease requires multiple special medications. The type of medications and how long your child has to take them depends on where the infection was acquired, what parts of the body are infected and the results of the various medical investigations. Children with tuberculosis infection are often seen by a specialist in pediatric infectious disease.

TB in a child is an important signal that an adult with tuberculosis, usually a close contact, has spread the infection to him. Therefore, an important aspect of tuberculosis treatment is to ensure that everyone in the family as well as all close contacts are traced, tested and treated appropriately by public health officials before they infect many others.

Typhoid Fever

What is typhoid fever? Typhoid fever is an infection caused by bacteria known as *Salmonella typhi*. It is usually contracted by eating food or drinking water contaminated by urine or feces of a person who carries the disease. Typhoid fever is found mainly as outbreaks in underdeveloped countries but returning travelers can bring it to North America.

What does typhoid fever look like? After a child ingests the bacteria from contaminated food or water, he usually has no symptoms for 7 to 14 days, although this **incubation period** can last up to 60 days. The infection then enters the bloodstream. At this stage, children develop fever and are unwell and tired with chills, headache, poor appetite, abdominal pain, dry cough and muscle aches. The tongue may be coated, the abdomen tender and the liver and spleen may be enlarged. Diarrhea can be a major feature of typhoid fever but sometimes people with it have constipation.

During the second week of the illness, the fever goes up. A rash can appear that looks like raised pink (rose) spots that are very small and are mainly found on the abdomen and chest.

Typhoid fever can affect different parts of the body and be very serious if not treated. Complications occur more commonly in patients who have been ill for longer than two weeks. Some of the more serious complications include bleeding from the gastrointestinal tract, perforation of the gastrointestinal tract and encephalopathy (a fluctuating level of consciousness).

Your doctor will take a blood and stool sample and culture it in the laboratory to see if the bacteria grow to diagnose typhoid. Neither of these is consistently helpful, as both tests can be negative in children who have typhoid fever.

How is typhoid treated? Typhoid fever requires antibiotics. The particular type of antibiotic will vary depending on where the typhoid was picked up. The antibiotics can be taken orally or intravenously, if necessary. Usually, the child starts to feel better within days of the start of treatment. Children who have bloody diarrhea will need fluid replacement by mouth or intravenous.

How can I prevent typhoid? For people living in developed countries, typhoid fever most commonly occurs when they travel to areas where typhoid is common. Travelers to such areas need to take care with food and water. If not drinking bottled water then you should boil it prior to drinking it. Fresh vegetables or fruits that have been washed in local water are potential sources of infection. Food needs to be thoroughly cooked. A vaccine is available for typhoid fever and recommended for travelers to areas where typhoid is common.

Urinary Tract Infections

What are urinary tract infections? A urinary tract infection (UTI) refers to an infection of the bladder or kidneys. Pyelonephritis is an infection in the kidney. Generally, infants and young children who have a fever with a urinary tract infection are considered to have pyelonephritis.

UTIs are common in childhood. Up to 10 percent of children have had a urinary tract infection by their teenage years. Except in the newborn period, UTIs are twice as common in girls as boys. Furthermore, about 5 percent of children aged 2 months to 2 years who have fever but no other symptoms or signs of infection have a urinary tract infection.

Many different bacteria can cause urinary tract infections. One common one is *Escherichia coli* (E. coli). This germ usually lives in the bowels and can enter the opening of the urinary tract, the urethra, from the diaper area, or it can spread to the kidneys through the bloodstream. Girls have a shorter urethra than boys, which may be one reason why urinary tract infections occur more commonly in females. There is generally minimal connection to hygiene or cleanliness, although little girls should be taught to clean themselves from "front to back."

What does a UTI look like? The symptoms of urinary tract infection in infants and children are variable. Children might have to urinate often

or urgently, or develop bedwetting when they have a urinary tract infection. Older children may complain of pain when urinating or have an ache in their lower back. Some children might cry when urinating, or have foul-smelling urine. Children might or might not have fever. They might vomit, be irritable or be more listless than usual. Sometimes, they have abdominal pain or even diarrhea.

How are urinary tract infections diagnosed? UTIs are diagnosed by testing a specimen of urine. The sample can be tested right away using a special stick dipped in the urine that can detect the presence of white blood cells, red blood cells and bacteria-producing nitrites. This is a screening test that helps to predict the likelihood of a urinary tract infection. The sample is then sent to a lab where it is placed in an incubator to confirm whether any bacteria grow from the urine. This test, called a urine culture, will definitively confirm the presence, or absence, of infection. Usually, it will take one to two days to get a urine culture result.

The way the sample is taken is very important for proper diagnosis. To obtain a urine sample from young infants, a catheter is placed through the urethra into the bladder. Another method of obtaining urine is to place a needle through the lower abdomen into the bladder. This procedure, called a suprapubic aspiration, sounds a lot worse than it is! A bag can be placed over the penis or vagina to collect urine. The problem with bag specimens is that they often get contaminated with the normal bacteria that live on the skin. This makes interpreting test results from bag specimens difficult. Older children, who are able to use the toilet, can give a "midstream" sample, taken midway through urination, for culture.

Why did my child get a urinary tract infection? Most children who get urinary tract infections are otherwise healthy. Urine normally contains no bacteria but, sometimes, bacteria can get into the urethra and infect the urine in the bladder from the skin around the rectum and the genitalia.

Some children may have a problem with their urinary tract system that places them at risk of getting urinary tract infections. One condition is called vesicoureteral reflux (VUR), or urinary reflux (see pages 252–53). VUR occurs when urine flows backward from the bladder to the ureters and/or kidney instead of forward into the urethra. This is thought to be something that a child is born with and might run in families. There are different severities of vesicoureteral reflux. Milder cases of VUR usually clear up with time but children might require a small daily dose of antibiotics to keep the urine sterile and prevent infections. The concern with vesicoureteral reflux is that it can result in urine "sitting around" and getting infected, which can cause repeated urinary tract infections and consequent scarring of the kidney. Scarring leads to loss of kidney function and, potentially, problems in the future, such as hypertension.

Circumcision has been linked with a reduced risk of urinary tract infection in boys during the first year of life. However, because the chance of getting a urinary tract infection is still low, circumcision is not recommended as a method of preventing urinary tract infections in otherwise healthy boys.

Some children have an abnormal pattern of voiding urine that may place them at risk for developing urinary tract infection (voiding dysfunction). Constipation has been linked to an increased risk of getting a urinary tract infection.

There are some uncommon conditions that can also predispose a child to urinary tract infec-

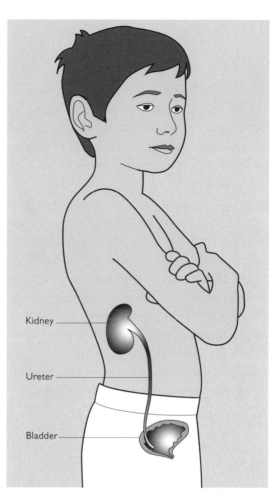

THE URINARY TRACT
A urinary tract infection (UTI) is an infection of the bladder or kidneys.

tions. Examples of these include a neurological problem involving the spinal cord, for example **spina bifida**, or an immune system problem.

What tests are done after diagnosis of a urinary tract infection? Children under 5 who have a urinary tract infection will often need some other tests. The purpose of these tests is to identify children who are at risk of developing more infections and scarring of the kidney, which could lead to kidney damage and long-term problems.

An ultrasound of the abdomen is usually done to look at the urinary tract system, which includes the kidneys, ureters and bladder. The main reason to do this test is to ensure that the system is connected properly and was formed properly during birth. It can also show whether any blockages are present or whether any collection of infection is present.

Another test, called a voiding cystourethrogram (VCUG), is also usually done after the first urinary tract infection to look for vesicoureteral reflux. A VCUG is done by placing a catheter into the urethra and injecting dye into the catheter. X-rays are then taken to see which way the dye flows in order to diagnose vesicoureteral reflux.

A DMSA scan is a nuclear medicine test that can demonstrate areas of recent infection in the kidney (pyelonephritis). And, months after the infection, the DMSA scan can be used to identify any scarring that might have occurred as a result of the infection.

How is a UTI treated? Urinary tract infections are treated with antibiotics. If a child looks very unwell, or can't take any fluids orally, he might be started on intravenous antibiotics and admitted to hospital. Most children can take antibiotics orally. Children usually feel better after taking at least two days of antibiotics. A repeat urine culture is generally not necessary if the child has improved as expected with the antibiotics.

Children who are at risk for recurrent urinary tract infection might be placed on low-dose daily antibiotics to prevent future infections. This is called "antibiotic prophylaxis." This is indicated for children with vesicoureteral reflux, who will have repeat testing to see whether the reflux has improved or resolved. This is usually done annually.

Many health care providers recommend a common-sense approach to prevention of urinary tract infections. These include good hygiene such as front-to-back wiping after urination in girls, correcting constipation and avoiding bubble baths.

It is important that children who are at risk of having recurrent infections, or who have had scarring of the kidney from a previous infection, be tested early for urinary tract infection when they have fever.

West Nile Virus

What is West Nile virus? West Nile virus (WNV) was first discovered in Uganda in 1937 and has since been found in parts of Africa, Asia, the Middle East and Europe. Only recently has it become a problem in North America. In 2004, across the United States, there were 2,470 reported human cases and 88 deaths. WNV is transmitted by mosquitoes but not every mosquito carries WNV and not every person bitten by a mosquito will get infected with WNV. The virus is most active from early July to mid-November in the northeastern and midwestern states, from mid-May to mid-December in the southern states, and in late summer in the western states.

What does WNV look like? Only one in five individuals infected with WNV will actually develop symptoms. If symptoms do appear, they usually show up between 3 and 14 days after an infected mosquito has bitten the person. They are often flulike and can include fever, aches and fatigue, weakness, headache and a rash. In a very few cases, approximately 1 in 150, the virus can cause a serious illness, such as **encephalitis**, **meningitis** or paralysis. Serious illness from WNV is more common in adults than in children and most children who get WNV will have only a mild illness. Children with weak immune systems or those who already have a serious underlying illness are particularly susceptible to the more serious effects of WNV.

How is WNV treated? Currently, there is no treatment or vaccine to prevent the disease. The best protection against West Nile virus is to avoid mosquito bites and reduce mosquito breeding spots. Insect repellents containing DEET are most effective at preventing mosquito bites and are safe if used appropriately. Do not use on children under the age of 6 months and apply only once daily in those under 2 years. It should be used sparingly at the lowest concentration recommended; 10 percent or less in the under-12-year-old group and 30 percent or less for those over 12. DEET is not harmless and there are potential complications, such as skin and respiratory irritation and seizures, if it is not used correctly. Regularly drain standing water from items like toys, flower pots, cans, buckets, barrels and pool covers, and clean out clogged gutters.

Avoiding mosquito bites:
- Reduce the amount of time spent outside during the dawn or dusk hours when mosquitoes are most active.
- Use barriers, like mosquito nets or screens for baby strollers.
- Make sure windows and doors are properly screened and screens are in good repair.
- Wear protective clothing when possible: light-colored clothing with long sleeves and

PRECAUTIONS TO TAKE WHEN USING INSECT REPELLANT:

- Apply to your hands and then put it on the child's skin, avoiding his eyes, mouth and palms.
- Do not allow young children to apply DEET products themselves.
- Avoid repellant on cuts or irritated skin.
- Reapply after swimming.
- Wash treated skin and clothing with soap and water after returning indoors.
- Store DEET out of reach of children.

cuffs, long pants tucked into socks or shoes, and hats.
- When outdoors in parks or rural settings, apply insect repellents containing DEET.
- Insect repellents that are used on children should have a small concentration of DEET, depending on the age of the child. These products should not be used on children younger than 6 months old.

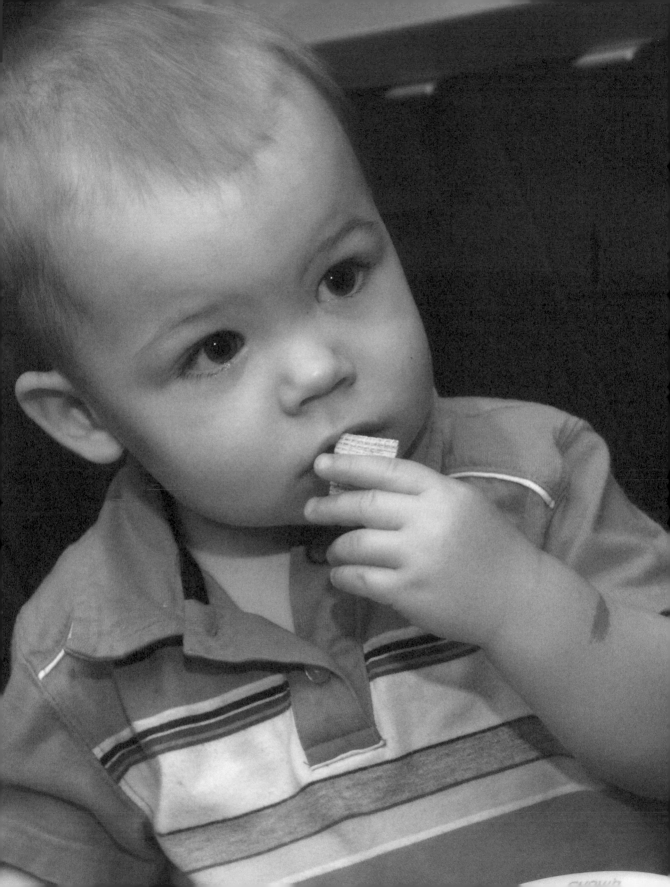

Growth and Nutrition

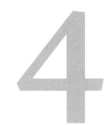

Failure to Thrive

What is failure to thrive? An infant's weight is an excellent marker of overall nutrition and health. Failure to gain weight well in the early months and years can have a negative impact upon the development of the infant's brain and nervous system. "Failure to thrive" is the term for when an infant fails to gain weight appropriately.

An accurate measurement of your baby's weight should be obtained at birth and at each well-baby checkup. The health care provider should plot these measurements on a standard growth chart. There is a possibility that your baby has failure to thrive if her weight is less than the third percentile for her age and sex; that is, if she weighs less than 97 out of 100 similar infants. Your doctor might also suspect failure to thrive if repeat weight measurements indicate that your infant's weight has fallen over two major percentiles (for example from above the 75th percentile to below the 25th percentile) over a period of several months.

Infants gain, on average, about an ounce (approximately 20 to 30 g) per day in the first six months of life; and then approximately half an ounce (15 g) per day from 6 months to a year. During the second year of life, infants continue to gain weight, but not nearly as rapidly as in

the first year of life. You or your doctor should be concerned by any unexplained weight loss at any time.

An infant's length must be considered along with her weight. A few growth patterns affecting the infant's weight and length should be distinguished from poor weight gain alone. For example, some babies are born, either at term or prematurely, proportionately small for both weight and length. If these babies continue to grow well and if it seems they are "catching up," you should not consider they have a problem with poor weight gain even if they are below the third percentile. Some babies are born at an average weight and length, and by the second year of life their weight and length are proportionately small. This often occurs if the infant's parents and extended family are short. This growth pattern should not be considered to be a problem, but rather reflects the genetic makeup of the child.

What could be causing failure to thrive? For decades, pediatricians have noted that a specific medical cause can seldom be identified for infants with failure to thrive. It is often a complicated matter to find the cause of the inadequate weight gain and, in fact, there may be several interacting factors. It is thought that the central issue for these infants is inadequate nutrition. Several reasons

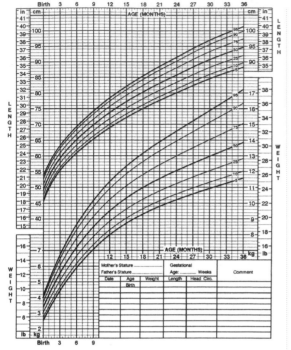

NORMAL GROWTH CHART
GIRLS (BIRTH TO 36 MONTHS)

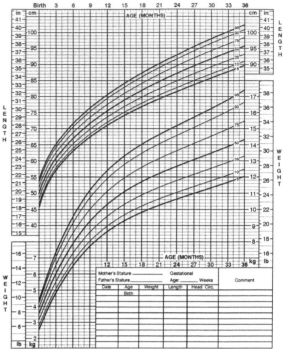

NORMAL GROWTH CHART
BOYS (BIRTH TO 36 MONTHS)

may contribute to this. The infant's temperament may play a role; for example, she might be a fussy or irritable infant. There might be problems in the interaction between the infant and the person who primarily feeds the infant. Or, the infant might not provide cues or the primary feeder might not identify cues that the infant is hungry. The baby might push away or refuse to feed, or the caregiver might have trouble feeding the infant.

On a rare occasion, a baby's formula has been prepared inadequately, so that the infant is receiving an insufficient number of calories. Sometimes, solid foods have been introduced too late and the child refuses to eat them. Decades ago it was noted that infants living in institutions who did not receive adequate nurturing did not gain weight well. Today, some

infants gain weight poorly if stressors in the home interfere with nurturing the infant. For example, a caregiver who is depressed or stressed might have difficulty spending time to nurture and feed the baby. These are complex issues that require time, trust and openness between the doctor and the family.

Less commonly in failure to thrive, there is some medical condition that produces inadequate weight gain. In such cases, there is usually some symptom or signal to suggest that a specific illness is present. Vomiting might lead to inadequate caloric intake. The vomiting might be due to an intestinal tract obstruction or severe gastroesophageal reflux disease. The baby might be having difficulty absorbing enough calories.

Malabsorption can occur as a result of medical conditions such as cystic fibrosis or **celiac**

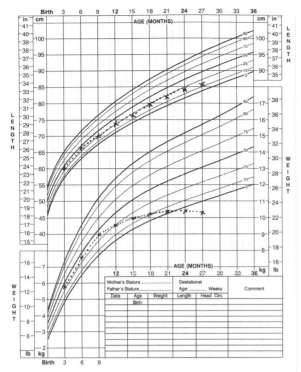

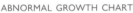

ABNORMAL GROWTH CHART

Sequential measurements of this child's weight reveal a failure to achieve expected gains. This pattern might be seen in diseases affecting food absorption, such as cystic fibrosis.

disease. Although most of the time diarrhea does not last long and is due to an **acute** viral infection, in some cases, infants develop longer periods of diarrhea that can lead to malabsorption. Also, there are some medical conditions that are associated with increased need for calories because the infant's metabolic rate has increased. This would include medical conditions of the heart, the lungs or the kidneys. Elevations in thyroid hormone are uncommon in infants but might result in an increased metabolic rate and poor weight gain. Common infections can also increase the infant's need for calories, especially if they are long-standing or go unnoticed, such as a urinary tract infection or recurrent ear infections. Less

common infections, such as tuberculosis or HIV, might lead to inadequate weight gain.

In brief, a lot of medical problems are capable of producing failure to thrive but, most of the time, there is no distinct disease.

Although infants might gain weight poorly during an acute illness, such as a viral upper respiratory tract infection or acute diarrhea, they should recover well with appropriate catch-up growth. This should not result in failure to gain weight adequately over several months.

What can be done about failure to thrive? Every baby should be weighed at birth and again at each visit to the doctor. Her length or height should also be measured. This will allow your doctor to assess her growth over time and monitor the relationship between weight and length. Inadequate weight gain should be identified early to allow for assessment and intervention.

Your child's doctor will undertake a detailed evaluation of the situation. She will review details of the pregnancy, labor and delivery; early newborn health and birth weight; and dietary and feeding history. The doctor will explore your baby's temperament and development, stressors or health issues in the family, especially for the caregiver who primarily feeds the infant. She will give your baby a detailed physical examination. With this information alone, the doctor can usually determine whether a medical cause is contributing to the inadequate weight gain. Laboratory tests are not always necessary, but may be requested if the doctor thinks that a medical condition is causing the problem, or if she is concerned that the poor nutrition has lead to a complication such as anemia.

If a specific medical cause is not found, you will have to pay close attention to nutrition and feeding. In some situations, you might have a consultation with a pediatric dietitian to provide recommendations for increasing the calories in your baby's diet. Techniques for feeding might also be explored. If the infant has developed severe feeding problems, you might have a consultation with a pediatric occupational therapist to improve the infant's oral-motor feeding skills. Additional treatment might be required, such as having the baby take oral iron supplements if she has developed anemia. Close follow up by all health specialists is necessary with regular measurement of weight and length until her growth has caught up adequately. Your baby's general psychological and motor development should be monitored and, if necessary, interventions such as an infant stimulation program might be considered. Of course, if a distinct medical condition is present, your baby will require appropriate specific treatment for that problem.

Abnormal Head Growth: Microcephaly and Macrocephaly

What is abnormal head growth? The circumference of a baby's head should be measured at birth and then regularly at each well-baby check-up. Your baby's brain grows tremendously in her early months and years: this is the major cause of the expansion of the bony skull. The place where the bones of the skull meet are called sutures and the soft spot on the top of the head, where several bones meet together, is called the fontanelle. The baby's brain is allowed to expand through bone growth at the suture lines. By 2 years of age, your baby's head will have reached two-thirds of its final adult head size. Therefore, head circumference is an important measurement of infant growth.

The measurement can be made with a tape measure placed just above your baby's eyes and around to the back of the skull. The largest head circumference should be measured. Growth charts are available, the same as for height and weight, to monitor head growth over time. As with height and weight, there is a range of measurements that are typical for children at the same age and sex. Measurements taken over time are most useful and will indicate if head growth for an individual child is progressing as expected. As with other aspects of your child's growth, family genetics are an important determinant of her head size and growth pattern. Microcephaly means possessing a small head. On a standard growth chart, the head circumference will be at or below the third percentile, which means that fewer than three children out of a hundred of that age and sex will have a head circumference that small. Macrocephaly means having a large head. On a standard growth chart, head measurement will place at or above the 97th percentile. Depending on the cause, micro- or macrocephaly could be noted on the first measurement performed just after birth or it may appear later on after the baby has had several head circumference measurements.

What could be causing abnormal head growth? Remember that there is tremendous variability in children's head sizes. This is largely the result of the genes that the children have inherited from their families. Generally, whether or not a child has a head that is slightly smaller or slightly larger than average should not affect health, development or intelligence. Micro- and macrocephaly refer to head sizes that are significantly smaller and larger than average. These are statistical definitions, merely measurements, and do not always mean the child has an associated health

HEAD CIRCUMFERENCE CHART

BOYS (BIRTH TO 36 MONTHS)

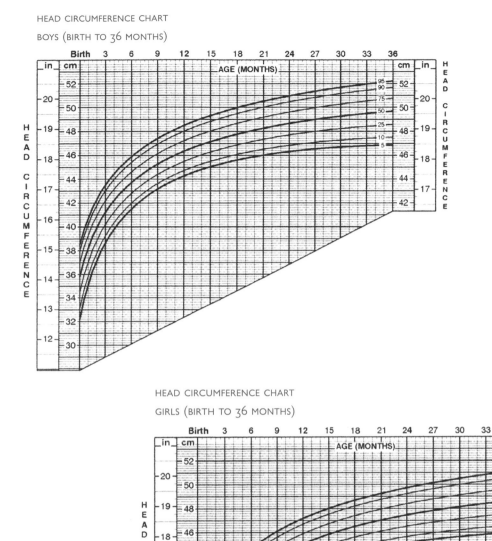

HEAD CIRCUMFERENCE CHART

GIRLS (BIRTH TO 36 MONTHS)

problem. However, it is known that children with micro- and macrocephaly have a higher chance for an associated health problem, and so this deserves further attention from a physician.

Microcephaly is most commonly associated with failure of the growth of or reduction in the size of the infant's brain. This can be due to an injury to the baby's developing brain before birth. Examples would include viral infections that the mother had during pregnancy (such as rubella or cytomegalovirus) or exposure to toxins during pregnancy, including alcohol, which can lead to fetal alcohol syndrome.

Abnormalities of chromosomes, such as **Down's syndrome** (also called trisomy 21), and other genetic syndromes can be associated with microcephaly. Some babies are born with abnormalities of their metabolic systems, for example **phenylketonuria**, which may lead to microcephaly. Other infants might have suffered a serious head injury due to a fall or an infection, such as **meningitis**, during the sensitive period of brain development and rapid head growth. This can result in the development of microcephaly. Some babies have an abnormality of the bony skull resulting in premature closure of the sutures that can impair the ability of the skull and the brain to grow. This is known as craniosynostosis. Sometimes only one or two of the sutures are involved, leading to an odd head shape as it expands unevenly.

Macrocephaly might be due to hydrocephalus. The brain is bathed in a fluid called cerebrospinal fluid. Hydrocephalus is due to an abnormal accumulation of cerebrospinal fluid. There are several causes of hydrocephalus. Babies can be born with abnormalities in the fluid drainage system that leads to a buildup of fluid. These babies will be born with macrocephaly. Some infants develop a mass, such as a brain tumor,

that blocks the passage of the cerebrospinal fluid. These infants will develop macrocephaly on repeated head circumference measurements. Babies who develop an accumulation of blood, for example due to a serious head injury, or an infection, such as meningitis, can develop an increase in pressure inside the skull leading to an abnormally large head. Some babies are born with bone abnormalities that lead to an abnormally thickened skull. Rarely, children are born with genetic conditions or abnormalities of their metabolic systems that lead to larger than normal brains.

How is abnormal head growth treated? As mentioned, your doctor should accurately measure your baby's head circumference at birth and at all well-infant visits. The measurements should be charted on a standard head circumference chart. This will allow for timely identification of children who are born with micro- or macrocephaly, or who develop an abnormal head size over time. Infants identified with an abnormal head size will need to be thoroughly assessed. The doctor will pay careful attention to details of the pregnancy, labor and delivery; family history; and your baby's general health, growth and development. She will take accurate measurements of height, weight and head circumference. A thorough physical assessment will include careful attention to any clues suggesting a genetic syndrome, abnormalities of the nervous system or infant development. The doctor might measure and record your and your partner's head circumferences, because the size of the head may run in the family. The doctor might recommend further tests, such as blood tests for genetic and metabolic abnormalities and diagnostic imaging such as skull x-rays, ultrasound, head CT scan or MRI. Depending upon the results, the doctor might request a referral to a specialist with expertise in neurology neurosurgery or genetics. Because there are so many possible causes of micro- and macrocephaly, the treatment and results will vary accordingly. All children will have very close follow up of their development and, if indicated, your doctor will refer them to developmental specialists and therapists.

Obesity

What is obesity? Obesity refers to the excessive accumulation of fat, rather than excessive weight. There is controversy about the best way to define and measure obesity. It is currently thought that the best measure is the body mass index (BMI), which shows body weight adjusted for height. Because children's body fatness changes as they grow, BMI for children is often called BMI-for-age, and is plotted on a series of gender and age specific growth charts. However, you can estimate your child's BMI, but not her BMI-for-age, by diving her weight in pounds by her height in inches squared, and then multiplying by 703 (or dividing her weight in kilograms by her height in meters squared). As with weight and height, BMI-for-age may be categorized according to percentile for the child's age and sex. Children at risk of being overweight are those whose BMI-for-age is between the 85th and 95th percentile for age and sex. Those who are overweight or obese are those whose BMI-for-age is at or above the 95th percentile.

Currently, about 15 percent of North American school-aged children and adolescents are at or above the 95th percentile and are, therefore, obese. This is a significant and concerning increase over the past 20 years. There are many known health consequences associated with childhood obesity. These include:

- heart-related problems, such as increased blood pressure and cholesterol levels;
- problems with blood sugar and insulin resulting in diabetes;
- mental health problems, such as low self-esteem and depression;
- breathing problems, such as asthma and **obstructive sleep apnea**;
- liver problems, such as fatty liver resulting in a type of hepatitis;
- problems with the hip bones;
- the risk of obesity persisting into adulthood.

What causes obesity? For most children who are overweight or obese, there is no single cause. Simplistically, obesity results when you eat more than you burn off in energy. Yet, it is likely that there is interaction among contributing factors such as genetics and other physical factors relating to that child, emotional and psychological factors and factors relating to the child's culture or social environment. Given this complex situation, there are several recognized risk factors for childhood obesity. You and your health care providers should place your emphasis on the prevention of overweight and obesity rather than treatment of obesity after it has occurred. Knowing the risk factors will help everyone focus upon healthy lifestyles to reduce these risks. Most of this focus has been on nutrition (caloric intake) and physical activity (energy expenditure).

Obesity in one or both parents of young preschool-aged children substantially increases the risk of the children becoming obese. Breastfeeding has been found to protect young children against developing obesity. Research has found that children whose parents are overcontrolling in regard to their eating are at higher risk of obesity. Your food choices will influence the food choices of your children. So if you eat a lot of junk food, don't be surprised to see your children do the same. Children whose families do not sit down together for meals might be at greater risk for developing unhealthy eating practices.

Sedentary children are at greater risk for obesity. Television watching has been found to be associated with obesity. Watching more than four hours of television per day and having a television in the bedroom are associated with obesity. Informal physical activity, such as walking to school, has decreased and this is thought to be associated with increasing obesity. Children and parents in some cities find it difficult to get to play areas, or might be concerned that play areas are too dangerous. And for many children, formal physical activity, such as school physical education programs, have been reduced.

There are other less common causes of overweight and obesity. Endocrine (hormonal) causes of obesity include deficiency of thyroid hormone, excess of cortisol hormone or polycystic ovary syndrome. Children with a deficiency of thyroid hormone might grow more slowly, and have constipation, decreased energy and increased need for sleep. Children might have an excess of cortisol hormone, either due to a medical condition or because of taking steroid medication. The excess weight may be distributed in the face, at the top of the back ("buffalo hump") and around the abdomen. Girls with polycystic ovary syndrome might have excessive facial hair, acne and abnormalities of their menstrual periods. A few rare genetic syndromes are associated with overweight and obesity, and these children usually have several other health and development issues.

How can obesity be prevented? Overweight and obesity are very difficult to treat and, in most cases, are due to an imbalance of your child's caloric intake (eating) and energy expenditure (exercise). Prevention begins with healthy nutrition and physical activity.

- If at all possible, you should breast-feed your baby for her first 6 months due to its protective effect.
- Once she is beginning solid food, encourage your child to have healthy eating patterns. Young children should be allowed to regulate their own food intake. Parents and other caregivers should be discouraged from "pushing" the young child to eat and paying too much attention to the child who is reluctant to eat.
- Parents and other caregivers should act as role models for healthy eating patterns, food choices and family meal times. Meals should be eaten without distractions, such as television, computers, homework or reading.
- Limit your child's pop intake.
- And, surprisingly, you should also limit her consumption of milk and milk products—no more than the daily requirements (2–3 cups per day). After 6 months of age your baby needs a number of nutrients—for example, iron, which is poorly absorbed from milk. Milk is also very high in fat and babies who fill up on milk will often refuse to eat their veggies, cereals and other food. Infants over the age of 6 months who drink too much milk to the exclusion of a more balanced diet will often be chubby and have a degree of iron deficiency anemia.
- Snacks should be healthy, such as fruit or vegetables.
- Get your children involved in regular physical activity, which can either be unstructured or formal. Encourage your children to walk or ride their bicycles to school. If you have safety concerns, there is often a parent or

caregiver in the neighborhood who is willing to walk or ride with a group of children to ensure safety.

- Restrict the number of hours of television and computer viewing.
- Consider becoming involved in school- or community-based programs aimed at improving healthy lifestyles in children.

How can overweight and obesity be treated? The treatment of overweight and obesity for both children and adults is very challenging. No single mode of treatment has been found to be successful for everyone. The appropriate goal for you and your child is to maintain (rather than lose) the weight. As she gets taller, her weight remains stable and her BMI is reduced. Weight reduction can have negative health consequences, including impairing her physical and brain growth.

The primary component of any treatment plan is modification of your child's diet. No single diet plan has proven to be superior. Nutritionists recommend a balanced, low-calorie diet following a national food guide of recommended daily requirements, and the gradual elimination of high-calorie foods. Some diet counselors utilize a "stoplight" approach: green foods can be consumed in unlimited quantities; yellow foods have average nutritional value and should be consumed with caution; and red foods should be restricted due to high fat or simple carbohydrate content.

The treatment plan needs an exercise component. No specific exercise has been found to be most effective, so exercise should be what your child enjoys. Your child should engage in both physical activity that is incorporated into her daily routine (for example, walking to school) and more vigorous physical activity. She should view exercise as fun—join a team, work out with the

family, play active games—all will add to her life immensely. Emphasize both increasing physical exercise and decreasing sedentary behavior. Once again, children will take their cues from you, so you should try to set a good example. Support and reinforce your child's changing behaviors. And she should actively participate in and accept responsibility for this change. Include behavior-modification strategies to support and maintain her changing diet and physical activity.

Treatment plans can be delivered through the school, in a community program, at a physician's office or in a specialized clinic. Although success might be best in a specialized clinic, this is frequently not available, and school and community programs can provide a readily accessible setting for many children and families. Only in rare cases should your child need medications and surgery. These should only be considered in consultation with a specialist. Overweight or obese children might require medical help with some of the complications, such as diabetes or high blood pressure. However, usually these problems improve or resolve with improvement in the child's BMI. Occasionally a medical problem is identified as the cause of the obesity, and medical treatment would be initiated accordingly.

Poor Eating Habits

What are poor eating habits? Infants and young children develop good eating habits as they develop other tasks such as sleeping and toilet training. Behaviors formed in the first one to two years of life have an important impact upon eating patterns throughout your child's life.

Eating abnormalities can have immediate consequences in infancy; for example, they can lead to poor weight gain or specific nutritional problems, such as an iron deficiency. Poor eating habits can lead to problems in later childhood and adolescence. These include obesity and eating disorders such as chronic dieting or anorexia nervosa. The relationship between development of good eating habits in infancy and good adult health is not known. However, healthy eating in adults can help prevent heart disease and some cancers.

When trying to understand poor eating habits, it is useful to consider what phases might be regarded as "normal," what parental and child factors are involved and, most importantly, how to prevent poor eating habits from developing.

What are normal eating patterns? In order to decide if a child really does have a problem with eating, let's first consider what normal eating patterns look like.

Initially, babies consume exclusively breast milk or formula. However, even at this young age, babies respond to internal cues of hunger and fullness and can control food intake by controlling the amount and timing of feedings. That is why it's recommended that young babies be fed "on demand." At around 5 or 6 months of age, you should introduce solids into the diet, and your baby has to adjust to multiple tastes and textures. As children get older, they give up some of the control of timing of meals as parents begin to set mealtimes in accordance with family and cultural practice. When they get hungry, children might request between-meal snacks on demand.

Research has shown that children can adequately regulate how much food they need on their own. When observed carefully, children's intake at individual meals is highly variable. However, the child's total daily food intake is quite similar each day. Often a child will eat a lot at one meal, followed by a small amount at the next meal, or vice versa. Therefore, it is believed that children can adjust their food intake according to the amount they have taken at the previous meal. The size of a meal consumed by a child is also influenced by the amount of calories in the meal. Children learn which foods make them feel full and adjust their intake accordingly. Thus, children might appear to eat erratically and are considered to be "picky," but they are, in fact, capable of adjusting their eating patterns according to their needs.

Children's preferences for certain foods are the most important factor determining their food intake. Babies appear to be born with a preference for sweet and salty tastes, and a dislike of sour or bitter tastes. By nature, infants and children tend to reject new foods except for sweet or salty ones. This initial rejection of a new food is normal among humans, but adults might conclude that the child is being picky. Studies have shown that a child will only accept a new food after tasting that food 5 to 10 times. Children also tend to prefer high-calorie foods; that is, foods with a high fat and sugar content. These foods are associated with a pleasant sensation of feeling full and satisfied, and might be sweet, which children naturally like. Furthermore, children learn to enjoy foods that are associated with pleasant social circumstances, such as holiday or birthday celebrations, or foods used as a reward. On the other hand, children can learn to dislike foods that they are encouraged or forced to eat in larger quantities than they would like.

Parents and family also determine children's food preferences. You need to offer a variety of healthy foods to your children, regardless of your own likes and dislikes. Children are also

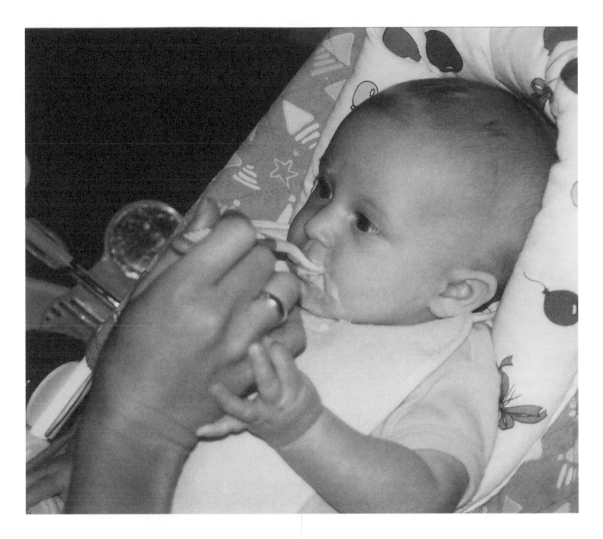

influenced by television advertisements for food. Research has shown that children exposed to advertisements select more foods with added sugar than those children who do not.

What do poor eating habits look like? It depends. Many healthy looking youngsters may also have developed unhealthy patterns of eating that will only become evident later in life. On the other hand, most thin children, even if they are picky eaters, are probably very healthy. In North America, malnutrition is much more likely to be a result of over-nutrition than under-nutrition!

Once again, it is important to determine if your child is truly a poor or picky eater or if she is exhibiting a normal phase of eating development. Eating that can appear "erratic" to adults can be completely normal. This might, in fact, demonstrate that the child is appropriately regulating her food requirements. Similarly, rejecting new foods on numerous occasions is also normal although it might appear that your child is being picky.

How should I manage poor eating habits? As with so many health issues that depend upon the

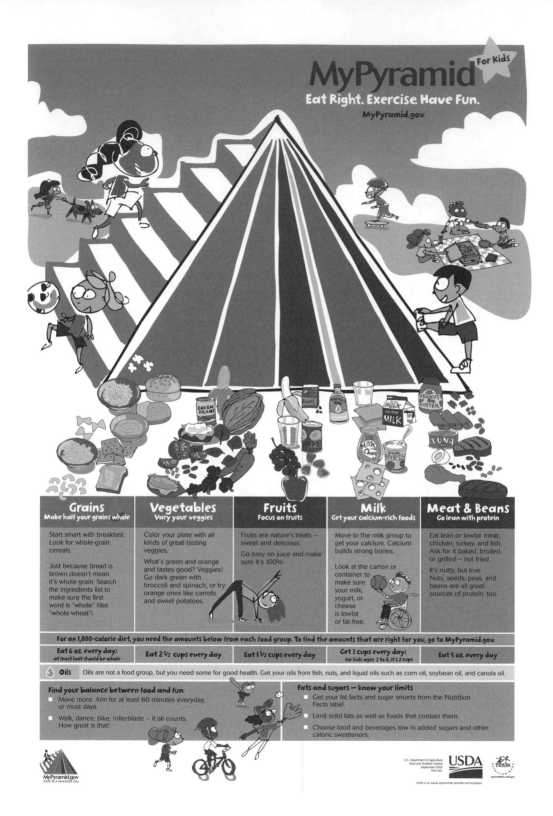

development of healthy habits, the prevention of poor eating patterns is most important.

- Babies, both breast- and formula-fed, should be fed on demand to allow them to regulate both the timing and volume of their feedings.
- When you introduce solids, you should influence the timing of feedings, with set mealtimes.
- Snacks, when necessary, should not interfere with the amount of food consumed.
- Provide plentiful and varied healthy foods from the various food groups, understanding that some of it will be consumed and some of it will be rejected.
- You should continue to offer new foods, even those that have been rejected several times in the past.
- Don't coerce or force feed and recognize that encouraging or discouraging a particular food can have the opposite effect.
- Recognize that all foods in moderation are good: there are no "good" foods and "bad" foods.
- Be aware of not influencing your child based on your own preferences.

Some babies continue to consume large quantities of milk after you have introduced solid food. This makes them feel full and satisfied and interferes with their interest in solid food. To avoid this, gradually decrease her milk intake to approximately 2 cups (500 mL) per day by 12 months of age. You can begin the transition to a cup as early as 6 months and by 12 to 15 months of age your baby should be drinking from a cup all the time, which might promote a greater appetite for solid food. Sitting in a high chair with the family at mealtime might also promote greater regulation of food intake. Giving your baby food in a variety of textures, rather than soft or pureed food, might also promote her interest in and acceptance of table foods.

Eating should be social and fun. Infants should enjoy their meals with the family, sitting in a high chair, and be allowed to enjoy the eating experience, even if it is a messy one. Children who repeatedly eat while "on the go" or in front of the television develop poor eating habits. In today's hectic life, enjoying a leisurely family meal together benefits everyone.

Once they are established, poor eating habits are hard to correct. Monitoring your child's weight and height is part of determining if her nutrition is seriously affecting her health. Even this can be difficult because children with a slim or small build might be scrutinized more carefully than others. Adults might think that these children have poor eating habits, when in fact their eating behaviors follow the norm for their age and their size is genetically determined. Recall your own childhood: "I was always skinny as a child." Recognize that your child's size is not related to poor eating habits.

If your child's doctor determines that her eating habits are affecting your child's health, she might recommend tests to examine, for example, her levels of iron or other nutrients. Your child can take supplements to correct these abnormalities.

Ultimately, however, it may be important to modify your child's eating habits. Using several of the techniques described to prevent poor eating habits, you can improve your child's eating habits over time. Patience is part of the equation here. Because the development of good eating habits is steeped in the development of a child's independence, don't let these changes become a battle for control. On some occasions, you might have to consult other health professionals, including dietitians, occupational therapists, social workers and child psychiatrists.

Short Stature

What is short stature? Short stature means that your child's height for her age and sex is smaller than it should be. It is statistically defined as a height that is three or more **standard deviations** below the mean and, therefore, on a standard growth chart, this measurement will place at or below the third percentile. This means that among children of the same age and sex, at least 97 out of 100 are taller than her. In addition, if your child grows slower than 2 inches (5 cm) per year, determined from serial height measurements, your doctor should also look into this even if her height is above the third percentile.

A baby's length should be measured at birth, and then at each well-infant and well-child visit. Her length is measured while lying down until at least 2 years of age, and in the standing position thereafter. Accurate and serial measurements of length or height are key to charting a child's growth and to identifying growth abnormalities.

Several factors contribute to determining a child's height at each age. Family genetics, as reflected by your height and that of her extended family, are important determinants of a child's growth under healthy circumstances. A baby's birth length does not correlate well with her eventual height. For example, babies who are genetically determined to be small can be born long, and conversely babies who are genetically determined to be tall can be born small. Many babies experience a shift in their grown pattern

from their prenatal growth pattern to their genetically determined growth pattern. This shift usually occurs by the end of the first or second year. By age 2, children maintain a fairly steady growth pattern. Then, between 4 years and puberty children grow at about 2 to 3 inches (5 to 7 cm) per year. At puberty, adolescents grow faster. The peak growth rate occurs earlier in girls than in boys. Adolescents can experience an early, moderate or late growth spurt. The period of maximal growth is closely related to the period of sexual maturity. Childhood growth occurs at the ends of the long bones called the epiphyses. When they have finished growing, the epiphyses fuse and no further growth occurs in the arms and legs. This occurs at about 15 years in girls and 17 years in boys.

What could be causing short stature? There are many, many causes of short stature. Remember that the definition of short stature is a statistical one that does not invariably mean that there is an associated health problem.

Two common causes of short stature are called familial short stature and constitutional delay. These are considered to be normal variations of growth patterns and are not a medical problem. Children who have always been short, but are healthy and growing at a steady rate have familial short stature. Their parents and other family members are usually short, the child's bones mature at a rate appropriate for her age and puberty occurs at a normal time. Children with familial short stature are healthy and reach their genetically determined final height.

Children with constitutional delay are of normal length at birth but shift to a lower percentile length in infancy. They then grow normally during their school years. At this time, their doctor might note that their bone maturity is delayed, indicating a good potential for growth later on. During early adolescence, these children continue to grow at a slow pace and enter puberty later than their peers. When puberty is complete, individuals with constitutional delay will attain a normal adult height. There is often a family history of a similar growth pattern.

There are many medical causes of short stature. Children with serious conditions of the heart, kidneys or lungs or those with inflammatory bowel disease often have associated short stature. Children with chromosomal abnormalities, such as **Down's syndrome** (trisomy 21), might be short. While your doctor will have identified most chromosomal abnormalities in infancy, girls with the chromosomal abnormalities that lead to **Turner syndrome** may not have been identified until their doctor recognizes their short stature and delayed puberty. Children with endocrine disorders, which refers to problems of naturally occurring hormones, can have associated short stature. This includes hypothyroidism (abnormally low thyroid function) and Cushing's syndrome (abnormally high cortisol levels). Growth hormone deficiency can occur but it is rare. Other rare genetic **syndromes** or bone abnormalities can result in short stature or dwarfism. Poor nutrition is rarely the cause of a child's short stature in developed countries, although it can contribute to her poor weight gain.

How should short stature be managed? All children's length or height should be measured accurately at all well-child visits. Your doctor will chart the measurements on a standard growth chart. This will allow for timely identification of children with short stature. Those children will be thoroughly assessed by a physician who will pay

careful attention to details of your pregnancy, labor and delivery; family history (including heights and growth patterns of parents and extended family); your child's general health, growth and development; and details pertaining to puberty in adolescents. The physician will accurately measure your child's height, weight and head circumference and will review previous serial measurements. She will do a thorough physical assessment paying careful attention to any clues of a genetic syndrome, endocrine disorder or chronic illness. In most cases, following this detailed examination of your child's medical history, family history and physical examination, she will make a diagnosis. The doctor might recommend further tests, such as an x-ray of the hand to determine the maturation of your child's bones. She might recommend additional tests to evaluate kidney function, evidence of a chronic inflammatory condition or thyroid dysfunction. She might recommend chromosome blood tests. Where an abnormality of thyroid or growth hormone is recognized, she will recommend a referral to a pediatric endocrinologist for further testing and treatment.

For children with normal variants of growth—that is, familial short stature and constitutional delay—the physician will counsel both your child and you that your child is healthy. Treatment for children with constitutional delay should be considered only in consultation with a pediatric endocrinologist.

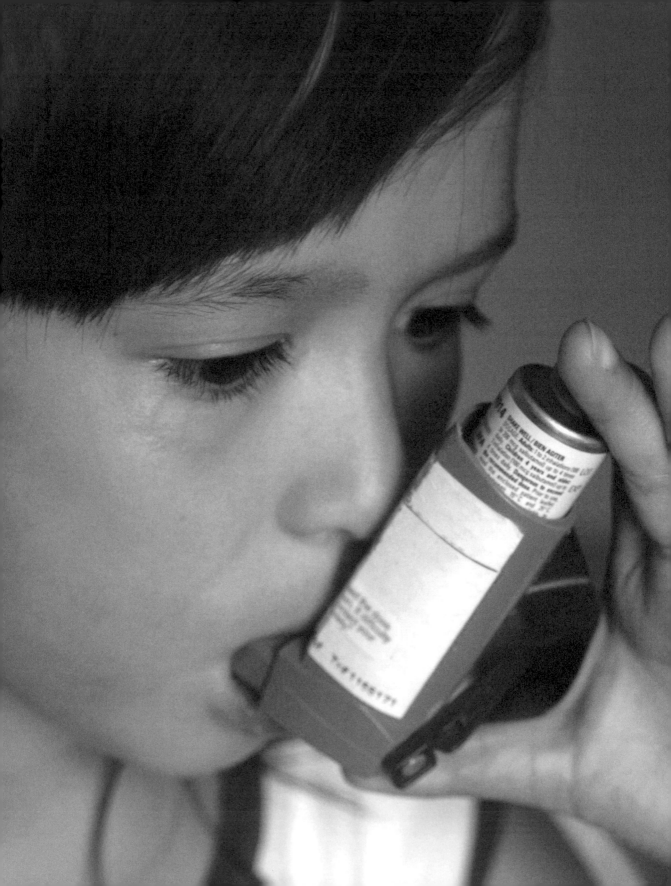

Allergic Disorders

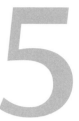

Asthma and Wheezing

What are asthma and wheezing? Wheezing is the sound that is created as air flows through obstructed airways, usually as the child exhales. Infants commonly have a single episode of wheezing. This is almost always associated with common respiratory viruses. These viruses can cause the symptoms of a cold and wheezing and difficulty breathing. Doctors call this constellation of symptoms in young infants **bronchiolitis** (see pages 81–84).

Asthma can be defined in many different ways. One practical and useful definition, especially in younger children, is recurrent wheezing and/or persistent coughing in a child who is at risk for asthma, and after other rarer conditions have been excluded. As children get older, you might consider more specific testing. Most commonly this would include pulmonary function testing, during which the child blows into a machine that measures the speed and amount of the air breathed out.

Asthma and wheezing are very common among children. It has been found that during the first six years of life, approximately half of all children will have had at least one episode of wheezing. Most of these children will outgrow the episodes of wheezing. Some, however, will have persistent wheezing, and those are considered to be asthmatic. Asthma is a leading cause of childhood chronic illness, occurring in up to 10 percent of children. Although not all asthma is severe, asthma and wheezing are the leading reasons for hospitalization of children.

The relationship between wheezing episodes in early childhood and the development of asthma has been well researched. These studies suggest that many factors can predispose children to developing asthma. They include an exposure to common respiratory viruses known to be associated with wheezing in early childhood, a tendency toward allergies (for example, eczema and hay fever), a genetic makeup (a family history of asthma and allergies) that predisposes a child to asthma, and exposure to environmental agents such as cigarette smoke. On the other hand, more recent research has suggested that early exposure to other common viruses might help protect children from developing asthma. For example, it has been found that children with older siblings and children attending day care are less likely to have asthma.

What does asthma and wheezing look like? Infants and babies experiencing their first episode of wheezing (bronchiolitis) will be breathing very quickly. They eat poorly, whether at the breast or by bottle. The virus that triggers the wheezing can also cause significant nasal congestion. Babies find it very difficult to close their mouths adequately for breast- or bottle-feeding when their nasal passages are obstructed. Infants will sleep poorly and appear irritable and unhappy. Because bronchiolitis is almost always triggered by a virus, the baby might also have an accompanying fever that will add to his irritability.

During an episode of asthma, two significant events occur in the lungs: the airways become constricted and inflamed. This leads to some degree of obstruction of airflow through the lungs, which results in difficult and fast breathing, a feeling of shortness of breath and wheezing. A physician using a stethoscope might hear wheezing, or it might be loud enough to be heard without a stethoscope. Children will also develop a significant amount of coughing that seems worse at night when the child is lying down. These symptoms can worsen during exercise, even mild exercise such as walking, or more moderate exercise, such as running in the playground. Exposure to cold air, such as going outdoors in the winter, can also worsen the child's symptoms.

Many children are very well between episodes. Some children have symptoms daily, with episodes of worsening symptoms. The episodes can be quite severe, sometimes called "asthma attacks." During such an episode, your child will breathe at a fast rate, his breathing will seem labored, with drawing in of the chest muscles between the ribs, and his abdominal muscles will be moving hard as well. He might have difficulty speaking due to breathlessness, he might express a feeling of not getting enough air and he can appear anxious and agitated. If the episode was precipitated by a viral infection, there can also be a fever. There is usually a significant amount

of coughing, which sounds wet and productive. The child might have difficulty eating, drinking and sleeping.

Children with milder episodes have the same symptoms but to a lesser degree. The child might be able to cope with the symptoms as long as he is quiet and inactive. He may not be able to play actively with other children or participate in physical education class or team sports. Coughing might disrupt his sleep and he might be more irritable and unhappy than usual. If these symptoms are allowed to persist without treatment, children can "adapt" by adopting a more sedentary lifestyle. One of the major goals of treatment is to ensure that children with asthma can enjoy the same active quality of life as all other children.

Episodes of asthma are often preceded by a cough and runny nose. If your child has recurrent wheezing and asthma, you learn to recognize these early warning signs and anticipate the development of more serious symptoms. This allows you to seek earlier assessment by your child's physician and/or to begin treatment early. Intervention should occur as early as possible in order to abort and control the symptoms. If you watch to see what might happen next, rather than taking action early, the result might be a more serious episode of asthma that requires more intensive treatment and a longer recovery time. You need to be aware that, rarely, delay in treatment has resulted in a child's preventable death.

How are asthma and wheezing treated? The first time your child has an episode of wheezing, take him to be assessed by his doctor. If your child develops recurrent wheezing and asthma, you will develop significant knowledge in order to monitor and assess, as well as treat your child. Your physician and asthma educators will provide

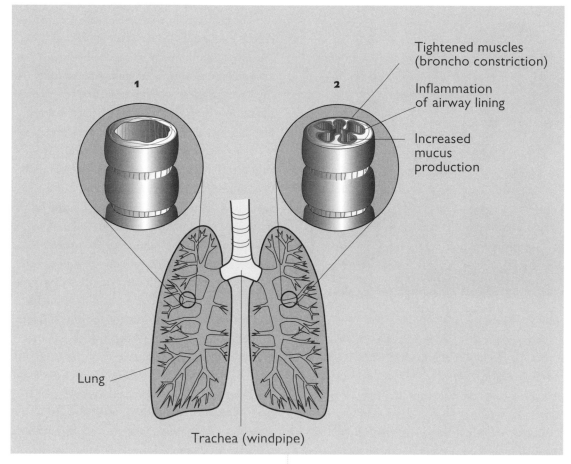

1

2

Tightened muscles
(broncho constriction)

Inflammation
of airway lining

Increased
mucus
production

Lung

Trachea (windpipe)

ASTHMA

*Picture 1 shows a normal airway (bronchiola). Picture 2
shows an airway during an acute asthma attack.*

you with formal education, and time and experience will guide you through subsequent episodes. You will develop a plan of action and work closely with your child's physician or an asthma nurse specialist.

There are many effective medicines to treat children when they develop episodes of wheezing. The choice of drug and how your child takes them depend upon the situation. In addition, your doctor might recommend other treatments, such as oxygen and fluids.

If your baby or young infant is having his first episode of wheezing (bronchiolitis), both his breathing and ability to keep feeding must be assessed. If his breathing difficulty is only mild and he is feeding adequately and is well hydrated, his doctor might not recommend any specific treatment. Because the episode of wheezing has been triggered by a virus, it should get better with time. However, babies with bronchiolitis sometimes get worse before they get better, and so close monitoring by you and your doctor is important. If your baby's breathing is more difficult, your doctor might recommend a bronchodilator medication that is inhaled through a mask to open up the constricted airways. Your baby might need some

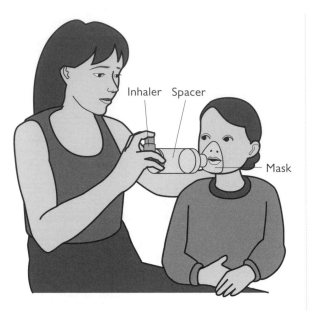

Inhaler   Spacer

Mask

HOW TO USE AN INHALER

A spacer—a portable device that attaches to the inhaler—is a common, effective method for improving the delivery of medication to the lungs. It should be used by all asthmatic children who require an inhaler.

extra oxygen, which can be inhaled through a mask. If he is feeding very poorly or appears dehydrated, he may require an intravenous to supply fluids. Babies and infants with more severe bronchiolitis are often admitted to hospital so that they can be closely monitored. When the episode is over, they usually do not require any further treatment.

Children who are known to have asthma, or who have had several previous episodes of wheezing, often have **acute** episodes of wheezing that require treatment. Because, as mentioned, there are two main events leading to the wheezing—constriction of the airways and inflammation leading to swelling of the lining of the airways with excessive mucus production—there are two main types of medication to combat these events.

The medications that open up the airways by relaxing tight muscles are called bronchodilators. The most commonly used bronchodilator is albuterol (generally called salbutamol outside the United States), which is inhaled through the mouth into the lungs. There is a liquid version taken by mouth but this is not felt to be effective.

The drugs that reduce inflammation are called anti-inflammatories. The most frequently used anti-inflammatory medications are steroids. They can be taken as a pill or liquid by mouth, or if your child is very unwell and unable to drink, they can be given intravenously. If the episode is milder, the steroid can be inhaled. Your child may require extra oxygen that is inhaled through a mask, and he might require an intravenous line for additional fluids.

Inhaled medications, both bronchodilators and steroids, are very important in the treatment of asthma and wheezing. Therefore, there has been a lot of attention paid to developing devices that will deliver the medicine effectively, directly to the airways. It is very important that these devices are used correctly. When used properly, the medications are very powerful and effective. If used incorrectly, your child might not receive any medication in his airways and the medication will be useless. A nebulizer is a device that changes liquid medication into a mist that is inhaled by the child through a mask. Nebulizers are often used in emergency departments and hospitals. Very young infants or children with developmental disabilities can benefit from using a nebulizer at home. At home, most children will use a metered-dose inhaler and a spacing device. The spacing device is critical because children are not able to coordinate the movements of pressing the metered-dose inhaler and inhaling the medications in the sequence required for effective delivery of the medication. The proper use of these devices is so important that you will have to take special learning sessions and practice using the device.

When the acute wheezing episode is over, which can take a few days to a few weeks, your doctor might suggest discontinuing the bronchodilator. The role of the bronchodilator is to open the constricted airways, and this medication works quickly and is short-acting. Therefore, it is appropriate to use this medication only when an acute episode occurs, and is inappropriate to use on a daily or long-term basis. Your doctor might recommend continuing the use of the inhaled steroid for its anti-inflammatory effect. Inflammation of the airways can persist after an acute episode of wheezing. In addition, children who have asthma that is difficult to control benefit from inhaling steroids daily. This works to control their daily symptoms and improve their quality of life by allowing them to be as active as their peers and to sleep well.

Concerns have been raised over the possibility of side effects for children receiving inhaled steroids on a long-term basis. Research has shown that these can be minimized by using newer steroid preparations and by keeping the dose as low as possible while controlling symptoms. Your doctor will monitor long-term use of steroids. Newer anti-inflammatory medications, called leukotriene antagonists, have been developed. These do not contain steroids and can be taken in pill form. Your doctor might recommend these newer medications if your child's asthma symptoms are not well controlled with inhaled steroids, or if he is experiencing side effects.

Other factors are important in controlling asthma symptoms. It is very important to eliminate children's exposure to tobacco smoke. Second-hand smoke is a powerful irritant to the lungs of all children but especially to those with asthma and recurrent wheezing. Most parents who smoke do not do so in close proximity to their children. However, research has shown that wheezing children can have high levels of tobacco by-products. Therefore, physicians recommend that you should discontinue smoking altogether, and ensure that other caregivers do not smoke. Additional environmental control measures include minimizing house dust mites and molds, removing pets if your children have animal allergies, controlling high humidity in the home and avoiding outdoor pollens.

Chronic Urticaria (Hives)

What is chronic urticaria? The more common word for urticaria is "hives." It is a common skin condition: as many as 20 percent of people will have urticaria at some time in their lives. Urticaria results from an allergic reaction that causes the release of **histamine** and other chemicals from cells in the skin. It is these chemicals that cause the typical skin lesions. Hives might occur only once but sometimes they disappear and then reappear repeatedly. When urticaria lasts longer than six weeks, it is termed "chronic urticaria."

What does chronic urticaria look like? The appearance of hives is very typical: well-defined, red, raised skin lesions of various sizes. These lesions are sometimes referred to as welts or wheals. Sometimes the individual skin lesions join together, giving the appearance of sheets of red, raised skin. The skin lesions are usually, but not always, very itchy. Individual hives can appear and then shortly thereafter disappear, with newer hives appearing.

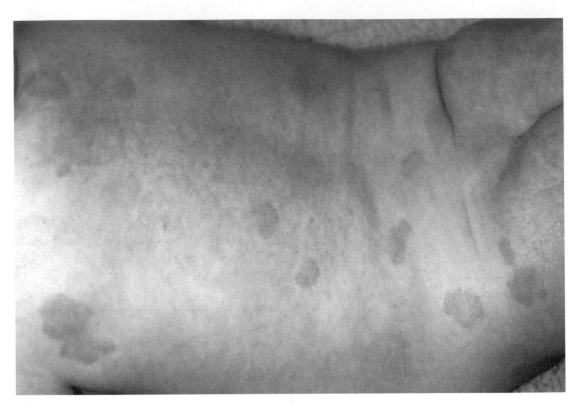

CHRONIC URTICARIA

Well-defined, red, raised lesions (also called welts or wheals) are characteristic of hives.

What could be causing chronic urticaria? Although medications, foods and viral infections are thought to be the common causes of urticaria, most often no specific cause is found. Occasionally, some children will get hives after exposure to cold. Allergy testing is not usually helpful, unless a specific medicine or food has been associated with the onset of the hives. Since urticaria gets better on its own with time and does not usually recur, specific tests are not usually recommended and minimal treatment is required.

How is chronic urticaria treated? In most cases, the only treatment required is an oral antihistamine to control the itch until the urticaria subsides.

Unless you noticed that the urticaria began following the introduction of a specific food, it is not worth eliminating different foods from your child's diet. If the urticaria becomes chronic and persistent, an allergy specialist might recommend treatment with antihistamines, steroids or other medications that suppress the immune system.

Drug Reactions

What are drug reactions? Some children will experience unwanted side effects during or after treatment with a drug. Most drug reactions are associated with the drug itself, and only a few are as a result of an allergic reaction. This is very important to remember, so that not all reactions to drugs should be labeled as allergies.

There are several reasons for your child to have had a nonallergic reaction to a drug. Your child might have received too much of the drug, resulting in an overdose. Your child may have received two drugs that interacted with one another. Some drugs, in addition to having wanted effects, have unwanted effects. For example, some antihistamines, in addition to improving allergy symptoms, cause sedation. Some children are born with enzyme deficiencies that affect the way their bodies handle drugs. Importantly, sometimes children develop symptoms of another illness while taking a drug and the symptoms are attributed to the drug in error. A common example of this would be a child who is prescribed antibiotics for a viral illness, and the viral illness is responsible for a skin rash. In some cases it is incorrectly thought that the antibiotic is responsible for the skin rash, the child is labeled as allergic to the antibiotic and subsequently loses the opportunity to receive this drug in the future when it is really necessary.

The common drugs to which allergic or immune-mediated reactions occur are antibiotics (drugs for treating bacterial infections) and anticonvulsants (drugs for treating seizures). If your child is allergic to penicillin, he is at higher risk of having an allergic reaction to antibiotics in a different but related category (cephalosporins). If you have an allergy to antibiotics, he is also at higher risk of having an allergy to an antibiotic.

What does a drug reaction look like? Skin rashes are the most common symptom of drug reactions in children. Many different types of skin rashes can occur. Often the skin rash is vague and nondescript, with no specific features. These rashes are difficult to distinguish from similar nondescript rashes seen in many viral illnesses.

Sometimes, however, the skin rash is very specific. An example of a specific skin rash would be urticaria. Urticaria (also called "hives") appears as well-defined, red, raised skin lesions of various sizes that are often very itchy. The lesions are sometimes referred to as welts or wheals. Another specific skin rash is one with the appearance of a bull's-eye, with a raised, red outer border, a pale inner ring and a dusky purple center.

Less common effects of drug reactions include abnormal blood counts, effects on the kidneys, lungs or liver, and the development of fever.

The most feared allergic drug reaction is anaphylaxis. Anaphylactic reactions occur rapidly. Your child might feel tingling around the face and mouth, have difficulty swallowing and experience tightness in the throat and chest. He might appear flushed and develop hives and wheezing. He might also develop abdominal cramps and diarrhea. Anaphylaxis is a life-threatening emergency.

How do I treat a drug reaction? It is often very difficult to distinguish allergic from nonallergic drug allergies. Because all drugs undergo rigorous testing before coming to market and many have been in use for many years, potential side effects (both allergic and nonallergic) are well known for many or most drugs. Your doctor will consider the following factors:

- the type of drug received by your child,
- previous drug reactions,
- family history of drug reactions,
- the type of reaction with details of the skin rash if present (whether it is a nondescript rash or a specific rash).

Even with this detailed assessment it can be difficult to establish if the reaction is due to an allergy. Furthermore, allergy testing for drugs is available for only a limited number of drugs.

Treatment depends upon what is causing the reaction. Doctors usually recommend discontinuing the drug, although in some circumstances it might be appropriate to continue taking it. If the doctor believes that the reaction is due to the drug itself (in other words, a side effect), it might still be appropriate to use the drug in the future, possibly adjusting the dose or the interval between doses. If your doctor believes that the reaction is allergic, your child should not receive that drug again, and he might recommend that other related drugs also be avoided. If your child has developed urticaria, it can be treated with antihistamines. If the reaction has been severe, or if allergy testing is indicated, your child should be assessed by an allergy specialist.

Adverse Food Reactions

What are adverse food reactions? Sometimes children appear to react badly to certain foods. Most of these adverse reactions are not due to a true allergy, but rather an intolerance to a given food or ingredient. For example, infants can develop a rash or diarrhea after eating fruits or drinking juices but these have not been proven to be caused by allergies. Often, people have difficulty distinguishing true food allergies from food intolerances. It can be hard to tell the two apart. As a result, as many as 25 percent of people believe they have food allergies yet research has shown that only about 5 percent of young children have food allergies and the percentage in older children and adults is even lower.

The most common food allergies are to cow's milk; eggs; legumes (especially peanuts and soybeans); tree nuts such as almonds, Brazil nuts, cashew nuts, filberts, hickory nuts, pecans, pine nuts, pistachios and walnuts; fish; crustaceans (lobster and shrimp); molluscs (mussels and scallops); and cereal grains. It is the protein component of these foods that triggers the allergic response. Young infants might be susceptible to food allergies because their immune systems and digestive tracts are immature. Approximately one-third of children will lose their food allergy after one to three years of a specific elimination diet, although allergies to peanuts, tree nuts and seafood are more likely to persist.

What do adverse food reactions look like? Due to different chemical reactions, allergic reactions can either be immediate or delayed. Immediate allergic reactions to foods usually occur within minutes to a few hours of eating. Allergic reactions to peanuts, nuts, fish and shellfish are usually immediate. The symptoms might be limited to the mouth and throat and include itching and tingling and swelling of the lips, tongue and throat. Sometimes, the symptoms are limited to the digestive tract, including abdominal cramps, vomiting and diarrhea. In some cases, the reaction will spread to the skin with the development of hives, the lungs with the onset of wheezing, and the nose and eyes with the presence of tearing and nasal congestion. In the most severe cases, your child can develop an anaphylactic reaction, with the above symptoms plus the development of low blood pressure. This is a life-threatening emergency.

Several delayed allergic reactions to foods can occur. In the first few months of life infants can develop inflammation of the digestive tract associated with protracted vomiting and diarrhea due to food allergies. Some babies become dehydrated and stool samples usually contain some blood. Most commonly, cow's milk and soy protein formulas are responsible, but other foods can cause these reactions in older infants and children. Elimination of the food generally leads to resolution of the diarrhea and vomiting in 72 hours.

Young infants can also develop a more localized area of inflammation in the rectum and around the anus, usually due to cow's milk or soy protein formulas. A breast-fed baby can also experience this type of food allergy because of proteins ingested by his mother and then transmitted in the breast milk. Usually your baby will not have diarrhea, but may pass bright red blood in the stools. Eliminating the cow's milk or soy from his diet directly or from the breast-feeding mother's diet will stop the passage of blood within several days, although complete healing of the rectum can take up to a month. The allergy can resolve completely after six months to two years of avoidance of cow's milk or soy protein.

Some young infants in the first few months of life develop more significant involvement of the digestive tract. In addition to protracted diarrhea and vomiting, the baby absorbs nutrients poorly, gains weight poorly and may become puffy and swollen because he is absorbing protein poorly. Again, cow's milk protein formula or whole cow's milk is the most frequent cause. With elimination of the food, his symptoms should gradually cease over days to weeks. Complete resolution can require 6 to 18 months of elimination of the food.

A serious and very specific food allergy is celiac disease. Children with celiac disease have a specific sensitivity to gluten, a protein found in wheat, oat, rye nd barley. Typically, his symptoms come on gradually between 6 months and 2 years of age after the introduction of solids.

Children with celiac disease have diarrhea, greasy stools, abdominal distension, gassiness and poor weight gain or weight loss. You will have to eliminate gluten-containing foods from your child's diet for life.

How are adverse food reactions managed? There might be some ways to prevent or reduce the possibility of food allergies in children. It has been suggested that breast-feeding exclusively can prevent some allergies, but this is controversial. Waiting to introduce solid foods to an infant's diet until after 4 months of age can also prevent some food allergies.

If your child has an immediate reaction to foods—especially peanuts, nuts, fish and shellfish—take him promptly to his doctor or your nearest emergency department. He might require medication to control the symptoms of the immediate reaction. Later you should ensure that he has a consultation with an allergy specialist who can perform allergy testing. If a food allergy is confirmed, you will have to strictly eliminate the food. Allergy needles are not necessary. You will have to read food labels in order to avoid the offending foodstuff. Your child's doctor might recommend that he have injectable epinephrine and an antihistamine available at all times in case of an emergency. If he has a severe food allergy, you and his caregivers at day care and then the staff at his schools will need special education regarding emergency measures. He can wear a MedicAlert bracelet to help identify the problem in the rare event that he loses consciousness due to a reaction.

If his reactions to foods is delayed, he should also be evaluated by his doctor. Usually no specific tests are useful to determine the cause of the allergy, although the doctor might request blood tests to evaluate the child's state of nutrition and hydration. Specific medications are usually not useful. Eliminating the offending food, for example cow's milk formula, might be recommended. In such cases, several specialized formulas are available that do not contain cow's milk or soy protein. Your child's physician might recommend reintroducing the food at some time in the future, according to the child's initial symptoms, resolution of symptoms and growth. If your child has celiac disease, your child's doctor or a nutritionist will develop a gluten-free diet that he'll be on for life.

Hay Fever (Allergic Rhinitis)

What is hay fever? "Hay fever" is actually a misnomer since there is no fever and the condition is not necessarily triggered by hay! The formal medical name for hay fever is "allergic rhinitis." Rhinitis means inflammation of the nasal passages, and allergic rhinitis is rhinitis caused by allergies. Most often, allergic rhinitis occurs each year in a seasonal pattern, when pollens are in abundance. Hence, it is called "seasonal allergic rhinitis." Allergic rhinitis that occurs at any time throughout the year is known as "perennial rhinitis." Children with hay fever frequently have a history of other allergic problems such as asthma and eczema. Often, many family members have allergic rhinitis, suggesting a genetic component to this condition. Allergic rhinitis usually begins in early childhood, and can improve in later adulthood.

What causes hay fewer? The main triggers for allergic rhinitis are airborne particles from the natural environment. Many flowering plants rely upon the wind to disperse their pollen, and some of

these can cause allergies. Tree pollens are the first of the allergy season, often appearing before the leaves unfold. Common trees, in the city and in forests, have pollens that can cause allergic rhinitis. These include oaks, maples, elms, birches, alders, ashes, mulberries and hickories. Grass pollens are the next to appear. In late summer, the final pollens to appear are those from weeds, specifically ragweed.

Several fungi, both outdoor and indoor, can cause allergic rhinitis. Outdoors, fungi grow on dead plant material. Activities that disrupt such material, such as cutting grass or raking leaves, can be associated with the release of fungi into the air. Indoors, fungi grow in humid environments, including poorly cleaned humidifiers.

Dust mites are tiny transparent bugs that are related to ticks. They feed upon skin scales shed by humans and require a humid environment. In homes, dust mites live in beds, carpets and upholstered furniture. Cockroaches and other insects can also produce airborne particles.

Animals can shed allergic particles into the environment that can become airborne and cause allergic rhinitis. The source of these **allergens** varies by animal. For example, the allergic particles from cats come from their skin, while the allergen from rats is from the urine.

What does hay fever look like? Symptoms of allergic rhinitis include nasal congestion, runny nose, a cough due to postnasal drip, sneezing and an itchy nose and eyes. Your child might develop "allergic shiners," which are dark puffy lower eyelids. He might also be observed giving an "allergic salute," which describes the upward rubbing of the dripping nose with the open hand. He might also have persistent mouth breathing that over time can lead to dental problems.

How is hay fever treated? Your child's doctor should evaluate him. If the history of the problem exposes a distinct relationship between the offending agent, such as ragweed, and the allergic symptoms, further tests might not be required. If a clear seasonal cause cannot be identified, or if the symptoms occur year round, your child might be referred to an allergist who could undertake specific allergy testing to identify the triggers.

- Avoid the offending agent.
- Use indoor air-conditioning.
- Reduce humidity in the home.
- Enclose bed mattresses and pillows in plastic.
- Wash bedsheets and blankets in hot water once per week.

Antihistamines are the most frequently recommended medications for allergic rhinitis. Newer antihistamines that don't cause sleepiness should be the first option. If your child has significant nasal congestion, decongestants might be recommended for occasional use. Steroids applied directly to the inside lining of the nasal passages as a spray are effective and should be considered if he has prolonged symptoms.

Immunotherapy, or "allergy shots," are injections that can be given every one to two weeks. The goal is to desensitize your child to the allergen by repeated mild exposure. This treatment option should be considered if the symptoms persist to an annoying degree in spite of taking medication on a daily basis.

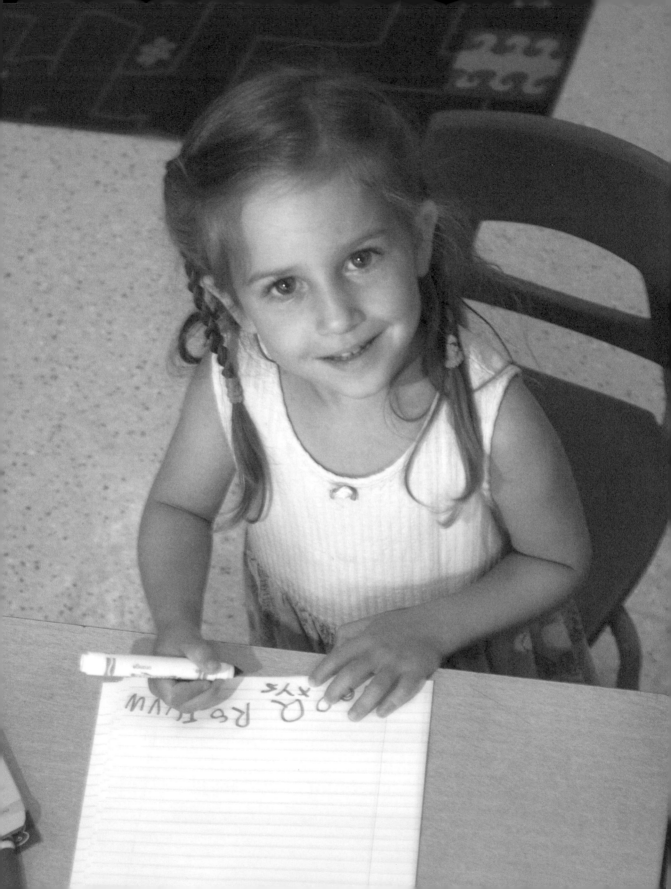

Development and School Problems

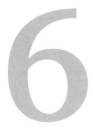

Developmental Delay

You might be wondering whether your child is developing normally. It is natural to compare your child with other children, but this can make you confused and concerned. How do you recognize problems early, without worrying excessively? It might help you to have some knowledge of normal developmental ranges and what to do if you think something is wrong.

There are several areas of development. Each one has a range of ages at which particular milestones are typically met. Children who do not achieve these milestones within the expected age range are said to have developmental delays. These delays can reflect a unique difference that resolves with age or they might indicate a problem that needs assessment and addressing to minimize long-term difficulties. Research indicates that early identification of developmental delays in children and prompt intervention improves the outcome.

What is normal development? Remember that each milestone has a range of ages at which it is achieved. The following summary provides average ages for the major milestones in each area of development in preschool-aged children. Once your child has begun school, developmental concerns typically focus on academic functioning (see ADHD and Learning Disabilities).

Gross motor development. Gross motor development refers to the way a child uses large muscles to move and balance. By about 2 months, most young babies are able to lift their heads briefly when placed lying on their stomach. Babies typically roll over by 4 to 5 months and sit unsupported by 6 or 7 months. Crawling occurs at variable ages, with some infants bypassing this milestone completely! By 9 to 10 months, infants are often able to pull themselves up to a standing position and the average age of walking is between 12 and 15 months. As parents of active toddlers know, the average 2-year-old can run, climb onto furniture, throw a ball, jump and walk up the stairs holding onto the railing or an adult's hand. By 3 to 3 ½ years old, she might be peddling a tricycle, progressing to a bicycle with training wheels around 4 years old and riding alone between 5 and 6.

Fine motor development. Fine motor development is the way a child uses the smaller muscles, such as those in the hands, to manipulate objects and to dress and feed herself. Infants of 4 months of age reach for and grasp objects, such as a block or rattle; by 5 months, they can pass the object

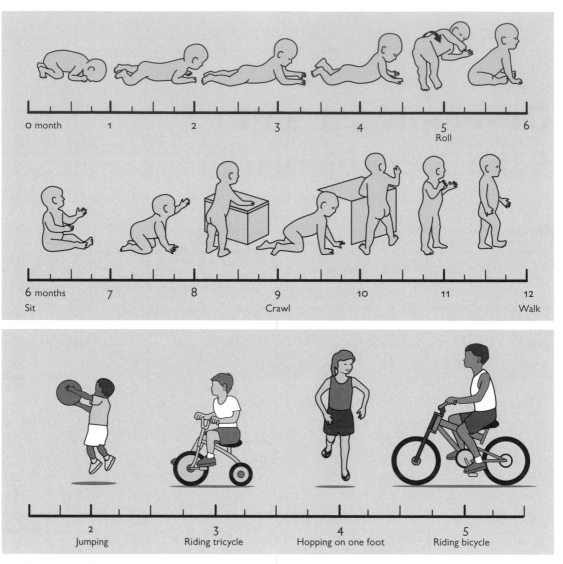

GROSS MOTOR DEVELOPMENT STAGES

Progression of gross motor milestones from birth to age 5 years.

from one hand to the other. Normally, infants at 9 or 10 months are able to pick up small objects with the thumb and forefinger and use this technique to bring food, and other objects, to their mouths—time to be aware of choking hazards! By 1 year of age, many children hold a crayon and scribble with it. They can begin feeding themselves with a spoon starting around 18 months, although it is not likely to be a neat and tidy experience. Two-year-old toddlers can often remove their shoes and socks. By 2 years, toddlers are typically able to draw straight lines and by 3 years, circles. By 4 years, children can often dress themselves, but need help with buttons and zippers until they are 5. Tying shoes is a skill usually learned around age 6 years, when children typically begin dressing themselves.

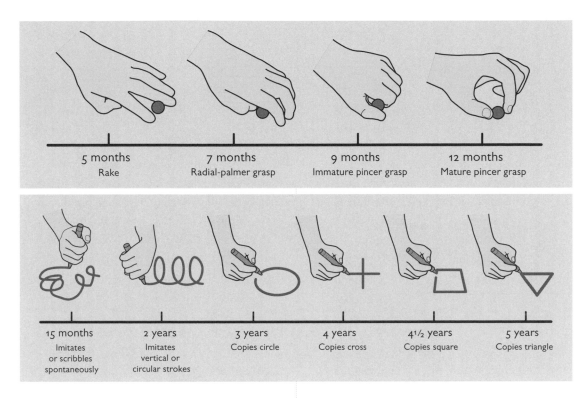

5 months	7 months	9 months	12 months
Rake	Radial-palmer grasp	Immature pincer grasp	Mature pincer grasp

15 months	2 years	3 years	4 years	4½ years	5 years
Imitates or scribbles spontaneously	Imitates vertical or circular strokes	Copies circle	Copies cross	Copies square	Copies triangle

Language development. Language development is usually divided into expressive language (what your child says) and receptive language (what your child understands). Cooing sounds, which are vowel sounds, such as the typical cute "ooh" and "ah" sounds that we all admire in babies are typical until they reach 6 months. By that age, most infants are able to babble, using vowel-consonant combinations, such as "bababababa," "lalalalala." The first word used with meaning, which is typically "dada," is usually spoken at about 1 year of age. By 18 months, toddlers usually understand words for their body parts and can point to their head, hair, eyes, nose, mouth, ears, belly button and toes. At 2 years, children generally use between 20 and 50 words, and are starting to put two words together, such as "more milk" or "my chair," although up to half of these words might only be understood by people who know the child. At this age, children

FINE MOTOR DEVELOPMENT STAGES
Progression of fine motor milestones from birth to 5 years.

can usually understand and follow simple instructions such as, "Go get your shoes." By age 3, three-word phrases to full sentences are used and by 4, almost all of a child's language can be understood by a stranger. Most 3-year-olds can identify colors and by age 4 to 5, letters of the alphabet. Most 4- or 5-year-olds can identify letters and print their name. Reading typically begins between 5 and 6 years.

Social development. Social development refers to the way children interact and behave. Around 6 weeks of age, babies start to smile in response to an adult's smile. By 4 to 5 months, babies are usually engaging with and may even laugh at an adult's antics. By 9 months, infants begin to learn to play and often enjoy playing "peekaboo." By 12 months, infants can imitate clapping hands and waving goodbye. Toddler temper tantrums are typical in 2- to 3-year-olds as they strive to demonstrate their new independence and voice their frustration, often loudly! Children of this age are usually interested in the activities of others and starting to use some imaginary play, such as pretending to talk on the telephone or put a stuffed animal to bed. By the age of 3, many children participate in more interactive play and understand simple rules in games such as tag and hide and seek. Toilet training has a wide range of normal, from 18 months to 4 years, even after which time accidents are common, particularly at night.

When should I be worried about my child's development? As mentioned, there is a wide range of normal ages at which major developmental milestones are achieved. Furthermore, each milestone should be considered in context with your child's overall developmental profile. A delay in achieving just one developmental target does not automatically indicate a problem. This might make it difficult for you to know when to be concerned. In general, if you are worried about your child's development, you should discuss your concerns with your child's physician. It has been shown repeatedly that parental concern is strongly correlated with identification of delays—your hunch is important!

What causes developmental delays? In many situations, particularly when delays are mild and isolated, the cause of the developmental delay is unknown. Heredity plays a role, as children often have a family history of learning difficulties or developmental delays.

What should I do if I suspect a developmental delay? If you suspect your child has a developmental delay, discuss this with your child's doctor as soon as possible. It is important that developmental delays be identified and treated as early as possible. Assessment of such concerns should include a detailed history from you and other caregivers. If your child is in preschool or day care, these sources should also provide information. Your child's doctor will do a physical examination and might assess your child's developmental skills herself. She will decide whether your child needs medical tests and/or more detailed developmental assessments.

In most cases, unless there are significant global developmental delays (meaning all areas of development are affected), a medical cause is not identifiable and few, if any, tests might be necessary. If there are specific medical signs, your child's doctor might discuss the options of genetic blood tests and/or radiology imaging of the brain (CT scan or MRI). However, in most cases these tests are not necessary and the focus is on management.

If your doctor suspects your child has developmental delays, she might recommend further assessment and management of the delays by another health care professional.

- Speech and language delays: A speech and language therapist should be consulted to provide further assessment and intervention. It has been shown that the most effective form of speech and language therapy for young children is that provided by their caregivers who are with them regularly, rather than provided directly by a therapist, who can typically offer service once per week. The therapist might recommend a

WARNING SIGNS OF POSSIBLE DEVELOPMENTAL DELAY

AREA OF DEVELOPMENT	WARNING SIGN
Gross motor development	Rolling prior to age 3 months Not walking by 18 months
Fine motor development	Holding hands tightly in fists for most of the time at 3 months Preferring right or left hand before 18 months old
Expressive language development	No words by 18 months Not pointing by 18 months Words difficult to understand at 3 years
Receptive language development	Not turning when name is called at 18 months Not able to identify body parts by 2 years
Social development	Not interested in other children at 2 years No imaginary play at 2 years

Hanen parent training program that teaches parents how to encourage speech and language development.

- Motor delays: Rehabilitation specialists, such as physiotherapists or occupational therapists, can provide further assessment and recommendations.
- Delays in social development: This may indicate the need for further assessment for a possible **autism spectrum disorder** (see pages 169–73) so that your child has the opportunity to respond to behavior management interventions.

If your child has identified developmental delays, everyone involved in her care needs to be aware of the level at which she is currently functioning. Expectations, disciplinary measures and home safety-proofing should be appropriate for her developmental level, rather than her chronological age. These measures, along with praise for accomplishments and development of individual strengths, can help promote her self-esteem and prevent secondary behavior problems.

Before she enters school, careful planning is necessary to ensure your child with developmental delays is receiving adequate support and appropriate programming. You should meet with the school principal in the winter or early spring of the year before she begins school to accomplish this. A psychology assessment might help delineate your child's strengths and weaknesses and provide recommendations to school personnel. If your child is already in school, all concerned with her care need a clear understanding of the identified delays and their impact on learning, and what interventions are available for support.

Although you might be disappointed and find it difficult to accept that your child has a developmental delay, with early help, you can help maximize your child's potential and minimize future difficulties.

Attention Deficit Hyperactivity Disorder (ADHD)

What is attention deficit hyperactivity disorder? ADHD is a developmental disorder that occurs to varying degrees of severity in 5 to 10 percent of school-aged children, typically boys. It is not a disease but rather a constellation of troublesome behaviors. Children with ADHD tend to be impulsive, distractible, inattentive and, fidgety. These behaviors usually interfere with learning and create difficulties in interpersonal relationships at home, in school and with peers.

There are different types of ADHD, depending on the number and type of specific criteria met. The "inattentive" subtype refers to children who are easily distracted, but less hyperactive. The "combined" subtype refers to children who have significant hyperactivity in addition to impulsivity.

Many children with ADHD have other areas of difficulty: 25 percent to 30 percent of children with ADHD also have learning disabilities, frequently difficulties in language-based areas such as reading. Many children with ADHD struggle with fine motor tasks, such as printing, drawing and writing. About half of affected children also have psychiatric diagnoses, including oppositional defiant disorder, conduct disorder, depression or anxiety. If your child has ADHD, it is important that any coexisting disorders be identified in order to put together the most effective management plan.

What causes ADHD? The exact cause of ADHD is unknown. It is clear that heredity plays a role, as ADHD is more common in families that have one other child or a parent with ADHD. It has been shown that children with ADHD have differences in the balances of chemicals in the brain called neurotransmitters. Although there is abundant information available on the Internet and elsewhere suggesting ADHD is caused by food sugars, dyes or additives, food allergies or environmental toxins, to date medical studies have not supported these claims.

What does ADHD look like? A child with ADHD is often described as forgetful and disorganized. He is easily distracted and has trouble maintaining attention in settings, such as a classroom, where there are many distractions. However, many parents describe that when their child is engaged in a chosen activity at home, such as watching TV or playing a video game, he is able to maintain focus well. Similarly, in a one-on-one situation, with frequent reminders to stay on task, a child with ADHD has little difficulty paying attention. Because he is easily distracted, a child with ADHD often fails to complete tasks, loses things and appears forgetful, careless or sloppy. Some children with ADHD, especially those who are not hyperactive, might appear to be daydreaming, disinterested or unmotivated because they are easily distracted.

A child with the combined type of ADHD will be hyperactive. He is frequently described as "always on the go," "as if driven by a motor." Fidgeting is common and his difficulty staying seated in the classroom can result in disruptions in class. Often children with ADHD have trouble playing quietly and they talk excessively.

Impulsivity can be another feature in children with ADHD. Difficulty controlling impulses can result in difficulty waiting for a turn, blurting out answers before the question is completed, and interrupting. Children with ADHD might leap before they look, leading to increased risk of injuries.

In the classroom, if the underlying problem is not well understood, children with the combined type of ADHD—with their hyperactivity and impulsivity—are often viewed as difficult children who are willfully disobedient. At home, problems following through with instructions, forgetfulness and impulsivity can result in conflict with parents and siblings. Children with ADHD talk before they think, resulting in fights with peers or difficulty maintaining friendships. However, most children with ADHD can function well when parents, teachers and siblings are provided an explanation for the symptoms and the appropriate management is put in place.

How is ADHD diagnosed? There is no blood test, x-ray or psychological test that can make the diagnosis of ADHD. The diagnosis is made by a physician or psychologist, based on the assessment of information provided by parents and school personnel describing the child's functioning at home and school. This information might be provided in the form of a detailed history, described in questionnaires, or can include checklists of criteria, such as the Conner's questionnaire. A defined number of criteria must be met in order to make the diagnosis. The child's difficulty in functioning must be present in more than one setting; for example, at home *and* at school. The diagnosis is usually made

after the child reaches the age of 6 years but the features of ADHD have been present long before.

In ADHD, it is difficulty maintaining focus and controlling impulses that lead to the subsequent problems in school and with relationships. However, children can appear distracted or behave in an impulsive manner for other reasons, without having ADHD. For example, children with learning disabilities or developmental delay might have difficulty paying attention to instructions they do not understand, or work they are finding hard to complete. Similarly, anxiety, hearing or vision problems, home stressors, such as conflict between parents, and psychiatric conditions, such as oppositional defiant disorder or conduct disorder, can also result in inattention and behavior problems and may therefore be confused with true ADHD. It is essential that the health care professional who makes the diagnosis of ADHD evaluate your child carefully for other possible causes of his difficulties.

How is ADHD treated? ADHD is a long-term problem for which there is no quick solution. A coordinated management plan with good communication among parents, teachers, physicians and mental health professionals is essential. The goals of treatment should be specific for each child and family, and clearly established before initiating a management plan. These goals can include:

- improvement in school performance, specifically completion of tasks and/or improved accuracy;
- decreased disruptive behaviors;
- increased independence;
- improvement in relationships with family members, teachers and peers;
- improved self-esteem;
- accident and injury prevention.

Patience, perseverance, close monitoring of the management plan and frequent reassessment are important.

The treatment of ADHD has been well studied for many years and includes medication and behavioral intervention approaches. Studies have shown that a combination of these two treatments is more effective than either alone and that medication use should be carefully initiated and monitored.

Medications. The decision to start your child on daily medication is often a difficult one. However, medication has been shown to be the most effective way to improve the ability to focus and reduce impulsivity in children with ADHD. Recognize that medications do not cure this disorder. The goals of medication treatment are to maximize the potential for learning and minimize negative interactions with adults and peers. Also, any associated problems must be addressed as part of the management plan.

Medications should be carefully administered, target symptoms should be recognized and evaluated and side effects monitored closely. The doctor will have to choose the dose of medication producing the maximum beneficial effect with minimum side effects. Some physicians elect to commence some of these medications as a **blinded trial** in which medication and sugar pills (a placebo) are each given for a period of time, and parents and teachers evaluate the effectiveness and side effects unaware whether the placebo or the real drug is being consumed. Thus, the drug can be evaluated in an unbiased manner. This has been shown to be the most effective way to initiate medication, although it might not be widely available.

The medications that have been most successful in treating ADHD are the "stimulant"

medications, such as methylphenidate (Ritalin) or dextroamphetamine. These medications are thought to work by restoring the normal chemical balance in the brain. Although Ritalin has received mixed coverage in the media, it is a safe medication that has few side effects and has been well studied in children. Short-acting Ritalin is typically taken twice daily, in the morning and at noon; or three times daily, morning, noon and after school. Whether your child should take the medications on the weekends and school holidays depends on the symptoms targeted and the treatment goals. If the main goal is to improve school performance and there are no significant issues at home, the medication can be taken on school days only. If there are issues related to impulsivity that are affecting relationships at home, or distractibility is impeding ability to complete homework, your child can take the medication on other days as well.

The most common side effects of stimulant medications include appetite suppression and sleep disturbance. Neither of these is typically a significant issue if the medication is taken with or after meals, and the last dose is at least four hours before bedtime. Your child might take newer forms of the traditional stimulants, such as methylphenidate, once daily in the morning. They have a more even effect throughout the day. Concern was raised in the past regarding growth suppression, but studies now show there is no significant difference in adult height in children who take Ritalin, compared with other children. Parents often fear that their child will appear "drugged" or like a "zombie." However, when appropriate doses of medication are used, your child will not be sedated. These medications are not addictive for children with ADHD.

If your child has ADHD, there are a number of other medications he can take. These medications are usually used if the stimulant medications are not successful, or where there are other associated disorders that might respond to medication. These medications include clonidine, antidepressants and **selective serotonin reuptake inhibitors** (SSRIs), such as sertraline, paroxetine or fluoxetine.

Behavioral Interventions. Living with and teaching a child with ADHD can, at times, be frustrating and difficult. It is important to remember that children with ADHD are usually not trying to annoy others, but are unable to inhibit their responses. Once you recognize and understand this disorder you can help prevent the cycle of negative interactions between your child with ADHD and his other caregivers or teachers. One of the most effective means of preventing loss of self-esteem and subsequent negative consequences is to promote an area of strength in your child—something that makes him happy and gives a sense of accomplishment. This could be a sport, music, boy scouts or girl guides, art or any other activity that he enjoys.

- Modifications in the classroom and at home can help minimize distractions and maximize independence.
- Children with ADHD often require organizational aids and reminders. You might pin reminders to his school bag or bedroom door to help him become more independent and prevent a fourth trip to school with something he forgot!
- Preferential seating, for example, at the front of the classroom, can help reduce distractions. Increased structure and routine can help.
- Use rewards and appropriate consequences consistently to increase appropriate behavior

and reduce targeted inappropriate behaviors.
- Good communication among home, school and health care professionals is essential in establishing the success of such management programs.

If your child has more severe behavior difficulties or psychiatric disorders, family counseling and management coordinated with a mental health professional may be of assistance.

Alternative therapies. A number of alternative therapies have been recommended for children with ADHD, including the use of megavitamins, essential fatty acids, restrictive diets, eye training exercises, eyeglasses, tinted lenses, chiropractic treatments and biofeedback. In carefully controlled trials none of these therapies has been demonstrated to be effective in children with ADHD. Some of these treatments, such as mega vitamins and restrictive diets, can even be harmful.

It is vital that ADHD be recognized and managed properly to prevent long-term difficulties with school functioning, poor self-esteem and trouble with relationships. With patience and the right kind of help, your child with ADHD can be successful, happy and independent.

Autism Spectrum Disorders: Autism, Pervasive Developmental Disorders and Asperger's Syndrome

What are autism spectrum disorders? The autism spectrum disorders are a group of similar developmental conditions characterized by difficulties or delays in the areas of communication, socialization, play, and behavior. Problems in these areas vary from child to child on a spectrum ranging from mild to severe. Children with more severe forms of the autism spectrum disorders might not talk, play differently, ignore other children and have repetitive behaviors, such as hand flapping. Children with a milder form of these disorders might speak and interact but, compared with other children their age, can seem unusual in how they converse or have some "odd" behaviors. Some children with autism spectrum disorders have severe cognitive delays —in other words, low intelligence—while others have a normal or above average IQ. The severity of the symptoms at the time of diagnosis does not necessarily predict how much a child will improve with treatment.

The diagnosis of each of the autism spectrum disorders is a clinical one. There is no blood test or x-ray that indicates whether your child has autism. A physician or psychologist makes the diagnosis by collecting information from caregivers, including parents, preschool and school, and from direct observation of your child. This person considers the overall development of your child and decides whether defined criteria are met. A certain number from a list of criteria must be met to make a diagnosis but a child does not need to have each and every feature listed to be diagnosed. These criteria determine a number of diagnoses that fall on the autistic spectrum, including autism, pervasive developmental disorder (PDD) and Asperger's syndrome. Careful and thorough assessment is needed to distinguish among autism spectrum disorders, language impairments, learning disabilities and other developmental disorders.

You might find the terminology used for the various diagnoses confusing. Indeed, the classification of the various subtypes of the autism spectrum disorders continues to be a work in progress. The term "autism" refers to the condition where a specific number of the features of disordered communication, socialization and behavior are apparent. "Pervasive developmental disorder" refers to individuals who have some but not all of the features of autism. "Asperger's syndrome" describes individuals who have developed language milestones at the expected time, but have difficulty initiating and maintaining conversation, are overly fixated on unusual topics of their own interest and have difficulty recognizing social cues.

What causes autism? At this time, there is no clearly defined cause for autism. In a small number of cases, there might be an underlying genetic problem, such as **fragile x syndrome** (see pages 240–41), that can be determined by a blood test. There does appear to be a genetic basis for autism, because the chance of having a child with autism is increased in families where a family member has already been diagnosed with an autism spectrum disorder.

In the past, parents were often blamed for causing the autism by inadequate or improper parenting, however, current research suggests that this disorder is something children are born with and that there may be very early signs in young infants. At this time, it does not appear that how your child is parented, stresses during the pregnancy or different forms of child care determine whether or not your child is on the autism spectrum.

There has been much recent discussion about immunizations and their relationship to autism spectrum disorders. Children with autism frequently make some initial progress in language and social development and subsequently regress, losing these skills. This regression frequently occurs between 12 and 24 months, during a period when children receive several immunizations. As parents and professionals have searched to understand the cause for autism, some have theorized that this association, particularly with the measles, mumps and rubella (MMR) vaccine is one of cause and effect; in other words, the immunization caused autism. Several carefully conducted studies have now been published that indicate that immunizations do not result in autism. New research suggests that signs of autism are present before the child receives the MMR vaccine.

What do autism spectrum disorders look like?

Problems with Communication. Children with autism spectrum disorders have difficulties in both verbal (use of spoken language) and nonverbal communication (use of eye contact, pointing, facial expressions and gestures). These children can have a range of impairments in verbal communication, ranging from not speaking at all to talking later than expected. They might speak unusually, for example in a high-pitched, songlike voice lacking variation in tone, or unusually repetitive. Some children can use words to label objects or to ask for something they want, but might not communicate shared interests, such as "Mommy, look at the airplane," or emotions, for example, "He made me sad." Children with Asperger's syndrome might speak at the expected age but have difficulty initiating, taking turns in and ending a conversation, and may become overly fixated on unusual topics of their own interest.

Impairments in nonverbal communication can also vary. A child with autism might use minimal eye contact or none at all. However, it should be noted that many children with autism spectrum disorders, particularly girls, can use some eye contact. Pointing is frequently delayed. Facial expressions and gestures can be limited or used less than expected in a child with simply delayed spoken language.

Problems with Social Skills. Children with autism spectrum disorders frequently do not play with other children as expected. Again, they can have a range of social impairments, from a complete lack of interest in playing with other children and a preference for playing alone to having difficulty taking turns or approaching other children in an unusual way. Often children with autism spectrum disorders do not share interests with others as expected. For example, they tend not to point to things that are interesting or bring things just to show their parents. This diminished interconnectedness is more apparent than an affected child's ability to request something that is needed. Imaginative play might be limited compared with other children of the same age. They may have difficulty expressing a range of emotions and recognizing and responding to other's emotions; for example, they may not respond when a parent or another child is crying and upset.

Unusual Play and Behavior. Often children with autism spectrum disorders are less interested in toys that other children enjoy. Typically, they play with them in unusual ways, for example, they might enjoy watching the wheels of a car spin repetitively. There may be unusual interest in certain sensations, such as the feeling of sand running through fingers, the look of running water, or the sound and sight of a plastic plate spinning. Some children with autism have an unusually intense interest in these sensations, and become focused on them. Other children can have an intense dislike of some sensations, such as the feeling of certain clothes or the sound of a baby crying. They might make repetitive movements, such as hand flapping, finger twisting, spinning, pacing or jumping.

How is autism treated? Unfortunately, there is currently no cure available for autism. However, there are treatments that can result in significant improvements. In fact, children who initially meet the criteria for a diagnosis of an autism spectrum disorder can, with time and therapy, no longer completely meet the criteria for diagnosis.

Early and intensive interventions are associated with better outcome. The forms of treatment of autism that are most effective include speech and language therapy and a specific form of behavioral intervention to develop communication, socialization and play skills, called Applied Behavioral Analysis (ABA) or Intensive Behavioral Intervention (IBI). Under the Individuals with Disabilities Education Act (IDEA), states are required to provide early identification and provision of services to children with a developmental concern. IDEA also mandates that states refer children, free of charge, for a comprehensive, multidisciplinary evaluation by a team who, with the family, decides on which services are needed for the child (via the Individualized Family Service Plan). Your child will probably be referred to a speech and language pathologist familiar with autism spectrum disorders. You or your doctor should also contact local agencies offering ABA or IBI. This type of treatment is very expensive but, sadly, access to publicly funded professionals offering these services might be limited in some communities. Some parents hire trained professionals to provide these services privately or learn how to do them themselves.

In general, children with autism spectrum disorders respond well to a predictable routine and schedule and preparation for change. You will need to plan for adequate support once your child enters the school system. You should obtain copies of written reports completed for any assessments, particularly a letter stating the diagnosis and recommendations, that you can provide to treatment and school personnel. You should meet with the school principal during the spring prior to first school attendance to plan for necessary classroom resources. School-aged children can benefit from a written or pictorial schedule and social skills interventions that include role playing and practicing social situations.

If your child with autism has difficulties tolerating specific sensations, such as food textures, clothing and noises, and his behavior seems to improve with certain kinds of touch such as light brushing or safe compression, sensory integration therapy is frequently recommended. Typically, occupational therapists provide this type of treatment. It has not been shown to change the core symptoms of autism; however, some parents feel it is helpful.

There is no medication currently available that results in improvements in the basic symptoms of autism. Some children with autism have particular difficulty with associated behavior problems that medication may be used to treat. For example, anxiety and obsessive or repetitive behaviors might be treated with a class of medications called **selective serotonin reuptake inhibitors** (SSRIs), such as sertraline and citalopram. Risperidone may be recommended for children with significant aggressive behavior. All of these medications have potential side effects and are typically reserved for behaviors that interfere with school or family life and when nonmedical treatments have been unsuccessful. Information about their safety when young children take them is limited.

You might find the array of treatments recommended by other parents and sources such as the Internet overwhelming and confusing. To date, treatments such as restricted diets, megavitamins, holding therapy and auditory training have not been shown to be effective in improving the symptoms of autism.

Living with a child who has an autistic spectrum disorder is an intense experience of total involvement. And it is frequently a draining experience. Once the diagnosis is made, things will never be quite the same again. You will need to connect with other parents to support one another, be helped by friends and family, and assisted by your community.

Intellectual Disability, Developmental Disability and Mental Retardation

What do the terms mean? Intellectual or developmental disability refers to intelligence that is significantly below average. Practically, by school age, this is determined by assessing the "intelligence quotient" (IQ) using standardized tests administered by a psychologist. The terms intellectual or developmental disability are synonymous and are used when the measured IQ of an individual is in the lowest third percentile for age, meaning that more than 97 percent of children of the same age score higher on IQ testing. Mental retardation is a term used when the IQ is below the third percentile and significantly affects a child's ability to accomplish daily functions.

What do intellectual disabilities look like? Most often, children who are diagnosed with intellec-

tual disabilities have a history of globally delayed milestones, affecting all areas of development. In some situations, motor development proceeds normally and parents and caregivers do not raise concerns until language is slow to develop. Subsequent delays in acquisition of number and letter skills are noticed. It is difficult to predict, particularly in very young children, what subsequent intelligence and school functioning will be. Typically, IQ testing to measure cognitive skills thinking is not done until children are in school and failing to progress as expected.

What causes intellectual disability? In approximately one-half of children with intellectual disability, there is an identifiable cause for the significant developmental delay. Possible causes include genetic problems such as **Down's syndrome**, brain infections such as **meningitis** or various neurological problems, and metabolic disorders in which the body is unable to make a chemical required for normal brain function. In the other half of children with significant intellectual disabilities, a medical cause cannot be found. What is clear is that intellectual disabilities and mental retardation are almost never due to poor parenting.

How should intellectual disability be managed? There are many possible causes for a child's learning problems, including learning disabilities, ADHD, hearing or vision problems and home stresses. The first step toward dealing with this problem is a thorough assessment to clarify the causes and contributors to school difficulties. If you suspect or have identified developmental delays, your child should receive a thorough medical assessment and careful planning for school placement and support resources. If your child continues to have difficulties learning at the expected rate, a psychologist will do a cognitive assessment to measure her intelligence quotient and determine specific learning strengths and weaknesses.

There is no medication that cures intellectual disabilities. Occasionally, medications can be used to reduce specific associated symptoms, such as aggressive behavior or inattention.

After cognitive testing has determined that your child has a significant intellectual disability, it is important that you meet with school personnel to discuss goals for the student and resources available in the school. Reassessment of educational goals should occur at least yearly. Your child might need placement in a special education classroom, for at least part of the day, where teaching can be provided at her level and more individualized attention is possible. You might be concerned about your child acquiring undesirable behaviors as a result of exposure to other students who have significant developmental and/or behavioral difficulties. However, placement in a regular classroom where other students are working on significantly different material is difficult for both student and teacher. In many cases, the child in a special education class can be integrated into the regular class for some period of the day, for example gym or art class. It is important that educational goals include life skills training, such as development of literacy and time and money skills relevant to getting around and accomplishing daily needs.

You are probably concerned about how your child will function as an adult. The degree of independence that a child with intellectual disability or mental retardation is able to achieve depends on the severity of the cognitive delay and is frequently difficult to predict in young children. More mildly affected individuals can learn to read and write, be relatively independent and actually hold a job. More severely affected adults can sometimes live semi-independently in small, supervised group homes, and participate in specialized vocational settings.

Parenting a child with a significant intellectual disability is undoubtedly challenging. It is important to remember that expectations, home safety-proofing and disciplinary measures should be those that are appropriate for your child's current level of functioning and not her chronological age. Under the Individuals with Disabilities Education Act, states are required to provide early identification and provision of services to children with developmental concerns. Every state sponsors a variety of agencies who provide support and guidance for families. With appropriate assistance, correct school planning and good communication between families, school personnel and health care professionals, your child's potential will be maximized.

Remember, the amount of joy a child experiences and gives to others does not depend on her intelligence. The goal of any parent or teacher remains the same regardless of handicap: to maximize your child's true potential.

Learning Disabilities

What are learning disabilities? Children with learning disabilities (LDs) possess normal intelligence but, because of difficulty with specific aspects of brain function required for learning, they perform at a lower academic level than expected. Learning disabilities are common, occurring in 10 percent of the school-age population. They often become evident around grades 2 or 3, when learning concepts becomes more complex or abstract and reading is required for learning.

There are two main types of learning disabilities:

- Language-based learning disabilities are the most common. They are characterized by difficulties with spoken language, understanding language, reading and written language. Many children with language-based learning disabilities have a history of language delays in early childhood. Dyslexia, which is also known as "specific reading disability," is a form of language-based learning disability.
- Nonverbal learning disability, is less common than language-based learning disabilities. Children with nonverbal learning disabilities typically have average reading and spelling skills but particular difficulty with mathematics. They have difficulty with visual-spatial motor skills, leading to struggles with spatial directions, copying shapes and printing and writing. Social impairment is common because of difficulty interpreting social cues, such as body postures, facial expressions and changes in voice intonation.

What causes learning disabilities? The cause of learning disabilities is not well understood. There appears to be a genetic component, as many parents who have struggled in school have children with learning disabilities. What is clear is that you are not to blame for these difficulties that your child was likely born with. In the majority of cases, there is no identifiable neurological abnormality in children with learning disabilities. No specific medical tests, such as brain imaging (CT scan or MRI) or blood tests are needed.

In the past, dyslexia, or specific reading disability, was thought to be due to difficulties with visual perception of letters. However, research now indicates that the primary problem is one of recognizing, processing and using the sounds that make up language, a process called **phonological awareness**.

How is a learning disability diagnosed? There are a number of possible explanations for why your child might be struggling in school. These include learning disability, intellectual limitations, attention deficit hyperactivity disorder (ADHD), problems with vision or hearing, anxiety, depression or family stresses. A careful and thorough assessment can determine the cause. This usually involves assessment by a physician. A children's mental health center might also be involved if there are behavior problems or family stressors that might be contributing to the school problems.

Any thorough evaluation of a child with a suspected learning disability must include a psycho-educational assessment including intelligence (IQ) testing. A psychologist completes this assessment. A formal measurement of academic skills—the grade level your child is functioning at in different areas—is also required. So is an assessment of your child's behavior in the classroom. An assessment by a speech and language therapist might also be indicated, particularly where there are language-based concerns.

What should be done to help my child? The recommendations for each child with a learning disability vary depending on the child's particular learning profile. The first step toward helping a youngster is obtaining a careful assessment to provide a clear understanding of your child's learning strengths and weaknesses. Once this assessment is complete, you should meet with school personnel to discuss the evaluation, including recommendations, and to develop an individualized plan for your child's education.

Depending on the type and severity of the learning disability, an individualized education plan (IEP) can include regular classroom placement with modifications to the teaching style and learning goals, withdrawal of your child from a regular classroom to provide specific remedial help, provision of an educational assistant in the classroom, or placement in a special class or school. You might wish to provide private tutoring outside of school, or to enroll your child in a private school. Whatever the setting, it is important that school personnel have access to and review any assessments completed, the educational placement is appropriate to your child's particular needs and proven teaching techniques are used.

Programs that target phonological awareness, the processing and use of the sounds that make up language, are necessary if your child has reading problems. Phonological awareness is different from "phonics," which refers to sounds and written language. A number of programs that focus on phonological awareness are available for use at home and in the classroom and are effective in improving reading if your child has dyslexia. Direct instruction reading programs can also help. A speech and language therapist or psychologist can provide specific programming recommendations.

If your child has fine motor difficulties that create problems with printing and writing, he might benefit from occupational therapy. The occupational therapist can provide exercises to improve fine motor skills and make recommendations for special equipment to support fine motor tasks. It may be necessary to modify timed assignments or tests if your child has difficulty producing written material quickly. If your child's difficulties in this area are severe, she might require oral rather than written exams or be allowed the use of a keyboard if her keyboarding skills are adequate.

If your child has nonverbal learning disabilities, she will benefit from a structured schedule with clear expectations and consistent routines. Explaining changes in routine ahead of time helps avoid difficulties with transitions. Explanations should be clear and direct and repeated to ensure she understands them. Social skills training can be very helpful. It also helps if you provide very structured, short, supervised play situations to ensure peer interactions are successful. The length of these sessions can be gradually increased and the amount of supervision gradually decreased. Previewing and preparing for new situations is also useful.

You and your child will need a good understanding of the areas of difficulty and recommendations for management. You will need to advocate for your child within the school system and keep good records of assessments and yearly individualized learning plans. Information related to local legislation governing education can help you to develop an understanding of the public school system and is available on government websites. Careful reassessment is recommended yearly and transition planning is essential when your child moves from one school to another.

Local support agencies, such as learning disabilities associations, can be of great help with advice about management options, educational materials and interventions such as social skills groups for children with LDs. With coordinated care involving families, schools and health care personnel, children with learning disabilities are able to succeed in school and achieve their long-term goals.

School Phobia and School Avoidance

What is school phobia? Children often complain about having to go to school, at least some of the time. Parents expect those comments and view them as normal. Sometimes there is a greater problem. Instead of the occasional complaint about attending class, children either refuse to attend school or create reasons not to go. This is termed "school avoidance." It's a common problem, occurring in approximately 5 percent of school-aged children. "School phobia" refers to a real anxiety about attending school and falls in the spectrum of school avoidance.

What does school phobia look like? If your child has school phobia, she might frequently miss extensive periods of time at school. She might complain of a number of physical symptoms that are actually related to stress or anxiety. She might be unaware of what is truly making her not feel well, and be unable to label her feelings or understand and articulate the cause. Just as adults get tension headaches, butterflies in the stomach or diarrhea when anxious or stressed, children may complain of not feeling well with vague symptoms, such as abdominal pain, nausea or headaches. Just like adults who really feel true pain with their stress headaches, children with these symptoms are not "faking," but generally truly feel unwell. When you seek medical attention for your child, the pattern of symptoms and physical examination findings does not fit with the severity of symptoms described. Often, the symptoms occur on school days and improve on weekends. Usually,

symptoms that would accompany significant medical illnesses—such as weight loss, fever and vomiting—are absent. In some cases, the symptoms can be quite severe and cause you, and even your doctor, concern that a medical diagnosis is being missed, leading to a series of negative medical tests. Eventually, with appropriate exploration of psychosocial stressors, the underlying issues causing the symptoms are found.

What causes school phobia or avoidance? School phobia or avoidance results from anxiety or stress related to attending school. Young children might not find the class environment as secure and loving as home. This is particularly true if your child is shy or timid. In some situations, it is related to a recent loss of a family member, or where there is conflict between family members in the home. Your child's reluctance to attend school might be due to difficulty with schoolwork due to unrecognized developmental delays or some learning disability. Sometimes teasing or bullying leads to school refusal.

How do I treat school phobia or avoidance? School refusal can be a difficult problem to solve and requires patience and perseverance. The first step is to obtain a medical assessment to ensure there is no underlying physical illness. Once you have established this, further exploration of the underlying reasons for the school refusal is essential to addressing the problem. You might have to involve a children's mental health professional, such as a psychiatrist or social worker. Developing a clear understanding of the problem will also likely require obtaining information from school personnel.

It is important that you support and believe your child, while recognizing that the underlying stressors causing the symptoms need to be addressed. It is also important that your child navigate the transition back to school as soon as possible. The longer the absence, the harder it will be for her to return. Good communication among families, school personnel and health care professionals is essential to developing a transition-to-school plan that makes sense for your individual child. In some cases, immediate return to full-time school attendance can be accomplished, while in other situations, a more graduated return is required. Although often difficult, you must remain firm in helping your child, who will likely continue to complain about symptoms upon her return to school.

Speech and Language Delay

It is both fascinating and delightful to witness children develop the ability to communicate with sounds, gestures and then words. Unfortunately, delays in developing language are common and these can have an impact on your child's behavior and relationships. How, then, can you know when to be concerned and what to do? Here is some information that might help.

What is normal language development? There is a range of normal for all developmental milestones in children, including speech and language milestones. The next few paragraphs provide average ages for the major milestones in each area of speech and language development in preschool-aged children. Following school entry, language development is mainly seen in the areas of reading and writing.

Speech Production. This refers to the way in which the sounds that make up language are made. This includes pronunciation (articulation)

and smoothness (fluency). It is not unusual for children who are in the early stages of language development to speak gibberish, which sounds like conversation, although the words are not identifiable. This typically occurs around the age of 18 months and is a normal stage of language development. By age 2, approximately half of your child's words should be recognizable by a stranger; parents are frequently able to understand much more. By the age of 3, approximately 75 percent of your child's words should be pronounced well enough for a stranger to understand, and by 4 years old, 95 percent. It is common for 4-year-olds to continue to use some sound substitutions, most commonly "w" for "r," for example "wabbit" instead of "rabbit." However, by age 6, all sounds should be made clearly and accurately. Stuttering refers to repeating of the initial sound in a word, for example "s-s-s-stop." Some stuttering around the time of rapid increases in your child's vocabulary is normal, particularly before age 4, as long as your child is not upset by it. (See Stuttering, pages 208–209.)

Expressive Language. Expressive language refers to what the child says, including the number and types of words, and how they are combined. Typically, young infants use cooing sounds, which consist of vowel sounds, including the cute "aaahs" that we all adore. Consonant-vowel combinations, or babbling, such as "bababa" and "dadada" usually begin around 6 months of age and are initially used without specific meaning. By 12 months, an infant is usually able to use at least one word with meaning, usually "dada" for dad. At 1 year, infants are also usually imitating sounds they hear their parents make, such as "uh oh!" More words are accumulated over the next year and by 2 years of age, toddlers are using between 20 and 50 words and starting to combine words, such as "my cup"—often used loudly and with great insistence! Sentences gradually lengthen, including three words by age 3 years. Children usually ask lots of questions when they are 3—the age of the "whys." As your child's language develops, she will often ask you to read the same story over and over again. She might come to know stories so well, it almost seems like she can read!

Receptive Language. Receptive language concerns what your child understands from speech. Generally, children understand more than they are able to say. Infants respond to sounds very early, usually by 1 month, and turn when their name is called by 6 months. At 18 months, most toddlers can identify their own major body parts, including head, hair, eyes, nose, mouth, belly button and toes. Most 2-year-olds are generally able to follow a simple command, such as "Go, get the keys." However, longer more detailed explanations or more complex instructions might not be understood. By age 3 years, most children are able to identify colors and by age 4, the alphabet. Children can answer "where" and "what" questions by age 3, but are generally not able to answer "why" questions until school age.

Nonverbal Communication. Children and adults communicate in several other ways that do not include words. This process is referred to as nonverbal communication. These forms of communication include the use of eye contact, gestures—nodding or shaking the head or shrugging shoulders—pointing and facial expressions. Young infants look at an adult's face and follow it with their eyes by 1 month. Young children frequently require a warm-up period before they make eye contact with an unfamiliar adult, but the use of eye contact,

once comfortable, to make requests, share interests and initiate play should be well developed prior to age 2 years. Pointing typically begins around 1 year of age and is used both to make requests and to share interest.

When should I be worried about my child's language development? There is a wide range of normal ages at which major developmental milestones are achieved. Furthermore, each milestone should be considered in context with your child's overall developmental profile. A delay in achieving just one developmental target does not automatically indicate a problem. This might make it difficult for you to know when to be concerned. In general, if you are worried about your child's development, you should discuss your concerns with your child's physician. It has been shown repeatedly that parental concern is strongly correlated with identification of delays—your hunch is important!

What causes language delays? In many situations, particularly when language delays are mild and there are no other areas of delay, the cause is unknown. Heredity plays a role, as children with language delays often have a family history of language delays, learning difficulties or developmental delays.

In all cases of language delay, you should have your child's hearing assessed. Mild hearing losses, often due to recurrent ear infections, can contribute to mild speech and language delays. However, it is important to recognize that most children who have ear infections do not have developmental delays. If your child has very frequent ear infections, more than six per year, it is especially important to have her hearing assessed and to consult with your child's doctor about the need to see an ear,

WARNING SIGNS OF POSSIBLE LANGUAGE DELAY

AREA OF DEVELOPMENT	WARNING SIGN
Expressive language development	No babbling with consonant sounds "bababa" by 9 months
	No words by 18 months
	Not pointing by 18 months
	Words difficult to understand at 3 years
	Stuttering after age 4 years that upsets your child
	or interferes with her ability to communicate
Receptive language development	Not responding to your voice or sounds by 6 months
	Not turning when name called at 18 months
	Not able to identify body parts by 2 years
	Not able to follow a simple instruction by 2 years
Social development	Not pointing to get your attention at 18 months
	Not interested in other children at 2 years
	No imaginary play at 2 years

nose and throat specialist to consider ventilating tube insertion, which can improve hearing and language development.

In many cases, isolated language delay, one with no other areas of developmental delay, simply reflects a normal child who develops a little later than average but has no specific difficulty with language development. These delays tend to resolve by themselves. In some cases, children with language delays have a specific language impairment. If this is the case with your child, she will require speech and language therapy and will be at higher risk for ongoing language-based difficulties, such as difficulties with reading and writing. Language delay might be part of a global developmental delay, or overall lower intelligence. Alternatively,

language delay may be a sign of **autism spectrum disorders**, particularly if you are also concerned about her interaction with peers and the use of nonverbal communication (see pages 169–73).

Sometimes, parents wonder if a younger child's language delays result from her siblings speaking for her. It has been shown that birth order does *not* account for significant language delays. Similarly, exposure to more than one language in the home can result in mixing of the two languages, but should not result in delays in development of the major language milestones. Although there are slight differences in the rate of language development between boys and girls, these differences are small and do not explain significant language delays in boys. Language delays are not the result of laziness.

What do I do if I suspect a language delay? If you suspect your child has a language delay, it is important to discuss this with your child's health care provider as soon as possible. Language delays should be identified and treated as early as possible.

In most cases, unless there are significant global developmental delays, no medical cause is found for language delays. Generally, medical tests are not necessary and the focus is on how best to help your child's language development.

A speech and language therapist can provide further assessment and intervention. In young children, it has been shown that the most effective form of speech and language therapy is that provided by their caregivers, who are with them regularly, rather than provided directly by a therapist, who can typically offer service once per week. You might take a parent training program. Professional speech therapy might be necessary for specific speech production difficulties, such as articulation problems or stuttering, that are causing your child distress.

There are many ways that you can help your child's language development. Talk to your child on a regular basis. Use simplified language that is at, or just above, your child's own language level. For example, if your 2-year-old is using only a few single words, lengthy explanations or stories are likely to be poorly understood and not stimulate a response. Instead, simplifying stories and prompting labeling of common pictures in a book ("Look at the dog!" "What's that?") are more likely to stimulate talking. Singing songs with your child, with pauses to see if your child asks for more or fills in the gap is fun for you and your child and can help with language development. Naming body parts or clothing as you dress, undress or bathe your young child is another way to introduce language into everyday activities. Repeating back what you hear your child say helps reinforce your child's language development.

Notice the impact of your child's language delay on her behavior. In many cases, particularly when expressive language is the only area of development affected, children can become frustrated as they attempt to communicate unsuccessfully with others. If your child has receptive language delays; that is, in the language you use with her, it is important to adjust instructions and explanations to correspond to her abilities. When severe, language delays can have an impact on a child's interaction with peers and interfere with social play. A caregiver can help by adding language to shared activities or repeating words that might not be understood easily by another child.

You will need to plan carefully before your child begins school to ensure she gets adequate support and appropriate programming. You should meet with the school principal in the winter or early spring of the year prior to school attendance. If language delays persist and affect her development of reading and writing, a psychology assessment might help delineate your child's strengths and weaknesses and make recommendations to school personnel. If your child is already in school, it is important to understand the identified delays, their impact on learning and what interventions are available for support.

Although it may be disappointing and difficult to accept that your child has a developmental delay, with early help, you can help maximize your child's potential and minimize future difficulties.

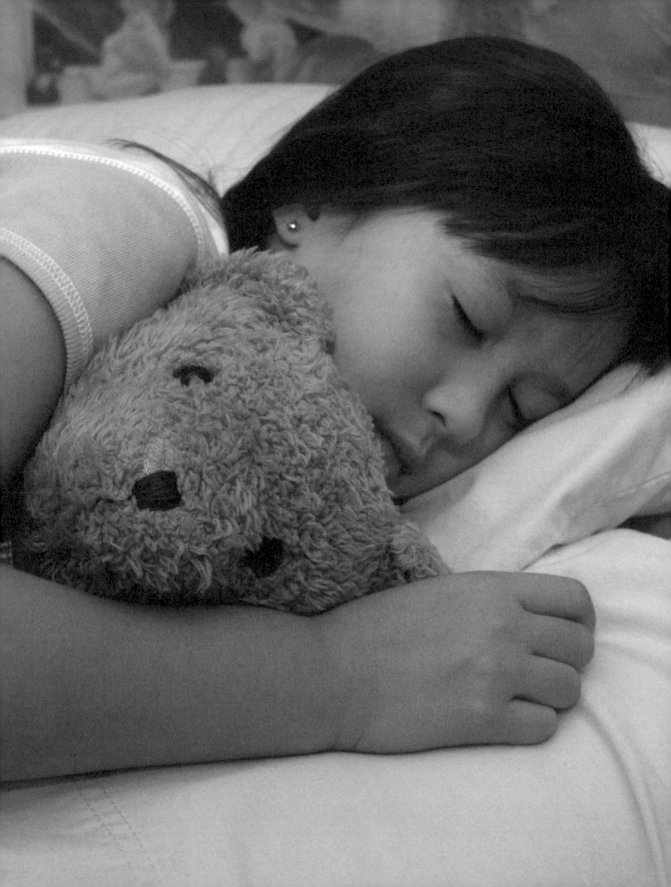

Sleep Problems

7

What are sleep problems? Most often, the sleep problems that infants and toddlers—and their families—experience revolve around difficulty settling down to sleep or repeated night waking. Many children have difficulty sleeping independently; it requires separation from a parent's warm, reassuring cuddle. Why would any child prefer leaving an enjoyable, stimulating environment, only to face the night alone? Parents also worry about other sleep-related problems, such as nightmares and night terrors.

Sleep problems are extremely common in children and can lead to parental exhaustion and family disruption. Although sleep-related issues can be very challenging for parents, modifications to bedtime routines, sleep timing and sleep environment can lead to resolution of the problem within a very short time. Once you understand what to expect, what is developmentally appropriate and why children have difficulties with sleep, you can solve these common problems. Strategies should be tailored to what is comfortable and manageable for your own family situation.

What is normal sleep? Depending on a child's age and developmental stage, there is considerable variation in the amount of sleep needed, as well as the pattern and cycles of sleep. At each age,

there is a range of normal; some children seem to require more sleep and others less. Similarly, some children seem to naturally fall into a regular pattern of sleeping, with few difficulties, while others require more help and support. Temporary disruptions in sleep often result from illness and changes in the child's environment or schedule.

In all of us, sleep consists of cycles that include periods of light sleep leading to deeper sleep, then to dreaming and, finally, waking. These cycles repeat themselves regularly throughout the night. Dreams occur during a stage of sleep called rapid eye movement (REM), sleep. Rest, the restorative phase of sleeping, occurs during non-REM sleep. Non-REM sleep tends to happen earlier in the night and REM sleep later. Most of us awaken during very light stages of sleep. In adults, these awakenings are usually brief: we usually look at the clock, turn over and go back to sleep. However, many children have some difficulty settling back down to sleep and need to be taught how to do so.

In general, babies sleep the most when they are newborn and gradually require less sleep as they get older. In the period immediately after birth, the normal amount of sleep can vary from 11 to 23 hours per day—a wide range of normal! The average newborn sleeps 16 ½ hours per day

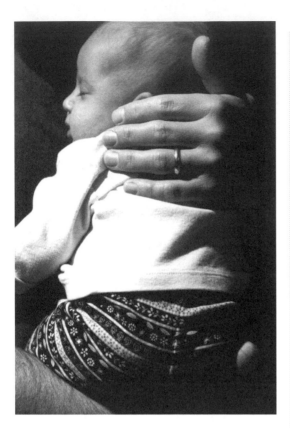

in sleep cycles that are quite short, generally around one hour per cycle. Sleep during this period of early infancy is typically divided into numerous brief naps, interspersed with short periods of wakefulness and feeding. Environmental cues, such as exposure to light, feeding, interaction, noise and play will help to group these short naps into fewer but longer periods of sleep.

In some babies, this clustering of naps results in the longest period of sleep occurring during the day rather than at night. This is called "day-night reversal." If your baby has this problem, you can try making environmental modifications, such as maintaining a dark, quiet environment with little interaction with the baby during the night, and a bright, stimulating environment during wakeful daytime periods.

By 3 or 4 months of age, many infants nap more regularly and are able to sleep through the night. The middle of the night feeding can usually be eliminated around this age. The average total sleep decreases to 12 to 14 hours daily. Two naps per day are typical for 6-month-olds.

At around 7 or 8 months of age, just when things seem to be settling into place, infants develop a greater awareness of separation. They begin to express their displeasure at being left by their parents. Falling asleep alone becomes more of a challenge. Most infants have a normal period of fussiness while they make the transition from wakefulness to sleeping. In fact, it is normal for them to cry for 10 to 20 minutes as they fall asleep.

Between 1 and 3 years old, one nap per day is typical and total sleep time including naps averages about 11 to 12 hours. After the first year, dreaming becomes more active. Increased awareness, in combination with an active imagination and an inability to clearly discriminate between fantasy and reality may lead to bedtime fears and nightmares in toddlers. Bedtime fears of the dark or "monsters" can appear as your baby's imagination starts to develop.

Sleep cycles gradually increase in duration until they reach an adult pattern by age 3 years, lasting around 1 ½ hours per cycle.

Difficulty Settling Down to Sleep

How common is difficulty settling? Trouble settling down to sleep is a very common problem. Up to one-third of children have some difficulty getting to sleep.

What could be causing difficulty settling? It seems easiest for most young infants to fall asleep when they are held, rocked or stroked, particularly when sucking on the breast or a pacifier. Toddlers and older children seem to fall asleep more easily when a parent lies beside them, singing or talking to them. Sometimes music or the television is playing while they are falling asleep. Children easily become accustomed to these sleep aids, or "associations," and develop an apparent dependency on them. They have difficulty and usually protest when these associations are unavailable and they are expected to fall asleep without them.

What is the best way to manage difficulty settling?

Routines and schedules help. The development of a consistent nap- and bedtime will help your child to know what to expect and seems to facilitate sleeping. Bedtimes will vary with the age of your child and your household routines. In general, it is best to pick a bedtime when your child often shows signs of being sleepy, but before he becomes irritable and overtired; then stick to that time. Naps should not be longer than two hours for infants and toddlers and the last nap should end before 4 p.m. to avoid interfering with his sleeping at night.

You might implement a structured bedtime routine lasting no more than 20 minutes. This routine for a young infant might include giving him a bath, putting on his night clothes, giving him a feed, and singing or talking quietly to him before putting your baby in his crib, drowsy but still awake. The bedtime routine for a toddler could includes a bath, dressing in pajamas, brushing teeth and reading a story. At the end of the story, you turn out the light, give him a good night kiss, and leave the room. Maintaining consistency in this routine will help your child settle down and make for a successful transition to sleep.

Provide a suitable sleep environment. In general, the environment in which a child falls asleep should remain the same throughout the night. Sleep and wake cycles are affected by a hormone produced in the brain called melatonin. Melatonin is released when the environment becomes dark and helps the brain to fall asleep. For this reason, most children and adults fall asleep more easily in the dark. Therefore, a dark, relatively quiet, and unstimulating environment will promote sleep. Infants under 6 months of age should be placed lying on their back for sleep. This sleep position has been associated with the lowest risk of crib death, otherwise known as **sudden infant death syndrome**. (see pages 78–79).

When separation awareness develops around 8 months of age, your child might need a "transitional object," such as a stuffed animal or blanket to cuddle or stroke. A dim night light often does the trick for toddlers who have bedtime fears.

Respond to crying appropriately. It is important and proper to respond to the cries of newborns and young infants in their first few months of life. These cries communicate a need; they are not manipulative behavior. By 7 or 8 months of age, however, a short period of crying prior to falling asleep is normal and not harmful. It's okay to let babies learn to calm themselves. But some parents have real difficulty not responding to their child's cries immediately. If your child has become conditioned to needing a parent's presence to settle down, you can reduce the acquired parental dependency. You might try responding to the night crying with gradually decreasing contact. One way to do this uses timed absences from the room while your child is crying and resisting separation. This involves calmly laying your child down, offering some brief reassuring words and then leaving the room for a few minutes before returning. Follow the same pattern, gradually increasing the amount of time spent out of the room until your child falls asleep. Consistency in this approach is essential. When this method is applied properly, children learn to settle to sleep alone in an average of four days.

Lengthy crying episodes at bedtime can be frustrating and upsetting for parents, particularly if they are exhausted and stressed. It is important to recognize that this is a normal developmental challenge and that your child is not being purposefully difficult. If you find yourself becoming angry with your child, put him in the crib, close the door and take a break. Having someone available to help, if possible, may make things more manageable, particularly if you have more than one child.

Deal with delaying tactics. Toddlers and young children can be very adept at avoiding and prolonging bedtime with requests for one more story, a trip to the washroom, a drink of water, one more kiss or another blanket. Children should be returned quickly, calmly and quietly to bed and told the door will be closed if they come out again.

Children can learn to separate. Parents who have been sleeping with their child or lying with him until he falls asleep must teach the child that he can settle himself without a parent's presence. Do this in stages, first by sitting in a chair near the bed until the child falls asleep instead of lying beside the youngster. Once the bedtime routine has been completed and your child is in bed with the lights out, you should sit in the chair, avoiding eye contact with the child, not talking and not making physical contact, simply being a reassuring presence. Move the chair gradually further from the bedside each night until it reaches the door. If your child gets out of bed, return him to bed and calmly tell him that you will leave the room and close the door if he gets out of bed again. Again, if you apply this approach consistently, children learn to settle to sleep alone in an average of four days.

Medications. Medications such as sleeping pills are very rarely required to treat sleep problems in children. Behavioral approaches, such as those previously described, are almost always successful when implemented consistently. Very occasionally, a short course of a sedative medication can be prescribed to help in changing a pattern that is particularly difficult to disrupt. However, long-term treatment with medication is generally not recommended. One exception to this general rule might be if your child has a developmental disability. These youngsters often have disordered sleep. Medications including sedatives such as chloral hydrate, certain anticonvulsants or melatonin may be useful for them and, therefore, recommended by a physician.

Co-sleeping

What is co-sleeping? Many parents and families choose to sleep in the same bed as their infants and young children. In many cultures, co-sleeping is the norm. Co-sleeping has been associated with increased success in maintaining breast-feeding and in most cases is not associated with long-term problems. Deaths from adults rolling onto and suffocating their children have received extensive coverage in the medical literature and the media. Yet, co-sleeping is probably safe, as long as the adult is not under the influence of drugs or alcohol, is a nonsmoker and not too obese. Co-sleeping should not happen on a surface where a young child could become trapped, for example between the mattress and a wall, on a couch or waterbed. Adults sleeping with young infants, particularly those under 6 months of age, should ensure that bedclothes and pillows that can smother a child are not in the infant's sleep area.

In certain circumstances you should take steps to move your child into his own bed. These would include if your sleep becomes disturbed, if it is part of an overall difficulty with setting limits for the child, if it is disruptive to your relationship with your partner or in older children who should be encouraged to sleep alone.

If you choose to sleep with your children, you should be aware that the child will likely come to depend on your presence to fall asleep, stay asleep and settle back to sleep. It is probably easiest to move from co-sleeping to putting your infant in a crib prior to 8 months of age, but there are interventions to help your child learn to fall asleep successfully at any age.

Night Awakening

What is night awakening? Night awakenings are very common in children. As children cycle through periods of lighter sleep, they often wake up. Children who have not learned to settle themselves to sleep might fully awaken and cry, call out for parents or get out of bed, depending on their age. Some parents are content to have the child sleep with them for the remainder of the night or move into the child's bed. However, for others, these disruptions in sleep are less acceptable. Whether or not night waking is viewed as a problem is really a matter of personal perspective.

How should night awakening be managed? Frequently, night awakenings occur when children have developed sleep associations, such as needing a bottle, soother or a parent lying beside them to fall back to sleep. The first steps toward solving this problem are to ensure a consistent, brief bedtime routine and to help your child learn to fall asleep alone.

- In general, the room should be kept dark and quiet.
- If possible, avoid rewarding your child for wakening by picking up, cuddling, rocking or playing with him.
- If your child older than 6 months is still drinking from a bottle during the night, he should be gradually weaned 1 ounce at a time, before other interventions are tried.
- If your infant is in a crib, you may want to wait for a short period before responding to his arousal: he might fuss a little but then turn over and fall back to sleep on his own.
- If you wish to check on your baby briefly, you should keep the interaction to a minimum, lie him down, and quietly tell him it's time to sleep.

A consistent approach of timed waiting to respond to crying (discussed in the section on settling) is very effective within only a few days, but consistency is the key! Although it is often hard, try to remain calm. Remember that the child is going through a normal developmental challenge and not being deliberately difficult.

Children who are older and sleep in a bed require a slightly different approach. Gradual withdrawal of your presence is frequently required. This can be accomplished using a chair sitting routine as discussed on page 186. Once again, if you wish to teach children to fall asleep alone, you must be very consistent in the implementation of this routine, minimizing interaction with your child and simply providing a reassuring presence that is gradually withdrawn.

Nightmares

What are nightmares? Nightmares are frightening dreams. They are not the same as night terrors, which are described in the next section. Nightmares are very common, occurring in 10 percent to 50 percent of children. They typically happen during the early morning hours. Because 3- to 6-year-olds possess vivid imaginations and have difficulty distinguishing fantasy and reality, they seem to experience the most nightmares. Some of the content of the dream might reflect daytime stresses or a frightening show that they saw on television. It does not necessarily indicate that your child is stressed or anxious.

How should I manage nightmares? When children are sufficiently frightened, they will have difficulty falling back to sleep after a nightmare. They can usually be reassured by your presence and brief comforting. A good bedtime routine with a quiet story can promote more restful sleep. And, screening what your child is watching on TV is a good idea for many reasons! If nightmares are persistent or frequent, it is worth mentioning to your doctor.

Night Terrors

What are night terrors? While nightmares are a problem of sleep, night terrors are a disorder of arousal. Night terrors are a phenomenon that occurs when your child partially wakes up during the transition from deeper sleep. They happen in approximately 6 percent of children between 18 months and 6 years of age. Night terrors are most likely to occur one to two hours after falling sleep. They occur in normal children and do not indicate an underlying problem. Stress, fatigue, a full bladder or loud noises can trigger a night terror in children who have them. Often, there is a family history of night terrors, sleepwalking or sleep talking.

What do night terrors look like? During a night terror, your child might appear frightened, pale and sweaty. Although his eyes may be wide open, he is not responsive to others in the room and might speak incoherently or scream. The child is not awake, and cannot be easily woken up. He might push a parent away, walk around or appear to see something that is not there. The episode can last as long as 20 to 30 minutes. You might find all this quite frightening. However, your child typically falls asleep quickly and does not remember the event in the morning.

How should I manage night terrors? Even those children who do experience night terrors, experience them infrequently. Nothing needs to be done. If they do recur, the environment should be free of safety hazards, particularly for children who walk around during the night terror. Talking to your child, hugging or picking him up won't do much good and can even reinforce the episode. Children do not usually remember night terrors, therefore talking to them about it or asking what happened is unlikely to be beneficial.

If the night terrors continue to be a problem, you can try to alter the child's sleep cycle. Arousing the youngster about 30 minutes before the night terror typically appears (usually around one hour after falling asleep) for one week might correct things. A 30- to 60-minute afternoon nap might also decrease the frequency of night terrors. Only rarely, very rarely, are sleep-altering medications needed.

When should I worry about night terrors? Children will outgrow their night terrors; they usually resolve by 6 to 8 years of age. If they persist in children older than 8 years, you should have the problem assessed by his doctor. Rhythmic movements occurring during these episodes might be a sign of seizures, and further assessment is recommended.

Sleepwalking

What is it? Sleepwalking is another disorder of arousal that is common in children. It is said that 15 percent of children sleepwalk at some point during childhood and 1 percent to 6 percent sleepwalk regularly. Sleepwalking is most common in children between the ages of 4 to 12 years and typically occurs one to two hours after falling asleep. It is not indicative of emotional problems in children.

What does sleepwalking look like? Children who sleepwalk often wander purposelessly throughout the house, appear uncoordinated and might try to do something that does not make sense, such as urinating in an unusual location.

You might not initially realize that your child is asleep and can have difficulty arousing him.

How should I manage sleepwalking? The most important thing is to keep your child safe. If your child is a sleepwalker, it is a good idea to install a lock out of his reach on outside doors and ensure windows are locked. Do not attempt to wake your child and guide him back to bed. Scheduled awakenings before the typical time of sleepwalking or a short afternoon nap might help frequent sleepwalkers. Where sleepwalking is severe or begins in adolescence, consult a doctor for further evaluation.

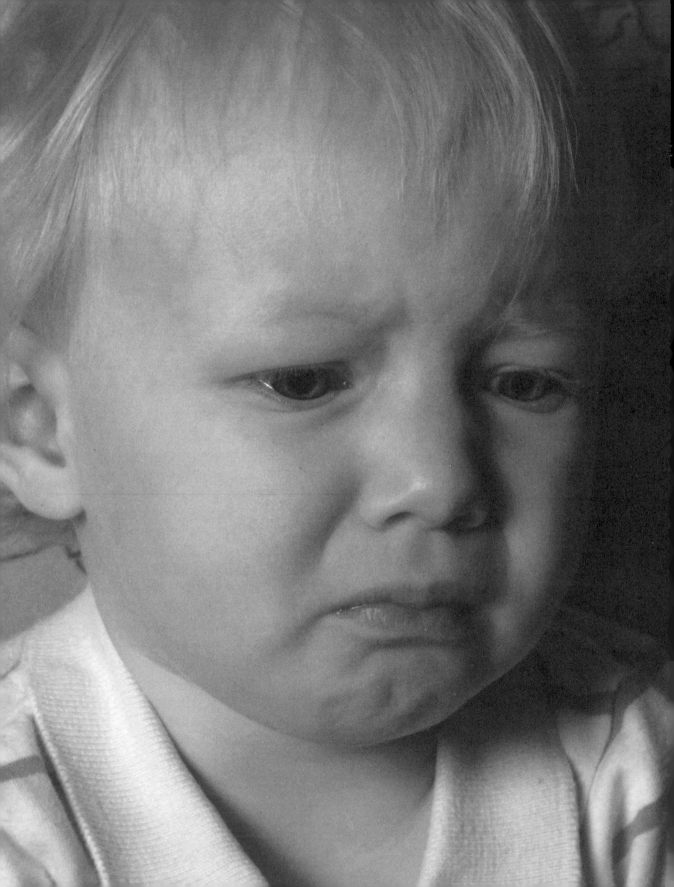

Behavior

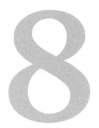

Temperament and Its Problems

What is temperament? Temperament refers to the part of a person's basic nature that determines how that individual reacts to people, places and things. Most experts believe that a child's temperament is already formed at birth, or at least within the first few months of life. Although environmental factors can modify temperament somewhat, these traits persist throughout life.

Temperament is neither "good" nor "bad." Yet, understanding your child's temperament and how he responds to certain situations can help your parenting. It is also important to recognize that parents, caregivers and educators also have particular temperamental characteristics that, in turn, can affect how they interact with children of different temperaments. The fit between a child's temperament and that of his parents can affect family life dramatically.

What does temperament look like? During the late 1950s and early 1960s, Alexander Thomas and Stella Chess completed the landmark studies that addressed childhood temperament. They identified nine temperamental traits:

- *Activity level:* how active or sedentary a child is.

- *Distractibility:* the degree of concentration and focus on an activity that a child is not particularly interested in.
- *Intensity:* how strongly a child responds to a given stimulus, either positive or negative.
- *Regularity:* predictability of bodily functions like appetite and sleep.
- *Sensory threshold:* how sensitive a child is to physical stimuli such as sound, taste and touch.
- *Approach/withdrawal:* how a child responds to new situations or strangers.
- *Adaptability:* how easily a child adapts to change in routine and transitions.
- *Persistence:* how long a child perseveres with difficult activities or tasks.
- *Mood:* how a child reacts to the world— is she generally positive or negative?

For any given child, the intensity of each of the traits tends to follow a pattern. Therefore, Thomas and Chess were able to identify three broad temperamental groups based on these nine characteristics. They labeled these profiles as: the "easy child," or one who adapts easily to new situations, has a good attention span and demonstrates regular body rhythms and a positive approach to life; the "difficult child" who is very intense, displays negative responses to change or new situations and has irregular patterns of sleep, eating, etc; and the "slow to warm up child" who initially shows negative responses to many situations, tends to be shy and cautious, but becomes accepting with repeated exposure to similar situations. Fortunately, most babies fall into the "easy child" category. But about 10 percent of children are burdened with a difficult temperament.

It is important to recognize that these categorizations should not be regarded as "good" or "bad." Yet, a child's temperament can become quite a problem if it conflicts with the expectations of parents, teachers or other authorities. For example, if you are intense or ambitious, you might have difficulty accepting that your child is easygoing and malleable. If you are extroverted and sociable, you might find it difficult to understand your child who is shy and withdrawn.

The greatest challenges tend to arise with the "difficult child." Often, an unfortunate circle of negative child-parent interactions develops. Conventional discipline can become increasingly ineffective. Although your love for your child remains strong, the pleasures of parenting can seem much diminished. Interestingly, those characteristics that are perceived as "difficult" in early childhood can become very positive features as your child matures. An intense and obstinate toddler can be very challenging but those very same traits in an adult can translate into an intense individual who is a high achiever.

How do I deal with a difficult temperament? There are no simple solutions. However, recognizing your child's temperament and learning how to nurture her strengths will create a strong foundation for a good parent-child relationship. Clearly defined behavioral limits and well-

established daily routines are helpful, if not essential. Give the difficult child some feedback and offer a preferred alternative to an unpleasant behavior. (For example, "Do you know you're shouting, dear? I can really follow you much better when you talk quietly.") Give rewards for specific good deeds and appropriately punish bad ones. Try not to discipline a child when you are tense or upset. Because parenting the difficult child can be exhausting, you must make sure that you have pleasurable times during the day to recharge your own batteries. Get help from a grandparent or spouse or enroll your child in a recreational program to help reduce the burden of parenting.

Sometimes the situation can be so difficult that parents can't really manage by themselves. In that case, it's obviously best to seek help. Don't be reluctant to call your health care provider. Many resources are currently available to help parents to identify and manage their own, as well as their children's temperaments.

Anxiety Disorders

What is anxiety and when is it a problem? Everyone needs to experience at least some degree of anxiety from time to time. It's a form of protection: anxiety serves as nature's alarm signal. In that sense, anxiety is not only normal, it is essential. The human body responds to potential threats both physically, by increasing the heart or perspiration rate, and emotionally, by feeling a sense of wariness and worry. Thus, it is natural for infants as young as 7 months to appear apprehensive when encountering strangers. It is also normal for toddlers to display some reluctance at being left alone in their rooms at bedtime. Unfortunately, in some children this sense of anxiety can be excessive or occur inappropriately. When that happens, the term "anxiety disorder" is applied. Anxiety disorders are common; approximately 5 percent to 10 percent of children will suffer from them at some time. When anxiety escalates and interferes with normal functioning and social development, you have to get some help for your child.

How are anxiety disorders classified? Health care providers tend to divide anxiety into various subtypes, although some overlap does occur and often children who initially have one type of anxiety disorder, such as separation anxiety, later develop another, for example, school phobia. Included in the types of anxiety disorders are:

- separation anxiety disorder,
- social phobia,
- generalized anxiety disorder,
- obsessive-compulsive disorders,
- specific phobias,
- post-traumatic stress disorder,
- panic attacks.

Anxiety can occur in specific situations, such as leaving a parent (separation anxiety), attending class (school phobia) or participating in social interactions (social phobia). It can be brought on by a particular trigger, such as hearing thunder or seeing a spider (specific phobias).

Sometimes, a child feels anxious pretty well most of the time. This is called a generalized anxiety disorder. Occasionally, temporarily manageable anxiety erupts abruptly, producing a panic attack characterized by sweating, a racing pulse, shortness of breath and panicky fear. Some forms of anxiety appear to be the result of a particularly stressful event, such as the death of a parent or witnessing an accident (**acute** stress disorders and post-traumatic stress disorders), while others coexist with another problem such as a learning disability, attention deficit hyperactivity disorder or depression. Finally, some anxiety disorders are defined by how an individual tries to deal with stress. In the obsessive-compulsive disorder, rigid and repetitive but restrictive routines are used to cope or the child can be immobilized by persistent ideas or fears.

How do I deal with anxiety disorders? If a child seems generally happy and is progressing well, mild transient anxiety can be satisfactorily managed by a little extra support, reassurance and encouragement. If your child has a temperament that tends toward the shy and timid, it is vital to recognize this and respond to her particular behavioral profile. In life, there are "waders," people who tend to slowly warm up to new situations, and there are "divers" who jump right in. Allow your timid child time to get comfortable in a novel situation. You and your child's teacher should nurture confidence by letting her build on life experiences. However, if you have concerns that your child seems unduly anxious, consult her pediatrician or family doctor. Many seemingly anxious behaviors, such as nightmares or transient anxiety when separated, are simply a normal stage of child development. Your child's doctor will reassure you in that regard. It is particularly important that you seek help for any anxiety disorder that significantly interferes with your child's enjoyment of life.

Many families have an easier time seeking advice for physical problems than emotional ones. That should not be the case. Get help.

Treatment of anxiety disorders needs to be a team effort, involving your child, the rest of the family, and her school, physician and therapist.

Therapy will consist of specific types of counseling and, if necessary, medication, neither of which should scare you, although it might at first.

One of the most successful forms of counseling for anxiety disorders is called cognitive-behavioral therapy. In this treatment method, your child will be taught to recognize and better understand the thoughts that result in anxiety. Using a variety of behavioral techniques, typically over 12 to 20 weeks, the therapist will help your child develop improved reactions to the triggers of anxiety. Cognitive-behavioral therapy has been shown to work particularly well for generalized anxiety, post-traumatic stress and obsessive-compulsive disorders. Other forms of therapy that can be tried include relaxation techniques, breathing exercises and systematic desensitization, which can overcome a phobia by gradually confronting the anxiety-provoking stimulus in manageable but increasing amounts.

Few parents want to see their child on drugs, especially pills designed to change behavior. Yet, there are times when the best way to deal with an anxiety disorder is with medication, in association with counseling. A group of drugs best known as SSRIs—**selective serotonin reuptake inhibitors**—have been shown to effectively treat several forms of debilitating anxiety. Among the more commonly prescribed SSRIs are fluoxetine, sertraline, paroxetine, citalopram and fluvoxamine. In many cases, SSRIs have replaced benzodiazepines such as diazepam, alprazolam and lorazepam as first-line treatment for anxiety disorders. On occasion, however, benzodiazepines might still have an important role to play, particularly as SSRIs take a few weeks to work and can actually be associated with a temporary initial increase in anxiety.

Some parents seem unconcerned about the possible side effects of "natural remedies" and might substitute herbal treatments for the doctor-prescribed medication. Unfortunately, the effectiveness of herbal treatments has not been established in large, carefully designed studies, and side effects, sometimes serious ones, can occur. Essentially, when herbs are used to treat illnesses, they should be considered medication. The same standards that are used for traditional drug therapy should apply.

What happens to children suffering from anxiety disorders? Transient mild anxiety in children tends to settle down after a month or two. Those who have significant anxiety disorders also tend to improve over time. But a significant percentage, as high as 30 percent, have been reported to subsequently develop another psychiatric problem, often a different form of anxiety. Furthermore, depression frequently coexists with, or follows, a diagnosis of anxiety and you and the team treating your child should monitor for and manage this in order to best support the anxious child. Finally, those children who display social anxiety are at risk of having difficulty in social settings when they get older. You should understand the importance of helping all children find a zone of comfort from where they can build self-confidence and develop healthy interpersonal relationships.

Bereavement: Dealing with Loss

Death of a family member or friend is one of the most stressful life events that any adult or child can experience. There are several factors that can affect how children react to loss, including age, temperament, the relationship with the deceased person and the stability of the family.

- Children under the age of 2 years have no thoughtful understanding of the concept of death. Very young children perceive death as a form of separation or abandonment, and their response to loss is despair, anger and withdrawal.
- Children aged 2 to 6 are unable to grasp the permanence of death. They believe that wishes come true and that death is reversible. Death can be confused with sleep.
- As children grow older, they gradually come to realize that death is irreversible and inevitable. By 11 years of age, most children have a fairly good understanding of the meaning of death.

How do I explain death to my child? Children should be informed about a death or impending loss with honesty, using language that is appropriate for their age and stage of development. You can incorporate personal family beliefs, such as the existence of heaven, into the explanation of death but do not deceive your child, no matter how good your intentions. Reassure your child that she was not responsible for the death, she could not have prevented it and she herself is not going to die soon. Bereaved children need to know that they will not be abandoned and that a consistent adult will take care of them. You and your family should be aware that showing your own emotions such as shock, anger, sadness and guilt are normal and can help the grieving process.

How do children show grief? As with adults, there is tremendous variation in how children express grief, according to multiple factors like culture, age and personality traits. Grief reactions are often intermittent in children, but they also can be very protracted. Normal grief reactions include crying, anger, sadness, physical symptoms such as abdominal pain and headaches, poor appetite, transient sleep disorders and changes in behavior. Seek professional help if these reactions persist for extended periods; or if a child appears very depressed, persistently angry or unhappy, or becomes socially withdrawn. Other manifestations that should concern you include a decline in school performance, eating disorders and delinquent behavior. Feelings of grief frequently resurface at the time of important milestones like birthdays, religious celebrations, graduations and anniversaries. This is a normal part of bereavement.

Should children attend and participate in funerals? Most experts agree that allowing children to attend the funerals of loved ones is helpful to the grieving process, provided that such involvement is supportive, appropriately explained and compatible with the family's values. Some children want to participate in the planning and associated rituals. However, a child should not be forced to attend against her will.

What kind of help is available for bereaved children? Family members, friends and teachers need to support the grieving child. Understanding and allowing for feelings of sadness and anger will help in the healing process. Many age-appropriate books are available to assist children with bereavement. All family members can be helped by drawing on religious support, as appropriate. Play therapy or art therapy can be helpful, especially for younger children or those who have difficulty articulating their feelings. Seek treatment from a health care provider or clergyperson for children whose grief is severe or persistent. Often, there are programs within hospitals or community centers that offer bereavement counseling for children.

Breath-Holding Spells

What are breath-holding spells? These are episodes during which young children stop breathing and actually lose consciousness for a very short period of time. The key feature of breath-holding spells is the fact that they seem precipitated by anger, fear or pain. Breath-holding spells occur in about 5 percent of children. They are most common in children between 1 and 4 years of age, although they can affect children as young as 2 months of age and as old as 8 years. The frequency of spells varies from several per day to once or twice per year. There is often a family history of breath-holding.

What do breath-holding spells look like? There are two types of breath-holding spells. The cyanotic form, or blue spell, is relatively common. Typically, the child first appears angry or upset, cries out and then holds his breath until she turns blue, becomes limp and loses consciousness. A seizurelike jerking might even occur. Such an episode lasts for several seconds, following which the child's color reverts to normal and she regains consciousness. Pallid spells are less common, and usually occur when a child is frightened or injured. The child becomes pale and limp, and loses consciousness. This type of spell is probably caused by an exaggerated neurological response that results in a sudden

slowing of the heart rate. Once the heart speeds up again, the child regains consciousness.

How do I treat breath-holding spells? Although you might find breath-holding spells terrifying, no specific medical management is needed. During the spells, it is important to ensure that your child does not hurt herself. It is prudent to take her to the doctor to rule out diseases that can have similar symptoms, especially if the spells are of the pallid type.

Most parents of children who experience breath-holding spells, especially those that occur frequently, will try to avoid situations that may provoke anger or injury. Prevention is obviously a good strategy, however, it is also important not to let these spells determine how you will guide or discipline your child.

What happens to children who have breath-holding spells? Breath-holding spells do not cause any long-term neurological or psychological damage, and all affected children will outgrow them by 8 years of age.

Bullying

What is bullying? Bullying can be defined as the repeated and systematic intimidation of others, either physically or psychologically. A bully is an individual who is "frequently cruel or overbearing, especially to people who are smaller or weaker."

Bullying can take on many forms. It can be physical, where the victim is physically assaulted or injured; or emotional, when bullies taunt, humiliate or belittle others; they also threaten and intimidate, or exclude a child from the peer group. Stealing other children's money or possessions is yet another manifestation of bullying. Physical bullying occurs more commonly among boys; emotional bullying is more frequent in girls. Although not always the case, bullies tend to be confident, aggressive individuals who come from homes where aggression is used to resolve conflict. Victims tend to be quieter, passive and less assertive children who do not retaliate, which makes them vulnerable targets. A small number of victims are children with poor social skills, who behave inappropriately and irritate other children.

Bullying can be difficult to detect because victims are typically afraid of being exposed to increasing injury and intimidation if they report the event(s). Since bullying is usually a hidden activity, victims frequently believe that adults are unable to protect them, especially in a busy school environment.

How frequently does bullying occur? The good news is that bullying appears to become less prevalent as children grow older. Studies from Norway have reported that the incidence of bullying is 16 percent to 17 percent in grade 2 and about 5 percent in grade 9. Other studies have suggested that bullying peaks in middle or junior high school years and declines in high school.

What happens to bullies and victims? The most extreme consequences of bullying are tragic: reports of beating deaths or high school shootings are chilling examples of human cruelty. There have also been several incidents of suicide by children who have been bullied incessantly. More often, the results of bullying are more subtle. Its victims are typically unhappy children, who are fearful, anxious and have low

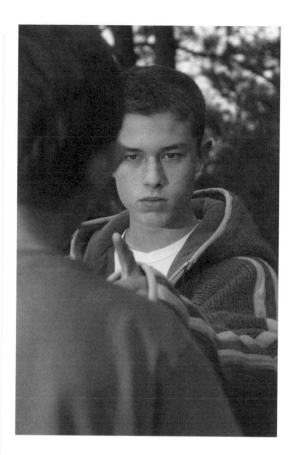

self-esteem. Victims of bullying might try to avoid school and social contact. In the longer term, they might experience difficulties socially, emotionally and academically. Prolonged bullying is associated with more severe adverse reactions on the part of the victim.

Bullies also experience adverse long-term consequences. They tend to grow into aggressive adults who have difficulties sustaining social relationships and are at significantly higher risk of becoming criminals.

Even the so-called bystanders are affected. Some develop fears about becoming victimized, while others may emulate and imitate bullying behavior, especially if the bystanders perceive that there are few or no consequences.

What can I do about bullying? Studies have shown that anti-bullying programs in schools can be extremely effective. School policies should provide strategies to deal with and prevent bullying.

- Define and enforce effective and consistent consequences for bullying behaviors.
- Teach the silent majority, "the bystanders" or children who are aware of bullying but who are afraid to intervene, the importance of assisting and supporting children who are victimized.
- Appropriate adult supervision greatly reduces the incidence of bullying.

The school environment should be one where bullying behavior is not tolerated. Good communication among teachers, parents and students is essential. So is setting a good example in the home.

Child Abuse

This is a very emotional subject. Few things evoke a stronger response than the thought of children being victimized or simply neglected. Because it is usually better to couple such strong emotions with the facts, here is some information to better understand child abuse and neglect.

What is child abuse? Child abuse can be defined as inappropriate physical, sexual or emotional treatment of a child by a parent or caregiver that causes or places a child at risk for short-term or long-term harm. This harm encompasses more than just physical injuries and includes developmental, emotional, psychological, social or behavioral problems.

Child physical abuse includes situations where a family member or caregiver commits an act of physical aggression against a child resulting in harm to the child. This can include the use of a generally accepted mode of physical discipline, but one used excessively. Spanking that results in buttock bruising is an example. Generally unacceptable methods of physical force, such as whipping, kicking or punching are also considered abusive. The amount and type of force applied during discipline that is considered acceptable in our society depends on the age and developmental level of the child, the risk of harm and whether injuries resulted. For example, spanking a 3 year old on the buttocks with an open hand may be acceptable, although not recommended. However, spanking a 2 month old who cannot learn from it, or using a belt at any age is illegal.

Child sexual abuse includes any use of a child by a caregiver for sexual purposes, including sexual touching, sexual intercourse, exposure to sexually explicit materials and exploitation.

Of course, children can be abused emotionally too. There is increasing recognition of the significant impact of emotional abuse on children. Emotional abuse is a pattern of destructive interactions between caregiver and child that might include repeatedly rejecting or degrading, threatening harm or isolating a child or encouraging a child to develop deviant behaviors. Direct or indirect exposure to violence within a family can result in significant emotional harm to a child and is considered a form of child abuse.

Sadly, child abuse is a common problem. Studies that survey adults anonymously for their recollection of prior child abuse indicate that physical and sexual abuse are actually more common than many other childhood medical disorders we have all heard about, including asthma. Despite its frequency, child abuse remains largely a hidden problem that is difficult to recognize and address.

What does child abuse look like? Child physical abuse is typically suspected when injuries occur that are unusual in their location, size, pattern or the age of the child, or do not seem to fit with the explanation that is provided for the injuries. Studies show that bruises and fractures are rarely seen in children who are not yet able to move around independently. Accidental bruises are uncommon in well-cushioned areas, such as the cheeks and the buttocks. Bruises on the ears do not typically result from accidental falls. Life-threatening injuries are rarely the result of common household falls. All of these are considered "red flags" that can indicate abusive injury and indicate the need for further assessment.

Many forms of child sexual abuse do not result in injuries or physical symptoms in children. For example, inappropriate fondling of a child most often does not leave physical marks that a caregiver or medical professional can see. Very rarely, girls can acquire a sexually transmitted infection from sexual contact with an adult, resulting in vaginal discharge (although there are several other possible explanations for vaginal discharge in children). Vaginal bleeding resulting from injuries related to sexual abuse is also very uncommon.

In most situations, it is something a child says that indicates that inappropriate sexual activity has taken place. Studies show that it is very common for children to disclose sexual abuse long after it has occurred, even in supportive and open families. In some situations, a child may not recognize that the contact that has occurred is inappropriate, due to her age or

developmental level, and lack of social awareness. Other factors that can contribute to a child's reluctance to disclose include feelings of guilt or shame, fear of repercussions for herself or her family that might be related to direct threats by the offender, or an attempted previous disclosure that did not go well.

Parents and professionals often become concerned about behavioral symptoms, such as bedwetting, stool withholding, nightmares or crying and clinging at the time of access visits with a parent in a separation or divorce situation. There can be many factors that contribute to these common behaviors in children, which are, in the great majority of cases, not due to child abuse. If these symptoms are particularly severe or begin abruptly, you should consult a health care professional familiar with assessment and management of child behavior symptoms for further assessment of the behaviors, caregiver responses and changes in the child's environment.

Sometimes, sexual behaviors in children, such as masturbating, touching a child or adult, or looking at another's genitalia might make you think sexual abuse has taken place. There is a wide range of normal sexual behavior in children. The presence of these behaviors does not necessarily indicate a child has been exposed to inappropriate sexual contact. For example, children commonly touch their own genitalia at home. Curiosity and lack of social awareness often leads young children to look at nude people, or touch women's breasts. If your reaction is strongly negative, you might be reinforcing these behaviors, particularly in young children.

Certain types of sexual behavior are uncommon in children and might make you more concerned that your child or a child in your care has been sexually abused. These include trying to have intercourse, asking others to do sex acts or inserting objects into the vagina or anus. In some situations, the level of concern is dependent on a child's age; for example, children under 5 may innocently undress to show each other their "private parts," but an older child would typically be aware that this is not appropriate. A thorough assessment of the behaviors in the child, the child's developmental level and other behavioral concerns or physical factors may be required to determine whether sexual abuse has occurred and what to do about it.

In some situations, children might appear less affected by child abuse than an adult would expect. A significant proportion of children who have been abused have no resultant behavioral or emotional symptoms. Studies show that there is no one typical symptom that follows child abuse. In fact, it seems that many children who experienced sexual abuse were not traumatized by it. A number of factors affect a child's response to abuse, including their relationship to the abuser, the frequency and severity of the abuse, the child's age and developmental level, injuries sustained and the response of the adult who received the child's disclosure.

What should I do if I suspect child abuse? It is natural for parents and professionals to find it difficult to consider that a child could have been abused. Often, they come up with other possible explanations. However, recognition of this common problem is of vital importance in preventing further injury to children.

In any situation where child abuse is suspected, you have to make a report to the local child welfare authority, such as child protection services or a children's aid society. It is not necessary for the abuse to be proven; a suspicion is enough to indicate the need for this report. Based on the information provided, child welfare authorities will determine whether they need to investigate. This investigation typically includes collection of information from relevant sources, which might include interviews with the child and caregivers, information provided by health care professionals and assessment of the environment in which the event might have occurred. A decision will be made regarding the risk to the child and the need for further intervention. In the majority of cases, child welfare workers recommend changes to the caregiving environment or provide supportive intervention. Children are removed from their parents' care in only a small minority of cases, where there is deemed to be imminent and significant risk to a child.

Accidental injuries can and do frequently occur in children. Careful assessment is required to distinguish between injuries resulting from accidents, those due to underlying medical conditions and those caused by a caregiver. When child abuse is suspected, a medical assessment should include a careful and detailed medical and injury history and a physical examination. Special tests, such as blood tests, tests for infections or x-rays, might be required to look for a medical disorder or other injuries.

The best form of management of child abuse is prevention. Parenting can have its difficult and frustrating moments—all parents feel challenged at times.

- If you find yourself angry with your child, ensure she is safe, remove yourself to another room, and take some time to cool down.
- If family or friends are available, do not be afraid to ask for their help to get some time to yourself.

- There are many community resources available to provide information and support. Talk to your doctor or local parenting center about stresses and parenting difficulties.
- Learn about your child's development and what to expect at different ages to help you understand your child's behavior and develop effective management strategies.
- Studies indicate that the most effective means of disciplining children do not include physical force, such as spanking, but rather the use of consistent, developmentally appropriate behavioral strategies.

If you suspect a friend or family member is having difficulty coping, talk to her about it and help her get professional support.

If your child has been physically or sexually abused, have a health care professional conduct an assessment of the impact on your child. Children are variably affected by abuse and many factors determine the symptoms that your child might experience. A children's mental health professional familiar with the effects of child abuse will provide support for children who have experienced abuse and for their families. Studies have shown that the most important factor in determining long-term outcomes for children who have experienced abuse is the response of the adult to whom the child discloses. A supportive, believing and protective response has been shown to improve the long-term outcome for these children. It is important to avoid asking the child lots of questions about the events, even though this can be difficult for caregivers who want to know what has happened. Frequently, children report information in small pieces over time, checking for adults' responses before they continue. The best

things you can do for your child in this type of situation are:

- listen,
- support her,
- indicate that you believe her,
- emphasize that what happened is not her fault,
- prevent further abuse, and
- find the right resources to address the problem.

Depression

What is depression? We all get depressed from time to time. Depression, both in children and adults, is characterized by persistent feelings of unhappiness. It becomes a mental illness when it causes significant distress and interferes with an individual's ability to function. Furthermore, these depressive symptoms cannot be accounted for by medical illness, substance abuse or bereavement.

How common is depression in children? About 5 percent of children and adolescents suffer from depression. Children who are under stress or experience significant loss are at increased risk for becoming depressed. Learning or attention difficulties, conduct or anxiety disorders predispose them to depression. Homosexual, pregnant and incarcerated adolescents are also considered to be at higher risk than the general population. Children who have family histories of depression are at higher risk for depressive illnesses.

What does depression look like? The symptoms of depression in children can differ from those of

THE SYMPTOMS OF DEPRESSION IN CHILDREN AND TEENS

- Frequent sadness, tearfulness or crying;
- hopelessness;
- decreased interest in activities, inability to enjoy previously favorite activities;
- persistent boredom, low energy;
- social isolation, poor communication;
- guilt or low self-esteem;
- extreme sensitivity to rejection or failure;
- increased irritability, anger or hostility;
- difficulty with relationships;
- frequent complaints of physical illness such as headaches and stomach aches;
- frequent absences from school or poor performance in school;
- poor concentration;
- a major change in eating and/or sleeping patterns;
- talk of, or attempts to, run away from home;
- thoughts or expressions of suicide or self-destructive behavior.

adults. Some depressed children do not necessarily appear sad in an obvious way. Consequently, a caregiver might not recognize that a child's disruptive behaviors are actually expressions of depression. According to the American Academy of Child and Adolescent Psychiatry, you should seek help if any of the symptoms listed above persist.

What are the complications of depression in children? It is extremely important to recognize and treat depression because the complications can be tragic. Depression can be a fatal disease.

Untreated depression is the leading cause of suicide in teens and adults. Teenagers who suffer from depression are more likely to abuse drugs or alcohol. Early diagnosis and intervention is crucial.

How do you treat depression? Depression is nothing to be ashamed about: it is a disease. Depressed individuals of all ages need not accept the misery that accompanies depression nor let a misguided "stiff upper lip" stand in the way of treatment. You should seek help from a trained mental health professional if you are at all concerned that your child or teenager is persistently depressed. If you are worried about suicide, view the condition as an emergency and obtain help urgently.

The treatment of depression usually involves psychotherapy or medication, or a combination of the two. Psychotherapy should involve the affected child as well as her family.

Several medications are available to treat depression. A family of drugs called **selective serotonin reuptake inhibitors**, (SSRIs) are commonly prescribed. These medications are believed to be safer and more effective than some of the older medications, and are used extensively in adults. However, their use has not been well studied in children and youths. Furthermore, there have been reports that SSRIs might actually increase the risk of completed suicide in depressed adolescents. Other medications such as tricyclic antidepressants and lithium are sometimes prescribed, the latter being particularly useful in "bipolar" disorders in which uncontrollable mood swings tend to occur.

It is also important that your child's health care provider recognize and treat coexisting disorders such as learning disabilities, attention deficit hyperactivity disorder (ADHD) and anxiety.

Common Habits: Thumb Sucking and Nail Biting

THUMB SUCKING

Why do children suck their thumbs? Many infants suck their thumbs even before they are born. Sucking is a comfort for infants and young children. As the child gets older, thumb sucking often becomes a habit. Thumb sucking is normal: some children just have a greater need for oral comfort than others. Children who suck their thumbs aren't neurotic nor should the habit make parents neurotic!

Is thumb sucking harmful for my child? Not for young children. The American Academy of Pediatric Dentistry states that thumb sucking is not a concern until the permanent front teeth begin to emerge, which is usually after 5 years of age. If thumb sucking does persist, pressure on the emerging permanent upper front teeth can cause them to protrude, resulting in problems with her bite. Sometimes, children who suck their thumbs develop calluses or even infections where their teeth contact the skin of the thumb.

Is sucking a pacifier preferable to sucking a thumb? Thumb, finger and pacifier sucking all have similar effects on teeth and jaws. The only advantage of sucking a pacifier is that it is an easier habit to break because it can be physically removed from the child.

How do I treat thumb sucking? The majority of children who suck their thumbs actually stop on their own. It's probably best just to ignore the habit, especially in younger children. Once your child's permanent teeth have erupted, you can use behavioral techniques, such as distraction

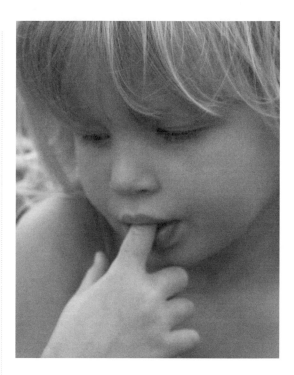

and encouragement (using "star charts"). Some parents apply bad-tasting, nontoxic solutions to the thumb as a deterrent. Occasionally it is necessary for a dentist to insert an oral device, which interferes with sucking, into your child's mouth. Hypnosis might work to stop your child sucking her thumb if she is already motivated to stop.

NAIL BITING

Why do children bite their nails? Nail biting is a very common habit that affects up to one-third of children aged 7 to 10 years. Sometimes it is associated with stress or anxiety, but more commonly there is no obvious reason for nail biting. The habit appears to run in families.

Is nail biting harmful for my child? Unattractive, yes, but harmful, not really. Occasionally the nail bed and cuticle can be damaged, or

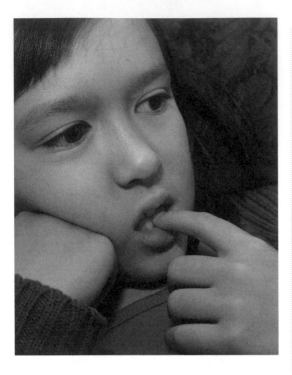

the skin surrounding the nail becomes infected. Children whose fingers and nails are frequently in their mouths can transmit infections to others.

How can I stop my child from biting her nails? As with thumb sucking, distraction and positive reinforcement are helpful techniques. Applying bitter solutions to the fingernails might serve as a reminder and a deterrent to nail biting. Many children will stop biting their nails of their own accord. However, it is estimated that the habit persists in up to 20 percent of adults.

Oppositional and Defiant Behavior

What is oppositional and defiant behavior? Oppositional and defiant behavior refers to the difficult, contrary and even hostile conduct that children can display. During such moments, the child is argumentative, disobedient or confrontational toward authority figures. All children are oppositional at least some of the time. Being occasionally challenging and defiant is regarded as part of normal development, especially in 2- to 3-year-olds, and in teenagers. Similar to most undesirable conduct, it is aggravated by hunger, fatigue, stress and anxiety. Sometimes, this type of behavior is so intense and pervasive that it has a significant impact on how a child socializes with her family, teachers and peers. Instead of being a trait, it becomes a "disorder."

How should I handle oppositional and defiant behaviors? Oppositional and defiant behaviors can prove extremely trying for parents, teachers and caregivers. You have to set clear and appropriate rules and limits, and consistently enforce reasonable consequences. Provide positive reinforcement and praise when it is due—try not to focus and dwell on the negatives. Time out is a helpful technique for both adults and children—take a time out for yourself if you feel that you are aggravating the conflict, and give your child a time out for misbehaving. Avoid angry verbal or physical retaliation: this teaches children that such responses are acceptable. Be a good role model for your children: they model their behavior on that of the adults around them.

When are oppositional and/or defiant behaviors a serious concern? These types of behaviors are considered an "oppositional defiant disorder" when they occur so frequently and persistently that they interfere with a child's social, family and academic functioning, *and* when they are obviously more severe than the behaviors of other children of similar ages. Oppositional defiant disorder occurs in 5 percent to 15 percent of school-aged children and is more common in boys. The cause is unknown, but genetic and environmental factors appear to play a role. Disruptive behaviors occur more frequently in children with difficult temperaments (see pages 191–92), and in dysfunctional families, especially where there is parental psychopathology, stress or substance abuse.

Some children with oppositional defiant disorder have coexisting disorders such as attention deficit hyperactivity disorder, learning disabilities, anxiety or mood disorders, or depression. It is therefore very important that you have children who show signs of oppositional defiant disorder fully assessed by a mental health professional. Identification and treatment of associated disorders can result in improvement in some of the difficult behaviors.

Occasionally, children with oppositional defiant disorder progress to conduct disorder, which is a very serious disorder, including aggression toward people or animals, destruction of property, lying, stealing and other criminal acts.

Treatment of oppositional defiant disorder is complex, and usually involves individual and family therapy, as well as social skills training for the child. All the significant people in your child's life, including teachers, should be included in the treatment program.

Be concerned if these behaviors are ongoing and interfere with normal day-to-day functioning:

- frequent temper tantrums;
- excessive arguing with adults;
- active defiance and refusal to comply with adult requests and rules;
- deliberate attempts to annoy or upset people;
- blaming others for his mistakes or misbehavior;
- often being touchy or easily annoyed by others;

- frequent anger and resentment;
- mean and hateful talking when upset;
- seeking revenge.

Phobias

What is a phobia? A phobia is a persistent, abnormal and irrational fear of a specific thing or situation that compels one to avoid it, despite the awareness and reassurance that it is not dangerous. Psychiatrists define two categories of phobias in children: specific phobias are excessive, persistent fear of an object or situation. There are five subcategories of specific phobias:

- animals;
- natural environment, such as heights or thunderstorms;
- blood, injection, injury;
- situational, for example airplanes or tunnels;
- and "others," for example, costumed characters.

The second category is social phobia, which is an excessive, persistent fear of social situations, such as public speaking; participating in public activities, such as going to public restrooms; and speaking to authority figures, such as teachers.

How common are phobias and what causes them? It has been estimated that 1 percent to 10 percent of children suffer from phobias. They occur more commonly in females of all ages. The cause of phobias is not well understood. In some children, phobias follow a traumatic or frightening experience, such as being attacked by a dog. However, the majority of people with phobias have not actually experienced an adverse event related to their fear. There does seem to be a genetic predisposition to developing phobias.

When should I be concerned that my child suffers from a phobia? Almost all children will report at least one specific fear at some time. For example, many young children are afraid of the dark or of clowns. This is a normal phenomenon. A fear becomes a phobia when it is long lasting (that is, at least six months), unreasonable and persists beyond an appropriate age. Exposure to the object or situation might cause severe anxiety, with symptoms like shaking, sweating, dizziness, shortness of breath or a fear of dying. These reactions are known as "panic attacks." Phobias are often more difficult to recognize in young children who can become extremely clingy or throw temper tantrums. Some children will develop an overwhelming need to avoid that object or situation. Phobias can, therefore, interfere significantly with a child's ability to function normally and participate in her regular activities.

How are phobias treated? If you think your child is suffering from phobias or panic attacks, contact her doctor. Sometimes, minor phobias can be dealt with by gradually desensitizing a child to the frightening object or situation. Mental health professionals manage many children with phobias. Treatment might include a form of psychotherapy called cognitive-behavioral therapy. This method minimizes anxiety by understanding its roots and then converts the trigger from one that provokes anxiety to a more appropriate response. Medications are frequently effective for prevention and treatment

of panic attacks but their use in children tends to be limited to more serious cases.

Separation Anxiety

What is separation anxiety? Separation anxiety refers to the emotional discomfort a child feels about being separated from familiar caregivers. This is a normal phenomenon in infants and, in fact, is one of the earliest behavioral milestones. Some degree of separation anxiety often persists in well-adjusted toddlers and young children.

When is separation anxiety regarded as abnormal? When separation causes severe, persistent anxiety in children and adolescents, it is known as separation anxiety disorder, which occurs in about 4 percent of children and young adolescents. The term "disorder" should only be applied when the symptoms last longer than a month, and cause distress or interfere with social or academic functioning, or employment.

What does separation anxiety look like? Children with separation anxiety disorder may have trouble going to sleep alone at night. Young children might experience nightmares or bedtime fears. Older children have exaggerated fears about getting lost, burglars or that their parents will be harmed, fall ill or die. Children with separation anxiety disorder can develop physical manifestations such as dizziness, nausea, palpitations and stomach aches. They might also display symptoms of depression, such as sadness or apathy. Separation anxiety disorder can result in difficulties with going to school, camp or sleepovers.

What causes separation anxiety? The causes of separation anxiety are not well understood. The temperament of some children is innately cautious. Sometimes, separation anxiety develops after a stressful event, such as a death in the family or a move. Physical or sexual trauma can also precipitate separation anxiety. The disorder sometimes runs in families.

What happens to children who have separation anxiety? "Normal" separation anxiety resolves by 2 years of age. The vast majority of children who have separation anxiety also improve over a period of several months. During times of stress, symptoms can recur. Some children later develop other signs of anxiety or panic disorders. Children with coexisting conditions such as oppositional defiant disorder (see pages 204–205) or attention deficit hyperactivity disorder may have more difficulty coping with separation anxiety. If the disorder persists into adolescence, it is associated with a higher risk of depression.

How do I prevent and treat separation anxiety? Children need to develop a sense of safety in people other than their parents, a feeling of safety in their environment and trust that their parents will return. Allow your cautious child time to warm up to a new situation. Prepare her for a transition to a new activity or event with a plan or schedule. Inform your child when you are leaving, and reassure her that you will return. When children are in stressful or unfamiliar situations, it is important that you be present to provide comfort and reassurance. Sneaking off without telling your child causes loss of trust and increased anxiety. When separation anxiety interferes with normal activities, treatment by a mental health professional may be necessary.

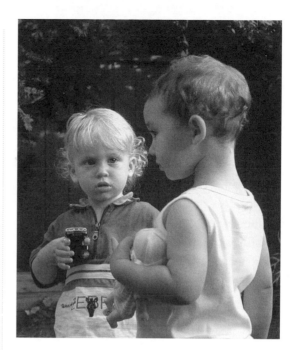

Sibling Rivalry

What is sibling rivalry? Sibling rivalry is the competitive, jealous and conflicting behaviors that occur among brothers and sisters. It is not a new phenomenon: some of the most appalling stories of sibling rivalry date back to biblical times. After all, in the Judeo-Christian tradition the very first siblings were Cain and Abel, and Joseph was sold into slavery by his jealous brothers.

What causes sibling rivalry? Many factors contribute to sibling rivalry. These include position in the family, age, temperament and gender. Sibling rivalry is a concern for almost all parents of more than one child.

How should I manage sibling rivalry? It is important for you to recognize that all children are individuals and, as such, have different needs. It is therefore impossible, and not in the children's best interests, to treat them equally. For example, it is reasonable to allow an older child to go to bed later than a younger sibling. Being fair is not the same as being equal.

You should set different expectations based on each child's unique personality traits and abilities, and not attempt to compare your offspring with each other. Avoid competitive activities between siblings, for example, racing to be ready first in the mornings.

Take the time to address and discuss your children's anger and resentful feelings. It is helpful to discuss and identify sources of conflict. Acknowledge that most people experience those emotions, but that we all need to learn how to resolve conflict and avoid malicious or violent behavior.

When possible, allow your children to settle their own disputes. It is often difficult for a parent to determine who "started" the battle, and many children perceive the parent is taking sides. You might try removing the source of conflict, such as a particular toy, if the young contenders will not share or take turns. Obviously, there are times when it is necessary to intervene, especially if children become physically or verbally abusive.

Praise your children when they interact well and support each other. Try and devote individual "quality" time to each of your children, on a regular basis, even if it is only for a few minutes a day. Let each of your children know that they are all special and loved.

Some circumstances are particularly difficult, for example, if one child is disabled and requires a lot of extra time and attention from caregivers, the other children can feel angry and resentful. Again, it is important to spend time with the "normal" child and, if feasible, to include her in the care of the child with special needs.

Being a good role model is of paramount importance. If you are constantly yelling at each other, it is not realistic to expect children to behave differently! Many useful books about managing sibling rivalry are available, targeted at both adults and children.

Stuttering

What is stuttering? Stuttering is a communication disorder characterized by excessive disruptions in the rate, rhythm and flow of speech. The professional term for stuttering is "dysfluency." Stuttering occurs in a variety of ways. Your child might repeat frequent sounds or syllables (for example, l-l-l-l-l-like). Or she might substitute a weak vowel (for example, luh-luh-luh-like). Or she might prolong a sound (ssssssssnake). Sometimes, the stuttering youngster just appears to get "stuck" on a word.

Is stuttering abnormal? It is common and quite normal for children between 2 and 5 years of age to stutter. Up to 5 percent of children are affected by stuttering for a while but it is persistent in less than 1 percent. Stuttering occurs three times more commonly in boys than in girls, and sometimes runs in families. The vast majority of children who stutter are healthy and developing at an appropriate rate for their age. The actual cause and mechanism of stuttering is not well understood.

When should I worry about my child's stuttering? Professional assessment by a speech and language pathologist should be sought if stuttering persists, or worsens over a period of several months. If your child is older than 5 or she demonstrates anxiety or frustration about her speech, especially if she starts to avoid situations where she is required to speak, you should seek help.

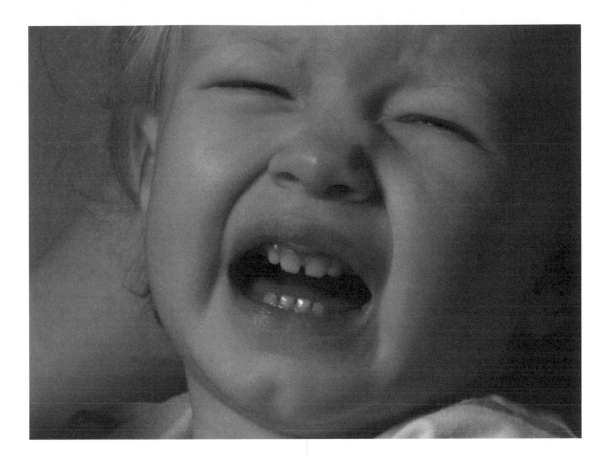

What can I do to help my child who stutters? There are several simple ways in which you can help. Your child should always be allowed to complete her thoughts or sentences, without interruption, prompting or correction. You should model slow and clear speech patterns. It is sometimes helpful to encourage nonverbal activities if your child has more severe difficulties.

Temper Tantrums

What are temper tantrums? Temper tantrums are a normal part of early childhood development. They are intense emotional outbursts during which children appear to be totally out of control; they scream, stomp, hit and throw themselves to the floor. Tantrums occur when a child is unable to express her needs in a socially acceptable manner. She becomes so frustrated that she loses her self control. Temper tantrums usually begin after the age of 12 months, peak between 2 and 3 years of age, and are seldom seen after the age of 4.

Why does my child have temper tantrums? Tantrums are usually precipitated by frustration; they can happen when your child does not get what she wants, when something has been taken away or simply because she does not understand what she is supposed to do. Tantrums tend to be more intense and frequent when a child is anxious, tired, hungry or sick. They are caused by an immaturity in self-regulatory skills and are

WHEN SHOULD I BE CONCERNED ABOUT TEMPER TANTRUMS?

You should seek professional advice if:

- temper tantrums continue to get worse after the age of 4;
- your child injures herself, or others, during tantrums, or destroys property;
- your child holds her breath, or faints, during tantrums;
- you are concerned about associated issues, such as nightmares, delay or regression in development, headaches or abdominal pain, eating or sleeping refusal, anxiety, or excessive clinginess.

more troublesome in those children who are intense by nature. Most young children do not have the verbal skills to express their needs and wants, so they have temper tantrums to communicate anger, frustration or loss of control. Temper tantrums can also occur because a child is seeking attention or testing the rules.

What should I do when my child has a temper tantrum? Most importantly, try to stay calm. Ensure that your child is not going to hurt herself, or anybody else. Appear to ignore the tantrum until she calms down. A short period of "time out" can help her regain control. Some children need to be held, gently but firmly, until they settle down. It is not helpful to try and reason with your child during the outburst. When she has calmed down, it may be constructive to discuss her behavior. Do not reinforce the

behavior by giving in to the tantrums, or offering rewards to stop. Hitting or spanking teaches children that violence is an acceptable way of dealing with anger—don't do it.

How can I avoid temper tantrums? Recognizing and avoiding situations that trigger tantrums generally helps to prevent or at least minimize tantrums. Try to ensure that children don't become overtired or hungry. Stick to routines as much as possible, and have realistic expectations of young children. Prepare your child for change or new situations. Establish the rules and enforce them consistently. For example, if you are taking a small child to the grocery store, do so when she is not tired or hungry, explain what you are planning to do and make it clear that she cannot have all the treats she wants. Provide positive reinforcement for good behavior. Offer choices when it is reasonable to do so. It is acceptable for a child to select clothes to wear that don't match, but crossing the street alone is not a reasonable option.

Tics and Tourette's Syndrome

What are tics? Tics are a particular type of involuntary rhythmic, repetitive event. Some of these are primarily movements, called motor tics, while others are sounds (vocal tics). Motor tics are classified as simple or complex. Eye blinking is a common example of a simple motor tic. Complex motor tics involve more than one muscle group, like facial grimacing or arm flapping. Vocal tics include throat clearing, sniffing and animal sounds like barking. Uttering obscene words or phrases (coprolalia), repeating one's own words (palilalia) and repeating another's words (echolalia) are much more unusual vocal tics.

Tics can be suppressed for variable lengths of time, anywhere from minutes to hours. Some children manage to suppress tics during school hours, and then have multiple frequent episodes once they get home. Typically, however, they cannot be stopped just by willing them instantly away.

Tics are common in children under the age of 10. Up to 20 percent of children will have a tic, which is usually transient. Motor tics are more common than vocal tics. Boys are affected more frequently than girls. In a minority of these children, their tics will persist and become chronic. Some tics progress to Tourette's syndrome.

What is Tourette's syndrome? Tourette's syndrome is a tic disorder that starts in childhood or adolescence, lasts for more than one year *and* is characterized by both motor and vocal tics. The motor and vocal tics do not necessarily occur at the same time, and their severity can vary significantly at different times. Tics can occur daily or intermittently. They can cause marked distress and interfere with social, occupational or other important areas of functioning.

The average age of onset of Tourette's syndrome is 6 to 7 years and, similar to tics, occurs more commonly in males. Tourette's syndrome is rare, affecting approximately 1 in 1,000 children. The tics are aggravated by physical factors like hunger, fatigue and anxiety, as well as by certain drugs or medications, particularly cocaine or stimulants. In the vast majority of children, symptoms improve substantially or disappear with time, usually after puberty. Approximately 5 percent to 10 percent will unfortunately experience persistent or worsening symptoms, continuing into adolescence and adulthood.

What causes tics and Tourette's syndrome? The exact cause is not known. It is believed that tics are caused by abnormalities in certain areas of the brain, and might be related to chemical imbalances in those areas. The chemical substance that has most frequently been incriminated is called dopamine. Genetic factors also seem to play a role.

Do children with tics and Tourette's syndrome have other problems? Children with isolated tics do not usually have associated conditions. However, many children with Tourette's syndrome also have attention deficit hyperactivity disorder (ADHD), learning disabilities and obsessive-compulsive disorder. Some children develop symptoms of depression, sleep problems, social difficulties and self-injurious behaviors because they are frequently teased and socially isolated.

Can tics and Tourette's syndrome be treated? Most children's tics are simple motor tics that are transient and require no specific treatment. When symptoms are disabling, your child might be helped by behavior therapy, relaxation techniques and medication. You might also consult one of a number of community associations established to provide education and support for affected children and their families.

Children with chronic tics or Tourette's syndrome should undergo comprehensive medical evaluation, for a number of reasons. First, it is important to establish that the symptoms are not caused by other neurological or psychiatric conditions, or by medications or illicit drugs. Secondly, coexisting disorders must be identified and treated.

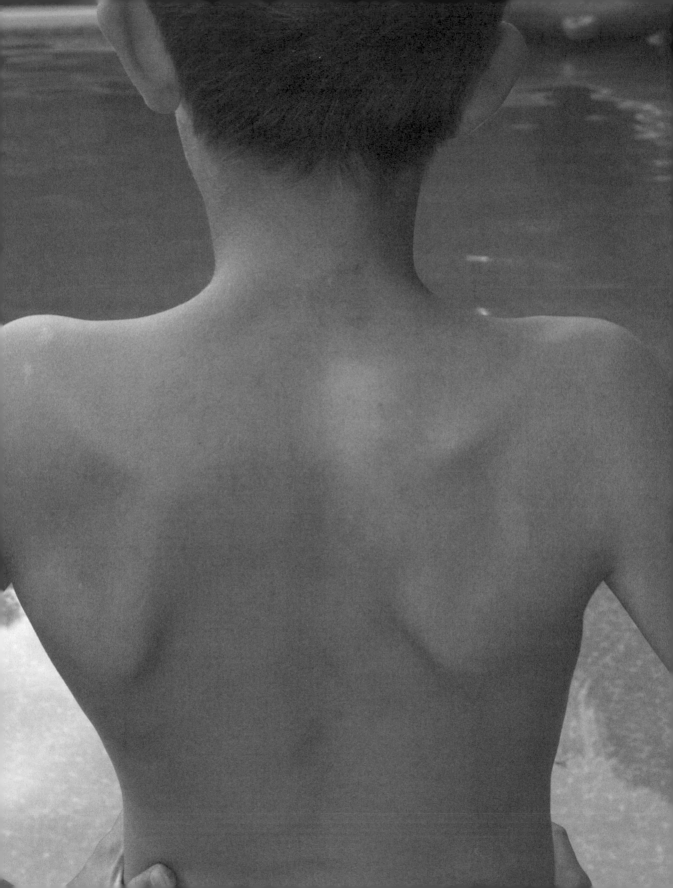

Orthopedic Problems

Growing Pains

What are growing pains? Nobody really knows what causes the recurrent pain so commonly attributed to "growing." The pain, however, is very real and also very common: it affects about 15 percent of children. Although painful, classical growing pains are harmless and not due to a specific disease. If you take your child to the doctor and he feels the history he takes is not typical, he must exclude serious problems.

What do growing pains look like? There is a typical pattern of growing pains making them fairly easy to recognize:

- The pain occurs mainly in the thighs or calves and is severe enough to make children cry.
- It is most common in children 3 to 5 and also 8 to 12 years of age.
- The pain tends to come and go but is worse at night.
- Usually it involves both legs.
- Typically, it occurs several times per week and lasts for months.

When should I take my child to the doctor? The following clues suggest that the pains may be more serious than simple growing pains:

- your child walks with a limp;
- there are signs of inflammation on her legs, for example, redness, warmth or swelling;
- the pain seems worse when the legs are moved or massaged;
- the pain is in one leg only, particularly if localized to a small area;
- the pain is worse with regular daytime activities.

How do I treat growing pains? First, reassure your child (and be reassured yourself) that the pain is temporary and that he will outgrow it. Massaging or pain-relief medications, such as children's acetaminophen or ibuprofen, should be effective. In one research study, children who were taken through some stretching exercises by their parents reported less pain than those who didn't stretch. However, it is not clear if the improvement was due to the emotional comfort of special time with parents or if there was really some physical relief afforded by the stretching.

Club Foot

What is it? The term "club foot" or, more formally, talipes equinovarus, refers to a condition present at birth in which the position of the foot is abnormal.

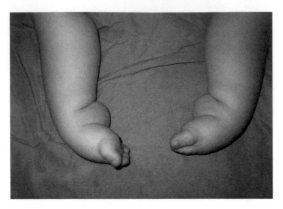

CLUB FOOT

The affected foot (or feet) is significantly inverted so that the outside edge of the foot points straight down and can't be moved back to the neutral walking position.

Specifically, the whole foot is inverted, that is, turned inward. The forefoot is angled inward (varus deformity) and the ankle is positioned so that the foot points downward, placing the toes lower than the heel (equines deformity). About 1 in 1,000 children are born with club foot. A small number of such children may have other health issues, such as **spina bifida**; however, children born with club feet are usually completely healthy otherwise.

What does club foot look like? The affected foot (or feet) is significantly inverted so that the outside edge of the foot points straight down and can't be easily moved back to the neutral walking position. If you can easily move the foot into the normal walking position, your child does not have club foot and no treatment is required.

How do you treat club foot? Early treatment shortly after birth is important to get the best results. The first step the orthopedic doctor will take is to gently move the affected foot toward the normal position and keep it there in a plaster cast for a couple of weeks. Every one to three weeks the cast is removed, the foot is positioned

more toward normal and the cast is reapplied. At about 3 months of age, an x-ray may be taken and a decision is made about surgery. About 75 percent of children with a club foot will require surgery. The operation involves lengthening the tendons on the inner side of the ankle and holding the foot in place temporarily with metal pins or another cast. Following casting, and in some cases surgery, your child may be given removable splints to wear up until age 1 or 2.

Despite your and your doctor's best efforts, some children with club feet will end up with a foot that works just fine but appears smaller and feels stiffer and a calf that is thinner on the affected side. About 25 percent of children may need another operation later in life. Most children with club feet, if treated early, will have feet that look and function entirely normally.

Why Aren't My Child's Legs Straight?

Children don't have perfectly straight legs. Some legs just curve more than others. This might worry you but, most often, it shouldn't. Usually, children's legs get straighter with age and very few require medical treatment. In fact, doctors now believe that for the conditions described below, trying to straighten legs or feet with braces, inserts or orthopedic shoes may be unnecessary, ineffective, uncomfortable, expensive and even harmful. This next section deals with common normal shapes of legs and feet to help you decide when, and when not, to worry. There are two basic types of problems: bones that seem to angle too much (knock-knees and bow-legs) and limbs that seem to angle excessively at the foot (metatarsus adductus), shin (anterior tibial torsion) or thigh (femoral anteversion).

KNOCK-KNEES AND BOW-LEGS

What are knock-knees and bow-legs? Bowing of the legs (genu varum) or knock-knees (genu valgum) are often seen as a part of the normal stages of growth in some children. Bow-legs are usually first noticed in infants and toddlers when they begin to walk. Bow-legs often overcorrect with time to become knock-knees. Knock-knees are usually seen in children between the ages of 3 and 5. The knock-knees then improve with further growth. They are usually not an issue by the time your child is 8 to 10. Although bowing and knock-knees are seen during normal stages of growth, bowing of the legs, rarely, can be due to a bone disease such as rickets. Rickets is seen most commonly in exclusively breast-fed infants who do not receive vitamin D supplementation. This is more likely to occur in dark-skinned families if the mother has avoided sunlight. If such is the situation, you should take your child to a pediatrician.

What do knock-knees and bow-legs look like? Most adults with straight legs can stand with their feet together and will find that their ankles and knees are pretty close to touching each other. If a person has bow-legs, there will be a big space between the knees. In knock-knees, the knees will touch but there will be a space between the ankles.

How are knock-knees and bow-legs treated? Generally, neither bow-legs nor knock-knees cause problems and therefore do not need treatment at all. Only rarely is a disease present.

However, if your infant or toddler shows the following signs, the bow-legs might be due to a rare problem requiring treatment:

- pain;
- a delay in reaching developmental mile-

stones such as sitting, crawling or walking;
- bowing only in one limb;
- worsening of the bowing instead of the expected improvement that occurs between the ages of 1 and 2.

Remember, although bow-legs typically should begin to improve in the second year of life, knock-knees might not begin to improve until after age 5.

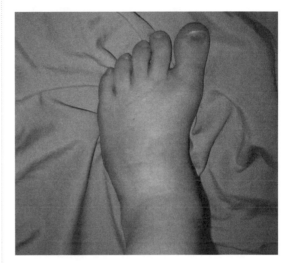

The forefoot angled inward, producing in-toeing.

TOEING IN AND TOEING OUT

Toeing In
What is toeing in? Some children's feet point inward and some don't. Most feet tend to straighten with time. In-toeing can result from any or all of the following:

- an in-turned forefoot, called "metatarsus adductus";
- an in-turned or slightly twisted lower leg, called "internal tibial torsion";
- an in-turned hip, called "femoral anteversion."

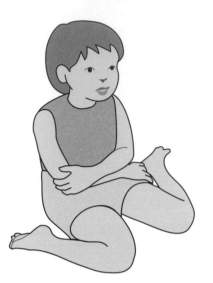

"W" SITTING POSITION
Discouraging your child from sitting in the "W" position may help to prefent further in-turning of the hip.

All of these conditions are normal variants and all straighten, often completely, as your child gets older.

What does in-toeing look like? Children with in-toeing have been described as "pigeon-toed" and walk with their feet pointing inward to varying degrees. Successful athletes are said to do well at sprinting if their feet turn in a tiny bit. You might want to have a look next time a track meet is televised.

How is in-toeing treated? Most in-toeing does not require bracing, special shoes, inserts or surgery. However, on occasion, metatarsus adductus will need correction if the deformity is very rigid. Some doctors believe that encouraging your children to avoid the "W" sitting position may do a little bit of good to help prevent further in-turning of the hip (see illustration above).

Toeing Out

What is toeing out? The reverse of in-toeing is of course out-toeing. Children with out-toeing also tend to improve as they get older. The usual cause is a twisting outward of the lower leg, called "external tibial torsion." This is a normal healthy variant. Only very rarely is out-toeing related to an orthopedic problem.

Consult your child's doctor if:

- Your child complains of leg or hip pain.
- The deformity worsens with age. It should get better.
- Your child seems to trip and fall much more than his peers.

Developmental Dysplasia of the Hip (Congenital Dislocation of the Hip)

What is developmental dysplasia of the hip? The hip is a ball-and-socket joint in which the ball-shaped top of the thighbone, the head of the femur, fits into the socket of the pelvis, or acetabulum. Developmental dysplasia of the hip (DDH), formerly known as congenital dislocation of the hip, is a malformation of the joint in which the hip socket is too shallow to properly contain the head of the femur. When this happens, the hip joint is said to be dysplastic and the hip is prone to dislocation. In severe cases, it can be crippling if untreated. The condition can run in families and is more common in girls and in children born in the breech (bottom first) position.

What does it look like? The signs of hip dysplasia in a newborn can be very subtle. Your doctor will examine your newborn's hips as part of the routine newborn assessment. If a subtle "clunk" from

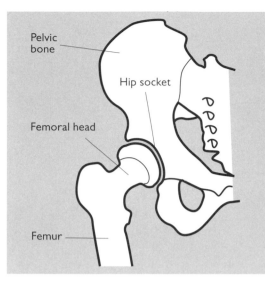

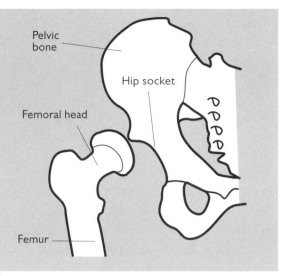

DEVELOPMENTAL DYSPLASIA OF THE HIP:
NORMAL HIP JOINT

The hip is a ball-and-socket joint in which the ball-shaped top of the thighbone, called the head of the femur, fits into the socket of the pelvis, or acetabulum.

DISLOCATED HIP JOINT

Dysplasia of the hip is a malformation of the joint in which the hip socket is too shallow to properly contain the head of the femur.

a possibly dislocatable hip is felt during opening and closing the hip joints, your child's doctor will likely repeat the exam in about a week to see if he can reproduce it. If the clunk sensation is still present, or if the finding was clearly out of the ordinary at birth, an ultrasound will likely be ordered to look at the depth of the hip socket.

    If the problem is not treated, in older infants, the stronger muscles and tendons around the hip joint tend to hold the hip in the dislocated position. This position does not allow the hip to function properly, making it difficult to open (abduct) the thigh; for example, when changing diapers. One leg can appear shorter since the dislocation tends to be upward. He might limp and the skin folds under the buttocks will be asymmetric. If your doctor feels that your baby might have a developmental dysplasia of the hip, he will make a referral to an orthopedic surgeon. Routine ultrasound screening for

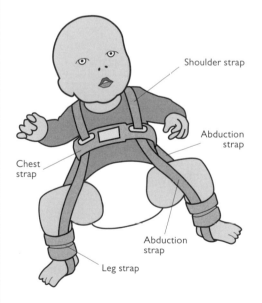

PAVLIK HARNESS FOR DYSPLASTIC HIPS

The Pavlik harness, which holds dysplastic hips in a "frog leg" position, allows the socket to develop deeply enough to hold the head of the femur in place.

DDH is controversial. It is certainly necessary in babies with an abnormal examination, that is, who have a palpable click or clunk feeling on hip exam.

How do you treat dysplasia? Dysplastic hips, when identified early, are treated for a period of months with a special removable harness or brace, such as the Pavlik harness, to hold your child's hips in a "frog leg" position. This allows the socket to form deeply enough to hold the head of the femur. When hip dysplasia is identified in the newborn period and treated with this special harness, chances are very high that surgery won't be necessary and your child will walk and run normally. When the hip problem is diagnosed after the first few months of age, surgery often becomes necessary. An orthopedic surgeon will perform a procedure to create a deeper socket.

Osgood-Schlatter Disease

What is Osgood-Schlatter disease? Osgood-Schlatter disease is a bone condition that is not dangerous but it is painful. The problem arises from a bump, called the "tibial tubercle," that is situated just below the knee on the upper part of the larger shinbone, the tibia. This is where the tendon of the large upper leg muscle, the quadriceps, connects to the lower leg. When the quadriceps muscle contracts, it pulls the tendon. This, in turn, pulls on the tibia and the lower leg is straightened at the knee. In some children, this repeated yanking causes some inflammation at the site of the tibial tubercle. Active, growing limbs are particularly vulnerable to this type of condition.

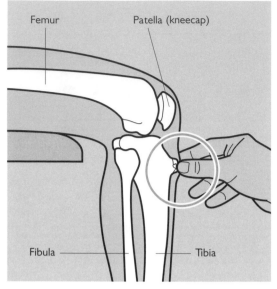

OSGOOD-SCHLATTER DISEASE
Pain and often a bump can be felt in the front of the knee just below the kneecap at the site of the tibial tubercle.

Osgood-Schlatter disease is most common in active preteen and teenage boys.

What does Osgood-Schlatter disease look like? Your child might notice a tender painful swelling on the front of the knee just below the kneecap at the site of the tibial tubercle. The pain is most intense when putting larger loads on the knee joint; for example, when squatting and climbing stairs.

How do you treat Osgood-Schlatter disease? Periods of rest can help with the pain. So do changes in certain activities that reduce the yanking on the tubercle; for example, switching playing positions in baseball from catcher to second base. Ongoing athletic activity is generally not harmful to children with Osgood-Schlatter disease and you should not discourage your child from this. Pain control measures are unlikely to speed the healing, but at least they will reduce the pain. Measures that may afford some pain relief include:

- icing after athletic activities;
- over-the-counter medications such as ibuprofen;
- knee pads to protect the area;
- low-impact strengthening and flexibility exercises.

With time, the symptoms eventually subside and the condition itself tends to disappear permanently with adulthood.

Perthes Disease (Legg-Calve-Perthes Disease)

What is Perthes disease? Drs. Legg, Calve and Perthes independently wrote about this condition about 100 years ago, but the full name is often shortened to "Perthes disease." It is a painful condition of the hip that most commonly affects 2- to 12-year-old boys. The round top of the thighbone that fits into the hip socket is called the head of the femur. It requires a steady blood supply for growth. If that blood supply is affected by illness or injured, part of the head of the femur is damaged and some tissue will die. The bone at the head of the femur may become slightly flattened and fragmented and hip movements become painful. Over time, usually in a few years, new bone replaces the old, dead tissue. Although healing occurs, some children will go on to develop arthritis of the hip as adults.

What does Perthes disease look like? Children with Perthes disease may develop a noticeable limp

without having injured their leg. They usually complain of hip pain or even of pain in the thigh or knee where the hip pain can be transferred. An x-ray might show the flattened and fragmented head of the femur. X-rays of the hip can help your doctor classify the disease into five distinct stages:

1) cessation of growth at the end of the head of the femur,
2) small fractures,
3) fragmentation,
4) re-ossification (new bone growth),
5) healed or residual stage.

How do you treat Perthes disease? The treatment of Perthes disease depends upon the risk factors for a poor result. Boys do better than girls and younger children do better than older. Observation alone with no active treatment is appropriate for children younger than 6 at onset. These children must be monitored closely, but generally do not develop arthritis or any other related problems.

In higher risk patients, the orthopedic surgeon will make sure the femoral head is positioned within the hip socket, either with surgery or a brace. Examples of high risk include:

- the head of the femur is not contained as it should be within the hip socket;
- the age at onset is 6 years or older (possibly 5 years in girls);
- there is extensive damage to the femoral head putting it at risk of dislocating out of the hip socket.

Although the x-rays of the hips of affected children usually never quite return to normal, most of the children with Perthes disease eventually walk and run without pain and do not develop arthritis in later life.

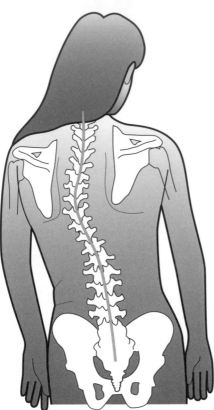

SCOLIOSIS

Scoliosis is a sideways curvature of the spine that usually affects preteens and teens.

Scoliosis

What is scoliosis? Scoliosis is a sideways curvature of the spine that usually affects preteens and teens. Usually, children with scoliosis have no other medical problems. Rarely, however, they might have an associated underlying bone or neurological disease that involves the spine. The curve can be quite subtle; however, it often worsens with time, at least until growth is fully completed. Scoliosis in its milder forms can be a cosmetic problem only. In severe disease, the child's lung function can be affected leading to heart problems. This latter scenario is extremely uncommon.

What does scoliosis look like? In the milder forms of scoliosis, if you look at a child's back when he is standing straight, you might not notice the curvature. However, if he bends over with his legs straight, one side of the back will appear higher than the other. Your child's doctor should screen your school-aged child annually for signs of scoliosis. If your doctor suspects scoliosis, special x-rays will be taken and the degree of the curvature, or "Cobb's angle," will be measured.

What does it not *look like?* The hunchback of Notre Dame had something called severe **kyphoscoliosis**. Kyphosis is a front-to-back curvature of the upper spine, whereas scoliosis is a side-to-side curvature. Kyphoscoliosis is a combination of both. A small amount of kyphosis in the upper spine is normal. Severe kyphosis is most commonly seen in the elderly in association with osteoporosis.

How do you treat scoliosis? There are guidelines about when to treat children with scoliosis. These guidelines take into consideration the age of the child and the degree of the curvature. If a child is close to the end of his growth, that is, past puberty, and the curve is mild, likely no treatment will be required. If the child is younger, or the curvature is more significant, treatment will be offered.

Most cases of scoliosis are mild and do not require treatment, only regular checkups to watch for how it progresses. Lightweight, removable braces that can be worn under clothing are the mainstay of treatment for more significant scoliosis. In severe scoliosis, your child might require surgery to fuse some of the spinal bones together. If the orthopedic surgeon feels that fusion is unlikely to be sufficient to correct and prevent further curvature, steel rods may need to be surgically placed parallel to the spinal column to support it. Most likely, if your child has scoliosis, he will never need surgery.

Spondylolysis and Spondylolisthesis

What are they? Spondylolysis is a disorder of the spine in which there is fragmentation in a spinal bone, or vertebra. Instead of a single vertebra being present, the bone is in two pieces. This fragmentation typically happens in a vertebra of the lower back where the bony ring surrounds the spinal cord. The problem occurs for unknown reasons and usually without any history of injury. Most often, spondylolysis doesn't hurt or cause any other symptoms. Sometimes, one of the fragments will slip forward. When this happens, the condition is called "spondylolisthesis"—definitely a tongue twister of a name. If the vertebra slips, your child will probably have significant symptoms. In rare cases, the slippage causes nerve compression. Note that a slipped, broken vertebra, in other words, spondylolisthesis, is not the same as a "slipped disk," but the symptoms can be similar. The disk commonly referred to is the cartilaginous shock absorber that sits between the vertebrae.

What does spondylolysis look like? In its mildest form, children with this disorder do not have any symptoms. The condition is discovered coincidentally when the child has an x-ray for other reasons. Children with spondylolisthesis, often adolescent athletes—commonly dancers, gymnasts or football players—complain of back pain. Very rarely, children with this disorder may have numbness,

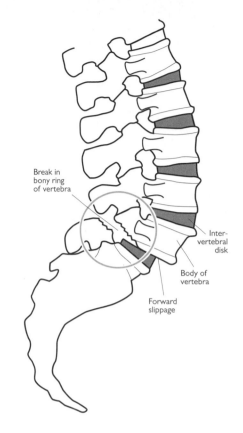

Break in bony ring of vertebra

Inter-vertebral disk

Body of vertebra

Forward slippage

SPONDYLOLISTHESIS
Spondylolisthesis is a condition in which a break in both sides of the ring allows the body of the vertebra to slip forward.

weakness in the legs or difficulty urinating. Back pain is a very common complaint in adults but less so in children. It should be taken seriously and prompt a visit to the doctor.

How do you treat spondylolysis and spondylolisthesis? Your child should take a break from sports and, when necessary, wear a brace to relieve the symptoms. He probably won't need surgery unless his symptoms are persistent or severe, or in the rare case where there are signs of spinal cord injury. He could participate in athletic activities guided by the degree of pain he experiences.

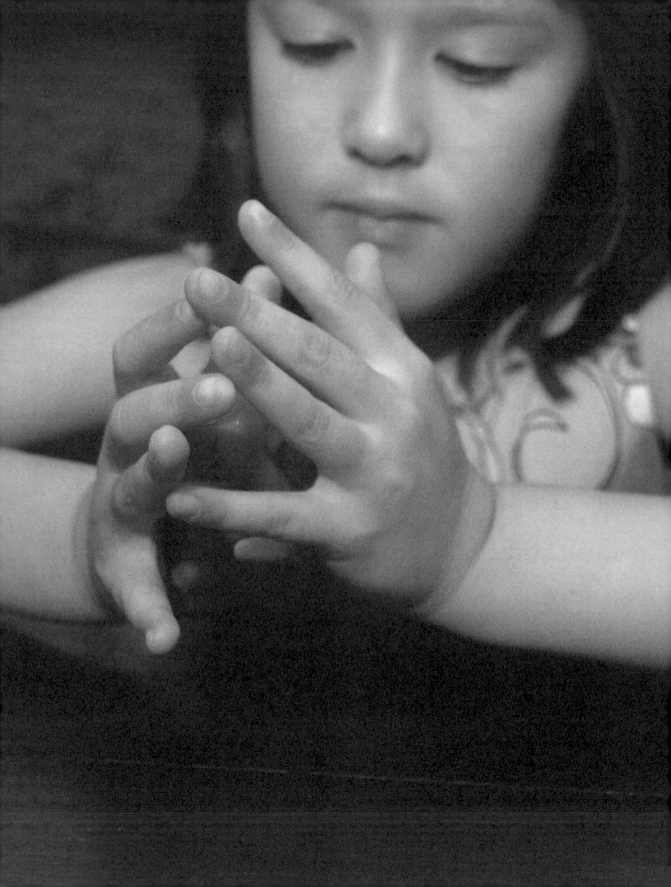

Rheumatological Diseases

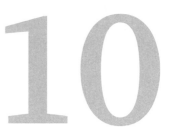

Autoimmune Disease

Human beings are equipped with a complex defence system to protect them from infection and foreign proteins. This immune system is truly a marvel, but an imperfect one. It occasionally makes mistakes. In some individuals, the immune system attacks the very body it is designed to defend.

The autoimmune disorders are a group of diseases in which parts of the body are damaged by a faulty or mistaken immune response. For example, this autoimmune process might occur as a result of an infection in which the immune system, when trying to destroy some germ, also damages normal body cells that resemble the germ immunologically. The result of this process might be just a mild and brief appearance of a rash that never returns. Or there may be severe and chronic disease. It is unclear why some forms of autoimmune disease tend to be brief and self-limited illnesses while others tend to be chronic or recurrent ones.

Autoimmune disease can involve almost every organ in the body. Yet, there are two target tissues that seem particularly vulnerable to an altered immune response: the blood vessels and the joints. Autoimmune disease that causes inflammation of the blood vessels is called a

"vasculitis" and those involving the joints give rise to some types of "arthritis." An example of this is rheumatoid arthritis where the joint injury is part of an autoimmune process, compared to osteoarthritis in which the damage is due mainly to wear and tear on the joints.

Henoch-Schonlein Purpura (HSP)

What is Henoch-Schonlein purpura? HSP is a type of vasculitis—an autoimmune disease primarily involving the blood vessels. There are different variants of vasculitis depending on which type of blood vessel is inflamed and where in the body the inflammation occurs. Certain forms of vasculitis are more common in adults and others more common in childhood. HSP is generally a childhood vasculitis in which the smaller blood vessels of the skin, joints, bowels and kidneys become inflamed. For some reason, it is the lower half of the body that seems to be most commonly affected. The exact trigger for HSP is unknown, although it sometimes follows a viral illness, for example the common cold. Toddlers and school-aged children are affected more frequently than infants or teens. HSP is generally a self-limited, one-time illness but recurrences can happen in rare cases.

What does HSP *look like?* The inflammation of the tiny blood vessels in the skin leads to leakage of blood and visible bruising. This bruising usually involves the buttocks, legs and feet. The bruises are called purpura. Often, the inflammation is great enough to produce a palpable swelling so that the purpura can actually be felt. Most children with HSP tend to have an arthritis, that is, inflammation in and around their joints, particularly the ankles and knees. Many affected children also have abdominal pain. At times, it can be severe enough to mimic appendicitis. Sometimes, the inflammatory swelling in the wall of the bowel can even cause part of the gut to actually telescope upon itself, creating a condition known as **intussusception**. (see pages 374–75). About half of the children with HSP will have traces of blood in their urine due to kidney involvement, but serious damage from the inflammation, or **glomerulonephritis**, is rare.

Other conditions can also cause purpura. If there is any blood in your child's sputum or if she has a nosebleed during an illness with what appears to be HSP, take her to her doctor so a more serious disease, Wegener's granulomatosis, can be ruled out. The doctor might take a skin biopsy as part of the diagnosis, but she will rarely need to if the signs and symptoms are classic. Generally, the doctor will order a blood count to make sure that your child's platelets (the cells of the blood that prevent bleeding) are not low. Low numbers of platelets are not seen in HSP but are seen in other conditions that can resemble it. She will also order a urinalysis and specific blood work to look at kidney function. In most cases, other than some traces of blood in the urine, these tests will be normal.

How do you treat HSP? Fortunately, the vast majority of children with HSP recover entirely in several days without specific treatment. The reported incidence is 15 cases per year for every 100,000 children. In fact, it is unclear whether any treatment affects the course of the disease. Pain relief is the main treatment, both for the abdominal discomfort and for the joint pain. Some children need to go into hospital for fluid replacement and nutritional support if they are vomiting or not eating and drinking. Some children will be bedridden briefly because of joint pain. Severe abdominal involvement, including pain or frequent vomiting, is sometimes treated with anti-inflammatory steroid medication. If there were traces of blood found on urine testing, your child will have surveillance urine tests to ensure that this gets better over a period of time, often taking as long as two years. Remember, complete recovery is the norm for this illness.

Juvenile Rheumatoid Arthritis (JRA)

What is juvenile rheumatoid arthritis? The term "arthritis" refers to a condition in which there is inflammation of one or more joints. There are many forms of arthritis, some of which are transient and some of which are chronic. Some are due to mechanical injury, others due to infection and some others due to unknown causes. Juvenile rheumatoid arthritis (JRA) is the common form of chronic childhood arthritis. It is caused by an autoimmune process of unknown origin. The resulting inflammation can damage joints and, sometimes, other tissues. In its severe forms, JRA will cause chronic disease and disability but it is not a fatal condition.

JRA is found in at least 1 child in 1,000. There are several types of JRA affecting children from infancy to adolescence. One or more joints might be involved and the joint damage varies in severity and persistence. Some children are affected for life while others have more mild disease that gets better. The tissues commonly involved depend on which type of JRA your child has. All forms involve the joints but some also affect the eyes. In one variant of JRA, systemic onset or Still's disease, your child will have a fever and perhaps also inflammation of the liver, spleen or the linings of the lung, heart or abdomen.

Affected children fulfill the diagnostic criteria if the arthritis began before the age of 16 years, has persisted for more than six weeks, and is not better accounted for by mechanical injury or another disease process.

JRA has traditionally been classified into different types depending on,

- the number of joints affected,
- whether or not certain markers on blood testing are present, and
- whether or not there is "systemic onset" disease as described above.

"Pauciarticular" arthritis refers to JRA in which four or fewer joints are affected. "Polyarticular" JRA refers to the situation in which five or more joints are affected. "Rheumatoid factor positive (RF+ve)" JRA is a type defined by the presence of a marker in the blood (rheumatoid factor or RF) in which the JRA closely resembles adult rheumatoid arthritis.

In addition to JRA there are other forms of chronic childhood arthritis including arthritis associated with psoriasis and arthritis associated with tendon insertion inflammation and back disease. More recent classification schemes include these other forms of arthritis and group them together with JRA as juvenile arthritis (JA).

What does juvenile rheumatoid arthritis look like?
Children with JRA can become symptomatic in infancy but more often the symptoms show up in childhood. Often, they have complained of morning stiffness. In young children, it tends to be the large joints such as the knees that become painful. Such children might refuse to walk. A visit to the doctor can reveal swelling and fluid (effusion) in the joint. In some children, only one joint is affected at first, making the diagnosis difficult because there are many conditions that can cause a single joint to become painful and swollen. A diagnosis of chronic JRA requires that the child has had signs and symptoms for at least six weeks.

Other children are taken to their doctor because of a rash and fever. This "systemic onset JRA" can continue to produce fever and rash for months or even years. Again, it is challenging at first for the doctor to make the diagnosis because both the rash and the fever tend to come and go. It sometimes seems that the rash appears in the evening just after doctors' offices close.

After a period of time of the child having persistent signs and symptoms of joint inflammation the doctor can more easily make the diagnosis. X-rays and blood tests can aid the diagnosis.

One blood test in particular is of special importance. The **antinuclear antibody** (ANA) is an antibody that is misguidedly aimed at elements in the nucleus of a person's own cells. If present, it identifies an increased risk of significant eye inflammation called "uveitis." The uveitis of pauciarticular JRA can actually produce more permanent damage, specifically impaired vision, than the arthritis itself, which frequently "burns out" (subsides) with no lasting joint injury. Normal healthy individuals and children with JRA who do not develop eye disease can still have a positive ANA test. So the test is most useful as a predictor if the test is negative. Children with a negative ANA are much less likely to have the chronic eye inflammation associated with JRA.

About half of the children affected by JRA will eventually become disease-free during childhood. This is particularly likely to happen with the pauciarticular form of the disease. Although JRA is not fatal, some children and adolescents may suffer considerably with both physical disability and psychological difficulties as a result. Some children might have significant restriction of movement of some joints and muscle weakness limiting activities of daily living. This latter scenario fortunately is not the usual one. Infrequently, there can also be small leg-length differences as the more affected leg can grow differently.

Older children with polyarticular (more than four joints affected) JRA resemble adults with rheumatoid arthritis. Knuckles swell, hand muscles diminish in size and strength, and the fingers bend slightly sideways.

How do you treat JRA? There is no cure for JRA, quick or otherwise. Fortunately, there is effective treatment to reduce joint inflammation and limit its consequences.

Your child can have anti-inflammatory medications, specifically corticosteroids, injected into an inflamed joint, which will offer prompt and often long-lasting pain relief and improved function. This is one of the key treatments for those children with only a few affected joints.

Non-steroidal anti-inflammatory drugs (NSAIDS) such as naproxen have been shown to be very effective at reducing pain and inflammation. The most common reason for treatment failure is stopping the medication before it has had a chance to work, which can take as long as six weeks. Your child might have an upset stomach and rarer side effects, but it is uncommon that he won't benefit overall from treatment with NSAIDS.

A number of other options are available for those children in whom NSAIDS and joint injections are insufficient to control disease. So-called disease-modifying anti-rheumatic drugs include methotrexate and sulfasalazine. These medications are used as "second line" therapy because their side effects are outweighed by their therapeutic effects only in the case of moderate to severe disease. Promising newer treatments, such as etanercept, which involve giving specific antibodies directed at interrupting the autoimmune process, hold promise for the future.

What can I do to help my child with JRA? You and your child can receive education and family support in the setting of a clinic specialized in the treatment of children with JRA. Studies have identified the main educational needs of affected families to be:

- understanding the particular child's prognosis;
- understanding and coping with the "empathy-resentment-guilt cycle" that family members of children with chronic illness can experience;

- learning how to deal with the school environment (to accommodate any physical limitations and the social consequences of the illness);
- learning how to manage joint pain and stiffness; and
- learning how to help preserve joint function.

Your child might have physiotherapy, often employing hydrotherapy (stretching and exercising in warm water), to help reduce pain and improve function without jarring her arthritic joints. She might wear splints at night and often during repetitive activities particularly if her wrists are affected, to reduce pain and ultimately improve range of motion. She does not need orthotics for her feet; these have not been shown to reduce pain or disability in children with JRA.

Your child should be screened regularly for uveitis if she is in the high risk group that has the pauciarticular form of JRA and a positive ANA blood test at a younger age. She will need to see an ophthalmologist every three months because there is effective treatment if uveitis is caught early.

Kawasaki Disease

What is Kawasaki disease? Kawasaki disease (KD) is another form of vasculitis, an autoimmune disorder involving the blood vessels. In this disease, both the small and medium-sized blood vessels are affected, particularly in children under 4 years of age. The exact trigger for KD is still unknown. The tissues commonly involved include the mouth, eyes, skin, heart and lymph nodes. The vast majority of children recover completely with proper treatment, but early identification and targeted treatment is crucial.

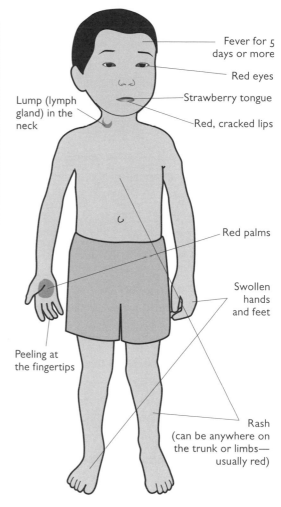

KAWASAKI DISEASE
The typical features of Kawasaki disease.

The worry for some affected children, particularly those who are not treated, is that they will develop long-standing damage to the coronary arteries, the arteries that supply the heart muscle. In fact, although Kawasaki disease is relatively uncommon, it has become the leading cause of acquired heart disease in children.

What does Kawasaki disease look like? At first, Kawasaki disease can mimic a common viral infection. However, it is much less common. It is the sustained fever, particularly in a young child with irritability and a rash that should raise the possibility of KD. To fulfill the widely accepted criteria for this diagnosis a child would have fever for more than five days *and* at least four of the following:

1) Eye changes: redness of the whites of the eyes but without any discharge.
2) Mouth changes:
   - dry, red, cracked lips,
   - "strawberry tongue,"
   - red mouth/throat.
3) Changes to the hands and feet:
   - redness on the palms and soles,
   - swelling or puffiness of the skin over the hands and feet,
   - peeling of dead skin of the fingertips, particularly around the tops of the fingernails. (Note: This is seen at a late stage; perhaps too late for treatment to be effective in preventing heart damage.)
4) A lump (lymph node) in the neck felt to be swollen to 1/2 inch (1.5 cm) in diameter or greater.
5) A rash, usually red with no crusting, blisters or weeping, seen anywhere on the trunk and limbs.

These signs do not all have to be present at the same time; for example the rash may have already faded away. Sometimes, KD is causing the child's symptoms but not all the criteria for making the diagnosis are present. This situation is referred to as atypical Kawasaki disease. Like full-blown KD, it can also be associated with inflammation of the coronary arteries.

How is Kawasaki disease treated? If untreated, the symptoms begin to disappear over two weeks. However, about 20 percent of children with untreated KD will sustain damage to one or more coronary arteries causing an aneurysm, a balloonlike widening that can predispose the child to blood clots inside the vessel. About 1 in 10 of this 20 percent will have a heart attack.

The outlook is much better with treatment. This consists of blocking the immune system with donated human antibodies, using intravenous **immunoglobulin**, also called IVIG. This slows down the overly active immune response causing the disease and will diminish the inflammation in the blood vessels. This treatment, in combination with high-dose aspirin has been shown to decrease the frequency of coronary artery damage and aneurysm from 20 percent to about 2 percent of cases, if given on time. After the **acute** symptoms, such as fever, subside, your child will be placed on a low dose of aspirin for a few weeks in order to prevent clots developing in her coronary arteries. To assess the status of these coronary arteries, children with KD undergo a safe, painless procedure, called an echocardiogram (an ultrasound of the heart), during the acute and convalescent phases of the disease.

Post-infectious Arthritis

What is post-infectious arthritis? One of the culprits thought to initiate autoimmune disease is infection. In response to infection, the body develops antibodies that help kill germs. Sometimes, these antibodies cannot distinguish between the infecting organism and the tissue that lines your child's joints. The result is "misguided" inflammation.

Post-infectious arthritis is a group of disorders in which certain infections or germs cause an arthritis because of this misdirected immune response. The classic example is rheumatic fever, in which your child's joints as well as her heart valves are attacked by her own antibodies following a very specific infection, group A streptococcus usually infecting the throat (strep throat). There are other diseases—such as the ones described earlier in this chapter, Kawasaki disease, Henoch-Schonlein purpura and even juvenile rheumatoid arthritis—whose cause is felt to be related to a faulty immune reaction, but the actual germ and process have yet to be fully identified. These conditions are thus known as autoimmune diseases but not as "post-infectious arthritis." Reactive arthritis is another term you might hear; it is often used to describe a group of post-infectious arthritis variants that tend to be chronic. These commonly follow a gastrointestinal or genitourinary infection. The most common form of post-infectious arthritis is also fortunately the one with the best outcome and is called transient synovitis. It is does not last very long and leaves no lasting effects.

What does transient synovitis look like? Transient synovitis most commonly affects the hips of toddlers following an upper respiratory tract infection such as the common cold. Your child might refuse to walk and will sit pointing to her hip or knee. (Hip inflammation often causes pain to be "referred" to the knee, and is interpreted as knee pain.) She might also have a **low-grade fever**. Consult your doctor to help make sure that the hip inflammation is not due to a serious infection called septic arthritis. If your doctor is unsure, she will draw fluid from the joint to be analyzed under a microscope.

How do I treat transient synovitis? Reassure the child, and yourself, that a full recovery in a matter of days is the rule. Let the child's discomfort determine the appropriate level of activity. Anti-inflammatory pain medications such as ibuprofen are usually sufficient to control the pain.

Reflex Sympathetic Dystrophy (Complex Regional Pain Syndrome)

What is reflex sympathetic dystrophy? Reflex sympathetic dystrophy (RSD) is a painful condition in which sensory nerves in the sympathetic nervous system are believed to transmit abnormal signals from a part of the body, often the lower leg. The sympathetic nerves are part of the autonomic nervous system that is responsible for controlling many involuntary processes such as the rate of flow of blood to certain parts of the body. In many cases, these abnormal nerve signals occur for unknown reasons (Type I complex regional pain syndrome) and in others, the syndrome follows a clearly identified injury such as a broken leg (Type II CRPS).

What does reflex sympathetic dystrophy look like? The hallmark of this condition is burning pain. In addition, the affected part has poorly regulated blood flow, so your child's limb might appear to be any or all of the following:

- discolored (for example, a foot might be paler or redder than the other foot, or it can even look blue);
- a different temperature, either warmer or colder than the other limb; and/or
- swollen and tender.

Psychological problems have commonly been associated with this condition, as a consequence rather than a cause of the disorder.

How do I treat reflex sympathetic dystrophy? Reducing your child's discomfort is the most important step. Pain control is best achieved by a combination of anti-inflammatory pain medications, such as ibuprofen, combined with physiotherapy. Some children get relief from a form of physiotherapy called **transcutaneous electrical nerve stimulation** (TENS). Injections that block the sympathetic nerves can help more severe cases. Drastic treatment measures have been tried to control intractable pain: these include cutting the sympathetic nerves (sympathectomy) and surgery to stimulate the spinal cord. In both of these procedures there is risk of complications. Moreover, there is a lack of evidence that such surgery does more good than harm.

In some cases of more severe RSD, the disease becomes a chronic and disabling illness despite treatment. However, the prognosis for children with milder signs and symptoms is probably very good. There might even be many children with milder symptoms who get better over weeks to months without ever having been diagnosed.

Systemic Lupus Erythematosus

What is systemic lupus erythematosus? Systemic lupus erythematosus (lupus or SLE) is a chronic autoimmune disorder that can involve many different parts of the body. SLE is so widespread throughout the body because the autoimmune process in lupus produces a wide array of antibodies. One of these antibodies attacks the patient's very own DNA. This is the substance that stores our genetic code. Therefore, it exists in every type of cell. In lupus, other antibodies can attack the cell membranes.

It is the blood vessels that seem most affected in SLE. Inflammation of the blood vessels, or vasculitis, can occur throughout the body. Blood cells, heart tissue, brain cells, skin and the lining of the body cavities and joints can also be affected to some degree. Over half of children with SLE have a kidney inflammation called **glomerulonephritis**.

SLE occurs less commonly in young children than it does in adults. Fewer than 1 child in 100,000 is affected by lupus. However, when lupus does occur in childhood, it can be more aggressive than adult-onset disease. Most affected children are teenage girls. The cause of lupus is still unknown. Many feel that an environmental trigger, perhaps a virus, in a person with a genetic susceptibility leads to the development of the autoimmune process causing lupus.

What does SLE look like? SLE has a wide spectrum of severity and involvement. It can be mild or severe, even fatal. It can involve only one organ or several. Often, in the early stages, SLE can be quite subtle: there may be only fatigue, weight loss or mild unexplained fever. Often, the doctor will only see a child with a persistent rash and arthritis.

A good way to think about what lupus looks like is to consider the list of problems encountered in the disease and if 4 out of the following 11 criteria are fulfilled, the diagnosis can be made.

1) A distinctive rash over the cheeks and nose in the shape of a butterfly. Note that the presence of a butterfly rash does not automatically mean a child must have lupus.
2) A disklike rash that starts out red and scaly, and later scars.

3) Sensitivity of the skin to the sun.
4) Oral ulcerations, painless erosions in the lining of the mouth or nose.
5) Arthritis.
6) Inflammation of the lining of the heart (**pericarditis**) or lungs (**pleuritis**).
7) Kidney inflammation with evidence of blood and protein in the urine.
8) Neurological symptoms, such as seizures, behavior changes, even psychosis.
9) Blood abnormalities (low red cell, white cell or **platelet** counts).
10) Abnormal immunologic tests, such as the presence of antibodies to DNA (anti-double-stranded DNA antibodies), to smooth muscle or to blood cells.
11) A positive **antinuclear antibody** (ANA) test.

Caution is needed when it comes to interpreting blood tests. SLE is a clinical diagnosis: a doctor uses signs and symptoms to diagnose the disease. However, you might have noticed that some of the criteria are blood tests. One criterion is the ANA test, which detects abnormal antibodies to the nucleus inside our cells. Why not simply rely on it? The answer is that most people with a positive ANA test do *not* have lupus. The test is sensitive but not specific, meaning that the test is only useful if it is negative, to help rule out lupus. The reverse is true of the anti-double-stranded-DNA test, which is specific but not that sensitive. Thus, many people with SLE have a negative anti-double-stranded-DNA test. The test is only useful when it is positive because it helps to confirm the diagnosis of lupus. Given that one test is not specific and another not sensitive, it is the signs and symptoms of lupus that are so important in making the diagnosis.

How do you treat lupus? Because lupus is a complex, multisystem disease, a team approach is often best for managing the disease. Your child, the family and the primary care physician are all part of that team that also consists of an autoimmune disease expert (rheumatologist) or a kidney specialist (nephrologist), or both. Many children need other specialists to become involved in their care.

Most individuals with SLE will require anti-inflammatory medication, usually oral corticosteroids, such as prednisone. Long-term treatment with prednisone has side effects. Part of the education program that you will participate in will include how to identify and manage these side effects.

In resistant cases that respond poorly to prednisone therapy, an immune system suppressor, such as cyclosporine, might also be required. There is evidence from adults who have lupus nephritis that cyclosporine might prevent kidney failure. Cyclosporine also has side effects and is usually not first-line therapy.

How can I help my child with lupus? The family becomes part of the team treating your child. You will receive education and support to help deal with this complex illness. Preventative measures, such as using sunblock and avoiding the sun can help prevent some of the skin manifestations of lupus. Children with kidney problems might require special diets.

Remember, most children with skin rashes similar to lupus do not have the disease. Most children with a positive ANA test also do not have SLE.

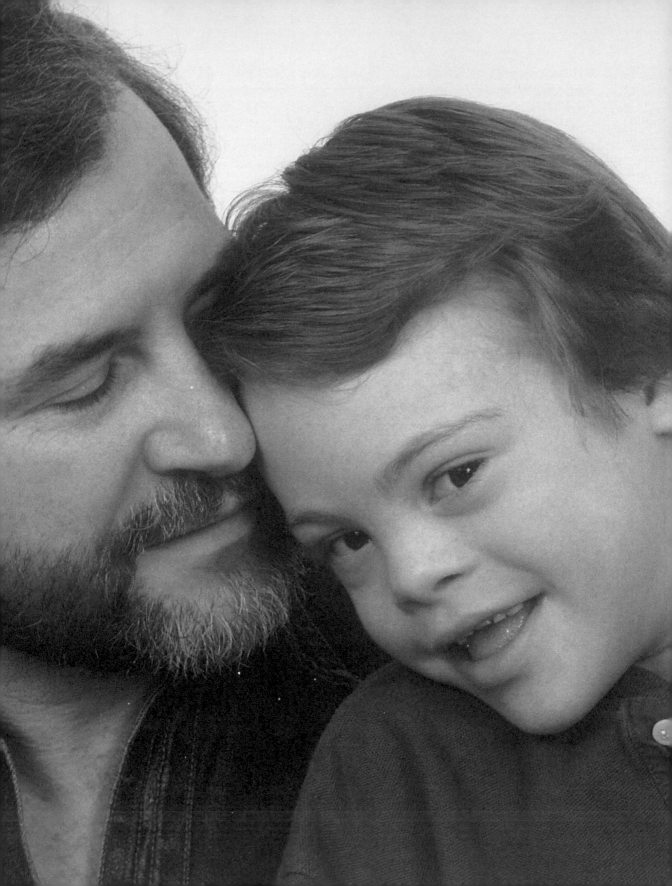

Genetic and Metabolic Diseases

An Overview

What are genes and the genome? Within every individual cell sits a structural blueprint that determines the very nature of our being. It is called the genome. This blueprint, or genome, is stored in chains of molecules called DNA that are arranged into individual units of code called genes. Each gene contains an individual instruction about the building of a specific protein. These proteins have a dual role: they are the building blocks of the cell's structure and the controllers, or "catalysts," for the chemical reactions that allow the cell to function. In every cell, there are literally thousands of genes that are packaged together in 46 chains of DNA called chromosomes.

Did you ever wonder why identical twins are as similar as peas in a pod? It is because each individual of the pair is built from the very same genome. Their genetic code is the same. The harder question is not why are two peas in a pod similar, but why are two types of peas different? Gregor Mendel, a part-time gardener and full-time monk, made astute observations about peas that led to the development of the body of knowledge called Mendelian inheritance. It turns out that sometimes things are a little more complicated in humans than peas, but Mendel had the right basic idea.

He concluded that there are two copies of each gene. Half a set of chromosomes comes from the mother's egg cell and the other half from the father's sperm cell. Eggs and sperm cells each contain 23 chromosomes that combine to total the 46 chromosomes in each of us.

One of each of the two genes can be "dominant" and the other "recessive." Take, for example, eye color. If both genes for eye color code blue, that person's eyes will be blue. If both genes are for brown eyes, the eye color will be brown. It so happens that the brown-eye gene is dominant over the blue-eye gene. Therefore, if a baby has inherited one brown-eye gene from one parent and one blue-eye gene from the other, then her eyes will be brown. But that baby still has one blue-eyed gene; that child is therefore a "carrier" of a blue-eye gene that can be the eye-color gene eventually transmitted to her offspring. Thus, if both parents are brown-eyed but "carriers" of a blue-eye gene, on average, one in four of their children will have blue eyes.

How can things go wrong? Genetic disease can occur in a number of ways. Each parent might carry an abnormal recessive gene. Because the gene is recessive, the parents themselves are healthy but there is a one in four chance that their child will receive two abnormal genes, one

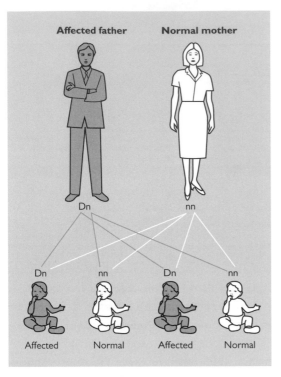

DOMINANT INHERITANCE

One affected parent has a single faulty gene (D) that dominates its normal counterpart (n). Each child's chances of inheriting either the D or the n from the affected parent is 50 percent.

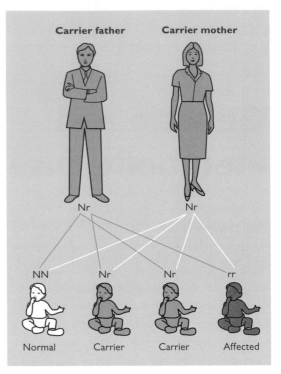

RECESSIVE INHERITANCE

Both parents, usually unaffected, carry a normal gene (N) which takes precedence over its faulty recessive counterpart (r). The odds for each child are:

1. *a 25 percent risk of inheriting a "double dose" of r-genes, which may cause a serious birth defect;*
2. *a 25 percent chance of inheriting two N-genes, thus being unaffected;*
3. *a 50 percent chance of being a carrier as both parents are carriers.*

from each parent. This produces a faulty genetic code and leads to an abnormal cell function, the expressed genetic condition.

Disease can also result from just a single abnormal gene, obtained from one of the parents, if that gene is dominant. Just as the brown-eye gene is dominant to the blue-eye gene, an unhealthy gene might be dominant over a healthy one. In this case, the healthy gene is not always enough to balance the abnormal one. Again, the faulty genetic instructions produce disease.

Genetic disease can be either sex-linked or **autosomal** (non sex-linked). Of our 46 chromosomes, two determine gender. Both might be an x chromosome, in which case the observable

characteristics of the child (**phenotype**) are female, or one may be an x and the other a y chromosome, which produces a male phenotype. A recessive gene carried on one x chromosome might only cause disease in males because males don't have the other x chromosome to balance the harmful gene. Thus the term x-linked recessive disease refers to a condition that affects males almost exclusively. An example is red-green color blindness. Individuals so affected can't tell the difference between red and green. The abnormal gene is on the x chromosome so that males are much more likely to be affected than females. Females would have to have inherited the abnormal gene on both of their x chromosomes whereas males only have to have the one abnormal gene.

What is "metabolic" disease? Genes control not only how we are structured, but also how we function. Abnormal genes that control biochemical function lead to so-called metabolic disease. Different genes code for the building of different proteins. As mentioned earlier, many of these proteins are catalysts for chemical reactions within our bodies. "Catalysts" are agents that guide a chemical pathway. If there is an inborn error in metabolism, abnormal chemical reactions can lead to a deficiency in a certain chemical product or an excess in a certain chemical precursor, or both.

Phenylketonuria (PKU) is an example of a metabolic disease in which the abnormal gene produces an abnormal protein that results in a chemical pathway being blocked. The blocked chemical pathway leads to an excessive buildup of the precursor chemical in the brain. If this is left untreated, the child will have significant brain damage and developmental delay.

A syndrome called congenital adrenal hyperplasia is an example of a genetic disease that leads to both a structural abnormality and a metabolic abnormality. The chemical pathway that occurs in the adrenal glands is responsible for converting one chemical that behaves like a male sex hormone into another chemical that is responsible for salt, potassium and water balance. The abnormal gene leads to an interruption in this pathway. The result is an excess in male hormone and a deficiency in the protein that

controls salt, potassium and water balance. This latter deficiency stimulates the body into further attempts to create the product and the adrenal gland begins to grow as compensation, a condition called hyperplasia. Thus, both a structural and metabolic abnormality develops. Affected girls may look like boys at birth because of the excess in male hormone; their adrenal glands are enlarged (the structural abnormalities), and they may have life-threatening potassium excess (the metabolic abnormality).

How do you treat metabolic diseases? It would be ideal if we could replace defective genes. So far, gene therapy is promising but only experimental. Gene therapy research has led to limited success to date. Treating the consequences of genetic disease is the current option available. Supplying the deficient hormone, such as cortisol in the case of congenital adrenal hyperplasia, or modifying the diet in PKU, can overcome the problems created by defective metabolic pathways. Parents should receive genetic counseling about the risk of having another child (which are not always as straightforward as Mendel's peas) with this condition and about the prognosis for their current children.

Cystic Fibrosis

What is cystic fibrosis? Cystic fibrosis (CF) is an inherited genetic disease in which the body produces abnormally thick secretions. These viscous secretions tend to plug up passageways in key areas of the body: most importantly the lungs and the pancreas. The secretions in the lungs are not cleared easily and thus inhaled microscopic debris and germs are not cleared easily. Despite taking antibiotics, a child with

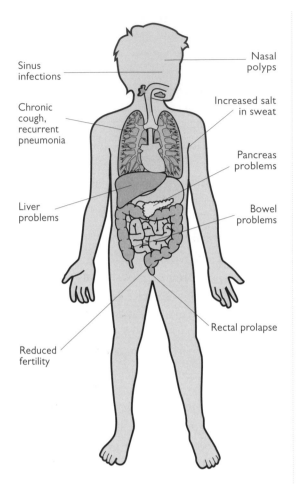

CYSTIC FIBROSIS

The typical features of cystic fibrosis.

CF experiences chronic infections that result in progressive lung damage.

The thick secretions also tend to plug up the duct that leads from the pancreas to the bowel. The pancreas has two main jobs: one is to make enzymes that digest food and the other is to produce insulin, the hormone so important for sugar regulation. The plug in the pancreatic duct results in digestive enzymes being unavailable to the bowel so that foods, especially fats and certain vitamins, are not properly absorbed.

As a result, without treatment, children with CF eventually become malnourished.

Cystic fibrosis is a genetic disease; it has an autosomal recessive form of inheritance. This means that both parents of a child with CF carry one normal and one abnormal CF gene. Because they each possess one normal gene, they are both healthy. Yet when each parent provides their child with the CF gene, the child possesses only two abnormal genes and, hence, has the disease.

There are actually several genes for CF, any of which, if paired with another CF gene, will lead to the disease. Researchers at The Hospital for Sick Children discovered the first CF gene in 1989. The abnormal CF gene is located at a specific site on chromosome number 7. The CF genes are among the most common recessive genes for significant chronic disease. About 1 in 30 people of European ancestry carry a CF gene. The gene is less common in people of African or Asian ancestry.

What does CF look like? Some children get hit harder with this disease than others. In less severely affected individuals, symptoms might not appear until adolescence. In most, the signs and symptoms appear in infancy. Many children with CF are diagnosed when their parents take them to the doctor because of diarrhea and poor weight gain resulting from a malfunctioning pancreas. In other children the first signs and symptoms are related to their problem with breathing. They will have a chronic cough, recurrent pneumonia and sinus infections. Other systems can be affected. Some newborns have such thick secretions that they have difficulty passing their first bowel movements. Older children can develop diabetes because the blocked up pancreas becomes damaged. The chronic lung disease can lead to heart disease.

Labels on figure:
Sinus infections
Chronic cough, recurrent pneumonia
Liver problems
Reduced fertility
Nasal polyps
Increased salt in sweat
Pancreas problems
Bowel problems
Rectal prolapse

Children with CF also have abnormal sweat. It contains more sodium chloride—salt. In fact, prior to the discovery of the gene for CF, the only way to confirm the diagnosis was the sweat chloride test. The sweat chloride test involves putting a chemical on a small patch of skin to promote sweating. The sweat is then collected and analyzed for its salt content. The sweat chloride test is still routinely used for diagnosis when CF is suspected. Genetic testing follows if the sweat chloride test is not entirely normal.

Cystic fibrosis can be devastating. First the family and the child have to deal with the shock of the diagnosis followed by the long journey coping with chronic illness. Psychological problems can develop in affected kids who may feel, and be treated as, very different from their peers.

How do you treat CF? A team specialized in the care of children with CF should provide you, your family and your child with education and support.

After the diagnosis is made, you will have to pay special attention to your child's nutrition. You will give your child digestive enzymes with her food as an oral medication that can treat the problem of deficient pancreatic enzymes. Your doctor will prescribe vitamins to ensure adequate amounts are digested.

Your child's lung problems will require physiotherapy ("chest physio") and your child will inhale a number of medicines. These inhalation therapies include aerosols of antibiotics to treat chronic infection, aerosols of anti-inflammatory corticosteroids to treat the inflammation associated with chronic infection and bronchodilators to widen the small airways that might be plugged with mucus. Other inhalations can help dissolve the mucus.

Despite these numerous and aggressive treatments for the lung disease of CF, some children might need a heart and lung transplant because of the ongoing damage.

There are some promising treatments on the horizon. Although it is much too early to place all hope on any one experimental treatment, the longer lifespan that kids with CF now have gives them a fighting chance that one novel treatment or another will be effective and available in their lifetime.

Down's Syndrome (Trisomy 21)

What is Down's syndrome? The word "syndrome" refers to a combination of signs and symptoms that characterizes a diagnosis. A syndrome usually arises from a single problem. Down's syndrome is one such, well-known, recognizable syndrome that arises as a result of an extra chromosome. Our genetic blueprint normally is stored on 23 pairs of chromosomes. In Down's syndrome, there are three, instead of the normal two, versions of chromosome 21. This extra genetic material from chromosome number 21 leads to all the features of the syndrome, the most important of which involve the brain and the heart. Trisomy 21 was first well described by Dr. John Langdon Down in 1866, hence the name Down's syndrome.

How does the extra chromosome occur? Trisomy 21 happens as a result of **non-disjunction**. During the development of mother's egg cells, instead of the 46 chromosomes dividing into two eggs with 23 chromosomes in each, the two copies of chromosome number 21 don't separate as they should and they both end up in one of the eggs. The egg missing chromosome number 21 is not compatible

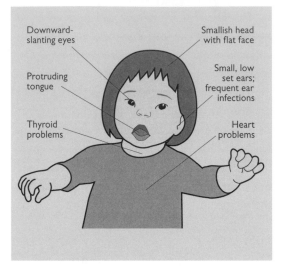

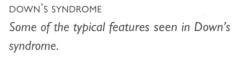

DOWN'S SYNDROME

Some of the typical features seen in Down's syndrome.

with life, but the one with the extra chromosome number 21 certainly is. Conception then leads to 47 instead of 46 chromosomes in the fetus, 23 chromosomes from the father and 24 from the mother. There is one extra chromosome number 21.

The risk of non-disjunction occurring when a woman's eggs divide increases with her age—the odds are 1 in 400 when a mother is 35 years of age but they increase to 1 in 35 when she turns 45. It is rare, but possible, that Down's syndrome arises from a defect in the father's sperm.

Another way an extra bit of chromosome number 21 can end up in an egg cell is the mechanism of "translocation." Here, part of the chromosome number 21, not all of it, moves to part of another chromosome and hitches a ride into the newly created egg. The result is extra genetic information originally from chromosome 21. Yet another variant of Down's syndrome is so-called **mosaicism**. In this situation, only some of the cells have the extra

bit of chromosome 21 but not all. Both mosaicism and translocation are quite rare mechanisms in which a child develops Down's syndrome. The usual mechanism is non-disjunction.

What does Down's syndrome look like? Every child is unique. Yet, those with Down's syndrome share certain physical traits and common medical problems.

Children with Down's syndrome share certain facial features immediately recognizable to the experienced eye. Many of these are quite commonly seen in unaffected individuals but a combination of them is seen more frequently in children with Down's syndrome. The child might have a subtly flattened and smaller head. There usually are epicanthal folds (skin folds in the side of the eyes nearer to the nose). The child might have Brushfield's spots, which are little white dots on the outside of the colored part of the eye. Typically, the eyes might slant, which led to the older, inappropriate term "mongoloid." The child's fingers and toes might be broader and shorter and there might be a wide space between the first and second toes. Half of these children have a single deep crease on their palms, called a simian crease, whereas most people have at least two.

Children with Down's syndrome are slow to reach expected developmental milestones. Still, they display a wide range of abilities. The average IQ of these children is in the mild to moderately delayed range. Usually, adults with the syndrome will require assisted community living. In addition to their intellectual challenges, they are unfortunately more prone to early Alzheimer's disease.

Hearing problems and frequent ear infections are a greater risk for children with

Down's syndrome than for the general population. Visual problems from cataracts are more frequent in newborns with Down's syndrome. Thyroid problems are more common as well. **Obstructive sleep apnea** and other sleep disturbances are also more frequent. Hearing, vision, sleep or thyroid problems can contribute to developmental delay. Although there is no cure for the intellectual handicap of Down's syndrome, the hearing, vision, sleep and thyroid problems they are prone to are indeed treatable and should not be missed so that the delayed development may be minimized.

The most immediate threat to a newborn with Down's syndrome is a malformation of the heart called endocardial cushion defect. This is an abnormality in the fetal tissue that forms the heart valves separating the atria from the ventricles. Approximately 40 percent of children with Down's syndrome will have a form of this malformation, often only a partial form, such as a trial or ventribular septal defect. This defect also varies widely in severity. Many affected children will require heart surgery to correct the defect.

Less frequently, children with Down's syndrome are born with a blockage in their bowels called **duodenal atresia**, which will require surgery to repair. A rare condition of the bowel, called **Hirschsprung's disease**, is also more frequent in children with Down's syndrome. Fortunately, this condition is also pretty rare in these children. Older children should be assessed before they participate in sports because of the possibility of a defect in the neck called atlanto-axial subluxation, which occurs in 1 percent of children with Down's syndrome. In this condition the first two bones of the neck can be unstable and injure the spinal cord. Children with Down's

syndrome have an increased risk of having a transient form of leukemia as infants that gets better by itself. Such children are unfortunately also more prone to other types of leukemia. Thankfully, nowadays, children with leukemia are commonly cured.

How do I treat Down's syndrome? Family support, education and prevention of complications are probably the three most essential ingredients for your child to have the best possible prognosis for her life. She should have a thorough history and physical exam, bearing in mind the potential complications, at each wel-child visit. Your doctor should individualize the plan for her care; however, certain principles apply to all children with Down's syndrome.

Although the features may be quite clear to the experienced eye, your doctor should order that your newborn have a confirmatory chromosomal test for Down's syndrome. A specialized hearing test should be performed. A lactation consultant might be called in to help with feeding. The routine newborn thyroid screen is extremely important.

A repeat hearing test at 6 months of age is recommended by experts. An ophthalmology referral should be sought at 6 months or earlier if there are any concerns that your child has abnormal eye movement or vision. The thyroid screen, which should be routine at birth for all babies, can be repeated at 6 and 12 months in children with Down's syndrome. Your doctor should plot your child's growth on special Down's syndrome growth charts. Your child can benefit from infant stimulation programs.

Your goals remain the same as all parents. You should strive to help your child reach her maximum potential and become as fulfilled as she can be. Because children with Down's syndrome tend to be good natured, parenting them is usually immensely rewarding.

Fragile X Syndrome

What is fragile x syndrome? When children who are slow to meet developmental milestones or have learning difficulties and are otherwise completely healthy are given diagnostic tests, there is usually no answer that explains the problem. Parents find this frustrating. However, sometimes, an answer does exist: the cause of the child's difficulties might be a genetic entity called "fragile x syndrome."

Understanding this **syndrome** might take a little concentration, but this explanation might help you. The chromosomes containing our genetic information are comprised of long chains of DNA in a specific sequence. Fragile sites of chromosomes are said to occur at places where they can break easily. In normal individuals, the fragile site of the x chromosome is in an area where a certain genetic code repeats itself up to about 30 or 40 times. In some people, for no apparent reason, there is a change, or mutation, in the genetic sequencing that results in the code repetitions occurring more often. These individuals are said to have a "premutation," which means that they are normal but carry the faulty tendency to excessive repetitions. Their offspring can have many more of these genetic code repetitions, hundreds in fact, and therefore display the features of fragile x syndrome.

Fragile x is the most common genetic syndrome identified as the cause for developmental delay in otherwise healthy children. This syndrome predominantly affects males and occurs in about 1 in 4,000 boys.

What does fragile x syndrome look like? Children appear quite normal at birth. As they grow, some affected children might have a slightly longer face with a prominent jaw and large ears. Older boys might have larger testicles. The differences in appearance are subtle and not readily recognized.

The difficulties associated with fragile x syndrome are quite variable. They mainly involve learning and behavioral problems. Girls can be affected but usually less so because they have a second normal x chromosome that provides some protection, although they have a 50 percent chance of passing the condition on to their children. Girls with fragile x tend to have learning disabilities and about a third are mentally challenged. Their attention span is often short and they tend to be shy, often anxious children.

Most, but not all, males with fragile x are intellectually disabled. They acquire speech later than their peers. They tend to behave unusually and about a quarter are actually autistic. Thus, they have poor eye contact and socialization, and difficulty with changes to their routine.

The diagnosis of fragile x syndrome is confirmed by specific blood testing that identifies the excessive number of repeated DNA sequences.

How do you treat fragile x syndrome? As with any child who is developmentally delayed, if your child has fragile x she should have an assessment and treatment plan offered by a group of health professionals who specialize in the care of developmentally delayed children. The treatment offered might include any or all of:

- infant stimulation programs,
- speech therapy,
- occupational therapy,
- behavior modification,
- individualized education plans, and
- counseling for both you and your child.

Klinefelter Syndrome

What is Klinefelter syndrome? Klinefelter syndrome is a relatively common genetic condition that results in infertility in males. It is caused by a problem, called non-disjunction, that occurs in the earliest stages of fetal development. In the normal situation, one of the sex chromosomes, either x or y, goes to each egg or sperm. With non-disjunction, one egg or sperm gets two sex chromosomes, and the other none. If an xx chromosome is fertilized by a y sperm, or an x chromosome is fertilized by a xy sperm, the result is a child with an abnormal xxy genotype. This differs from the normal xx genotype of the female or the xy of males. And, a total of 47 instead of 46 chromosomes are present in each cell. This xxy genotype results in the constellation of clinical features known as Klinefelter syndrome. This genetic finding is believed to be as frequent as 1 in 500, many of whom go through life without being diagnosed.

What does Klinefelter syndrome look like? Newborns appear as entirely normal males because of the presence of a normal y chromosome. Some of these children may have been identified incidentally before birth by an amniocentesis that was done for other reasons, and can grow up to have no obvious features of the syndrome. Other children, but certainly not all, might have some developmental delay or learning disabilities. The extra x chromosome will later lead to the development of some female characteristics such as broader hips and less facial hair. These boys tend to be tall and slim with smallish testicles and penis. The xxy genotype invariably produces infertility.

How do I treat Klinefelter syndrome? Emotional support is essential for the boy who can feel different from his peers. He should be reassured that he has a functioning y chromosome that will help him to develop into a young man. Adolescents with the syndrome can benefit from testosterone replacement. If your child develops some extra breast tissue, known as **gynecomastia**, he might have cosmetic surgery. If your child's language development is delayed, he might benefit from early speech therapy.

It can be difficult to know how much to tell your son, and how soon. Particularly because of the infertility, he will have to be told sooner or later about his condition. Some experts recommend telling him a little at a time but, if you feel uneasy with the process, you can get help with counseling from a clinical geneticist.

Neurofibromatosis

What is neurofibromatosis? There are two types of neurofibromatosis: NF-1 and NF-2. They share some common features, including tumors of

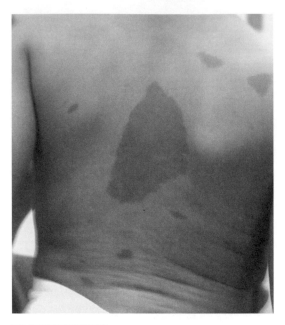

NEUROFIBROMATOSIS

A good example of the "café-au-lait" spot seen in neurofibromatosis.

nerve cells, but are clinically and genetically different diseases. In about half of new cases, the disease is inherited in an **autosomal** dominant pattern, which means one of the parents also has neurofibromatosis. In the other half, the newborn's gene has "mutated" and the parents are unaffected.

What does neurofibromatosis look like?

Type I (NF-1). This is the more common form, found in about 1 in 3,000 children. The gene for NF-1 is found on chromosome number 17.

Affected children have six or more "café-au-lait" spots, which are coffee-colored, flat birthmarks at least 1/5 inch (5 mm) in diameter in children and at least 3/5 inch (15 mm) in diameter in teens. They might also have freckles in their underarms or groin; benign "growths" in the iris of the eye, called "Lisch nodules" that go unrecognized

until the eye doctor has a look; and growths of the nerve lining that can be felt under the skin as little bumps. There can be growths in other areas as well, including the bones and the brain, especially in the nerve behind the eye (optic **gliomas**). The growths, or tumors, are usually benign, but malignancies are also more common in children with neurofibromatosis. Children with NF-1 are prone to seizures, learning problems, visual problems or a combination of these difficulties.

Type II (NF-2). The abnormal gene for this type is found on chromosome number 22, and occurs in about 1 in 40,000 people. What distinguishes this type of neurofibromatosis from NF-1 is the presence of tumors on the nerve cells along the inner ears called acoustic neuromas. The other tumors that are found in NF-1, both benign and malignant, can also be seen in NF-2. The "café-au-lait" spots are less common in NF-2. These children can also have eye problems, usually opacities at the back of the lens.

How do you treat neurofibromatosis? Education is important so that you and your child's doctors can anticipate the problems she might have and carry out investigations in a timely fashion if she develops symptoms. A scan of the brain at the time of diagnosis can not only determine whether the problem is type I or II but also see the extent of any growths for comparison with subsequent scans that may, or may not, be necessary. The value of repeated routine brain scanning is controversial. It is important to remember that most children with NF-1 have benign tumors, not cancer. Annual eye exams and careful annual physicals are very important.

Treatment is symptomatic: if there are seizures, you treat the seizures. Your child should be tested for learning problems early on and treated effectively.

Turner Syndrome

What is Turner syndrome? Normally, girls have a 46 XX genotype, in other words, they possess 46 chromosomes in total, of which two are X (sex-determining chromosomes). Girls with Turner syndrome inherit one normal X chromosome—but only one. They possess only 45 chromosomes and, therefore, their genotype is designated 45 XO. Some girls have a milder variant of Turner syndrome, called a mosaic, in which some cells have the 46 XX genotype while others are 45 XO.

Both X chromosomes are necessary for the development of a fully functional female reproductive system. Girls with Turner syndrome have small, nonfunctioning, so-called "streak" ovaries. Other organs can also be affected, including the heart and the kidneys.

What does Turner syndrome look like? Girls with Turner syndrome are short. Their slow linear growth starts to become more marked after 3 to 5 years of age and leads to an ultimate height averaging 57 inches (145 cm). Often, the diagnosis of Turner syndrome is not made until childhood when a girl is evaluated for short stature, or even in the teenage years when a girl does not go through the normal stages of puberty, with no sexual development of breasts or onset of menstruation.

Girls with Turner syndrome are much more likely to be born with heart and blood vessel abnormalities. The most frequent is an abnormality of the aortic valve, but some can have a particularly dangerous heart problem called coarctation of the aorta, which is a narrowing of the great artery carrying blood from the heart. This can be readily treated if identified early enough.

Turner syndrome is also associated with structural defects of the kidney. Other features of the syndrome that may provide earlier clues include edema, or puffiness, of the hands and feet at birth, that slowly gets better on its own. Some newborns with Turner syndrome have a slightly webbed neck, slightly more tissue on the sides of the neck that produces loose skin folds. Older girls will be short with a broad chest and small widely spaced nipples and a low hairline at the back. These features might sound dramatic but in fact can be subtle and are not obvious to the untrained eye. If someone notices these features in a newborn, your doctor should make sure your child has a prompt evaluation of her heart. Most children with Turner syndrome have normal intelligence, but learning difficulties are slightly more common. If your child is having trouble at school, she should be checked for hearing and thyroid problems, both of which are found more commonly in this condition.

How do you treat Turner syndrome? Probably the most important aspect of treatment is education and counseling. Peer and family support groups are available for girls with this condition. She will need counseling about infertility. Treatment with female hormones can stimulate the onset of puberty. Growth hormone therapy for her anticipated short stature is available. If initiated early on, many girls can achieve heights greater than 60 inches (150 cm). It does however require daily injections and is very expensive. Any significant cardiac and kidney problems will also need treatment.

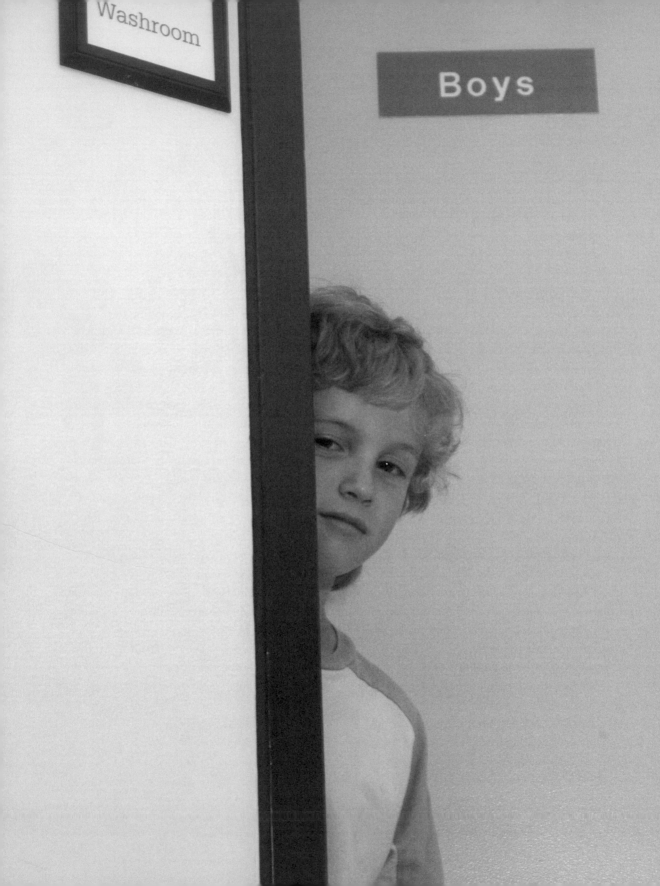

Urinary Tract and Genital Problems

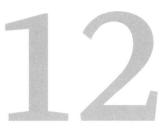

Blood in the Urine: Hematuria

What is hematuria? Hematuria means the presence of blood in the urine. It suggests blood has entered somewhere into the urinary tract, the path that urine travels starting in the kidneys, through tubes called ureters, into the bladder and out the body through the urethra. Blood in a child's urine might be plainly visible to the naked eye, turning the urine brown or red, or it might be found only when his urine is either tested by a "dipstick" (a chemically treated paper strip) or looked at under the microscope.

What causes hematuria? You might become alarmed if you see blood in your child's urine but often it is not a sign of a serious disease. In fact, the urine's dark appearance may not be due to blood at all. Red or brown urine can also be caused by certain foods (for example, beets, berries), food-coloring and medications. Sometimes other compounds being filtered by the kidney (proteins from muscle or blood cells) can cause the same appearance. Newborns often have a pinkish color to their urine because of the presence of urate crystals in the urine that could indicate that the baby is not receiving enough milk. Blood in the urine can appear brownish if it comes from the upper kidney or bright red if it originates from lower down in the urinary tract such as the bladder. **Glomerulonephritis**, which is the inflammation of the tiny filtering units of the kidney, is relatively common in children. It often causes the urine to look like tea or cola. This can occur after an infection, typically streptococcal throat and skin infections. It can also be part of a condition called Henoch-Schonlein purpura (see pages 223–24), which is an inflammation of small vessels of the kidney, skin, joints and bowel; or hemolytic uremic syndrome, a condition that affects the kidney and blood cells often after an episode of bloody diarrhea.

How do you treat hematuria? If you see blood in your child's urine, take him to see his doctor. A dipstick test and microscopic examination of a urine sample will help distinguish between blood and other compounds that can cause the urine to appear brown or red. Your doctor might order other tests, including blood tests and an ultrasound of the kidneys and urinary tract, depending on your child's situation. Very frequently, microscopic blood will be found in the urine when it is tested for other reasons or as part of a routine health examination. Microscopic blood in the urine generally is only a concern if it is persistent or associated with other signs and symptoms.

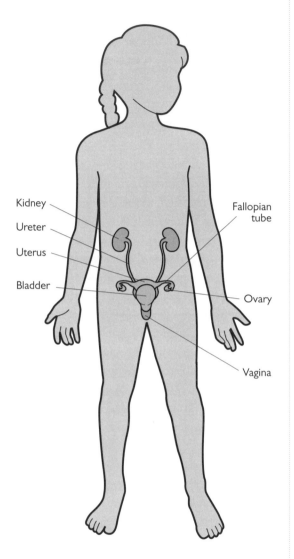

Kidney

Ureter

Uterus

Bladder

Fallopian tube

Ovary

Vagina

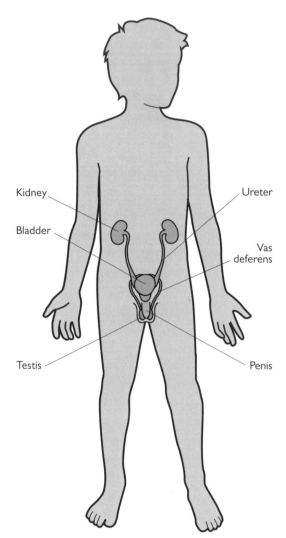

Kidney

Bladder

Ureter

Vas deferens

Testis

Penis

GIRL'S GENITOURINARY SYSTEM

The urinary system—kidneys, ureters and bladder—filters waste products, surplus water and excess salts from the blood. The genital system is composed of two ovaries, the uterus and vagina.

BOY'S GENITOURINARY SYSTEM

As in a girl's, a boy's urinary system comprises kidneys, ureters and a bladder. Urine and, after puberty, semen pass out of the body through the urethra and penis. The testes produce hormones that are responsible for the male characteristics that appear at puberty.

Glomerulonephritis

What is glomerulonephritis? Glomerulonephritis refers to those conditions that produce inflammation and damage to the filtering units of the kidney, called glomeruli. It can be a part of several diseases. Most children develop the **acute** form of glomerulonephritis. This is the sudden appearance of kidney inflammation in previously healthy children, often in response to a recent infection. The most common infections to cause glomerulonephritis are streptococcal infections of the throat (tonsillitis, or "strep throat") or the skin (**impetigo**). By the time kidney inflammation becomes apparent, these triggering infections have usually cleared up. Glomerulonephritis can also develop chronically, that is, slowly over years. Some types of chronic glomerulonephritis run in families.

What does glomerulonephritis look like? The acute type will turn your child's urine red or cola-colored due to the presence of blood. Because the kidney's filtering units are damaged, waste products and excess fluid accumulate in the body. The fluid retention is often first noticed in the face of young children: the eyes appear puffy, which, at first, is often mistakenly interpreted as an allergic reaction. Although easily overlooked, children urinate less than usual and begin to gain weight. Fluid retention will often cause high blood pressure that might lead to headaches. Rarely, severe retention of fluid might even lead to the accumulation of fluid around the lungs causing breathing difficulty. The accumulated waste products can also reduce the child's appetite and energy level.

Sometimes glomerulonephritis will be detected before any signs and symptoms develop. This is more likely to be the case in

chronic forms of nephritis. Perhaps you have taken your child to the doctor for another reason but he orders a urine test that shows microscopic blood or protein, or blood tests are done for other reasons.

How do you treat glomerulonephritis? Glomerulonephritis most commonly will show itself by a change in the urine color to a cola or tea appearance. You should take your child to his physician. The doctor will usually order tests of your child's urine and blood tests to evaluate how well the kidneys are working and to determine the reason for the kidney inflammation.

Most forms of glomerulonephritis get better on their own with time. Treatment is focused on managing the effects of the kidneys' reduced ability to filter blood: fluid retention, accumulation of excessive waste products and high blood pressure. If the fluid retention is significant, your doctor will ask you to limit your child's intake of liquid and salt. Medications to increase urine production (diuretics) and control blood pressure may be required. If your child has very high blood pressure, severe fluid retention or very marked reduction in the kidneys' usual function, he will be hospitalized.

Glomerulonephritis that occurs suddenly after a recent infection goes away by itself in most cases with the return of normal kidney function. However, blood in the urine often persists for some time and, if his urine is examined under the microscope, can be detected for years.

The chronic forms of glomerulonephritis, because of their more gradual onset, tend to be managed differently. First, your child's doctor has to make a proper diagnosis. Commonly, the first clue is the presence of blood or protein in the urine. However, small amounts of blood or protein in the urine do not necessarily signify kidney disease: the protein and microscopic blood can occur in the setting of common self-limited infections, fever and even vigorous exercise. On the other hand, when the blood or protein in urine is persistent or of a significant amount, they might indicate inflammation of the kidneys' filtering units. Some forms of this condition run in families with other relatives having a history of reduced kidney function, blood in the urine or hearing loss that is associated with kidney disease. If your doctor thinks your child has one of these conditions, he will probably refer you to a kidney specialist (nephrologist).

Hemolytic Uremic Syndrome

What is hemolytic uremic syndrome? Hemolytic uremic syndrome (HUS) is a condition where there is damage to the filtering units of the kidney, the glomeruli. The **syndrome** also includes destruction of oxygen-carrying red blood cells and platelets, which are the small blood cells that prevent bleeding. HUS is the most common cause of sudden kidney failure in childhood and can occur at any age but is most common

and severe in children younger than 5. HUS typically occurs following a bout of bloody diarrhea. An infection with a particular strain of the bacteria E. coli (type 0157:H7) is the most common cause of HUS but the syndrome can follow other infections or even occur without any prior illness.

What does hemolytic uremic syndrome look like? Children who get HUS from an E. coli infection typically show the signs and symptoms of the condition within 10 days of developing bloody diarrhea. The infection can be acquired from another infected person; eating undercooked beef; or drinking unpasteurized milk, apple juice products or contaminated water. It is important to realize that over 90 percent of children who suffer diarrhea from an E. coli 0157:H7 infection *do not* develop HUS.

The common signs of HUS are due to the damage done to the kidney and blood cells. Your child's urine may turn tea- or cola-colored, and he might urinate less often. He might develop puffiness around the eyes and swelling from fluid retention (see Glomerulonephritis, pages 247–48). The child might look pale from the destruction of red blood cells; fatigue and loss of appetite due to this anemia are common. Severe bleeding is unusual. Your child might experience headaches, often from high blood pressure; seizures, while less common, can occur.

How do you treat hemolytic uremic syndrome? Unfortunately there is no treatment that can be given to children already infected with E. coli 0157:H7 that will prevent the development of HUS. The best you can do is to minimize the risk of getting an E. coli infection by frequent hand washing, ensuring that meat is adequately cooked and avoiding contaminated water.

HUS is a serious illness: children who get it need to be treated in specialized pediatric centers. Up to 50 percent of children will require renal dialysis until the kidneys recover. They might need medication to control any high blood pressure and to manage the reduction in the kidney's ability to filter the blood and make urine. They might also need transfusions of red blood cells. Specialized medical care has greatly improved the outcomes for children with HUS. While death is now rare, these children might still have long-term effects on their kidneys.

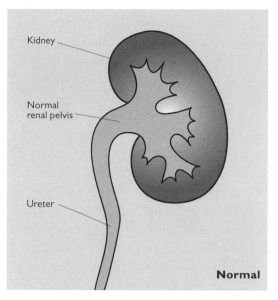

Hydronephrosis

What is hydronephrosis? After urine is made in the kidney, it passes through a funnel-like structure called the renal pelvis, down thin-walled tubes called ureters and into the bladder. The urine then exits the bladder through a thin tube called the urethra. Hydronephrosis is a fluid-filled enlargement of the kidney's collecting system, the path through which urine flows from the kidney down to the bladder. If the swelling of the collecting system is severe, it can cause a swelling or mass in the abdomen. One or both kidneys can be affected.

Prenatal hydronephrosis is common. An enlargement of the renal pelvis, called *pelviectasis*, is often found on routine ultrasounds of the developing baby. When the enlargement is minor, this finding will often disappear when an ultrasound is done after the baby is born. Babies who have pelviectasis but do not have a blockage or reflux generally will outgrow the pelviectasis over the first few years of life without any untoward effects on the kidney.

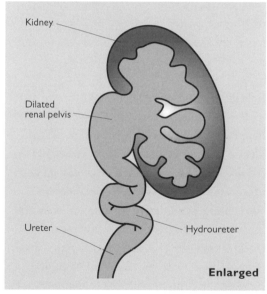

HYDRONEPHROSIS

Hydronephrosis is a fluid-filled enlargement of the kidney's collection system.

What causes hydronephrosis? Two of the more common causes of hydronephrosis are a blockage or narrowing of the kidney's collecting system and a condition called reflux. This refers to the unnatural flow of urine back toward the kidney when the bladder fills or empties. Blockages most often occur in one of three places: at the connection between the ureter and kidney (ureteropelvic junction), at the connection between the ureter and bladder (ureterovesical junction) and, in some male infants, where the lining of the urethra may have a valvelike pleat (posterior urethral valves). Reflux is found in about a quarter of cases after tests are performed on a baby or young child who has had a urinary tract infection. Most of these children have mild reflux that they generally outgrow. Hydronephrosis will be seen in those children whose reflux is stronger.

Sometimes, hydronephrosis is associated with a kidney or collecting system that was malformed during development. The cause of most of these conditions is unknown and could not have been prevented or anticipated.

How do you treat hydronephrosis? Tests are done to determine the extent and cause of the hydronephrosis. Your child's doctor will order an ultrasound of your child's kidneys to determine the degree of hydronephrosis. A **voiding cystourethrogram** (VCUG) is done to evaluate whether your child has reflux. This test involves inserting a small catheter into the bladder through the urethra with x-rays taken after liquid contrast is flushed into the bladder. Depending on these results, another nuclear medicine imaging test might be done to evaluate how the two kidneys are functioning and to determine whether there is a blockage in the urine flow. This examination involves an intravenous injection of a compound with pictures recorded as the compound is filtered by the kidney and travels down the collecting system.

Hydronephrosis that is mild and not associated with reflux or due to a blockage is most often simply left alone and monitored. It will usually get better on its own with time over the first years of your child's life. If your child has reflux, he will often need to take preventative daily antibiotics to avoid urine infections and their potential for scarring the kidneys. If your child has severe hydronephrosis that is associated with a blockage, he will probably require surgery.

Nephrotic Syndrome

What is nephrotic syndrome? The kidney is composed of millions of tiny filtering units called glomeruli. These filter blood in order to excrete the body's waste products into the urine. When these filtering units are damaged, protein leaks into the urine and the level of protein in the blood drops. This causes water to move into the body's tissues, which produces swelling. Nephrotic syndrome, or nephrosis, is a condition caused by large amounts of protein being lost in the urine due to disease in the glomeruli. In most cases, the cause of nephrotic syndrome is unknown. It is a common condition in childhood and affects boys more often than girls. It can occur at any age but is most common in preschool and early school-aged children.

What does nephrotic syndrome look like? Fluid retention and swelling are the most obvious signs of nephrotic syndrome. Initially, you might notice the swelling around his eyes when your child first gets up in the morning or after a nap. Later, the swelling can increase in amount and last longer. His ankles, feet and even the stomach will become swollen. This might make clothing seem tight, creating elastic marks on the legs and waist and make putting shoes on more difficult. Your child might gain weight and urinate less frequently. Children with nephrosis are often more tired and irritable, eat less and appear pale.

To diagnose nephrotic syndrome, your child's doctor will ask for a sample of your child's urine and check it for protein with a dipstick, which is a chemically treated strip of test material. This test is quick and simple. If there is a large amount of protein on the sample, the doctor might ask for a 24 hour collection of urine to obtain a more accurate result and will take a blood sample to check for the level of protein in the blood and to determine how well the kidneys are working.

How do you treat nephrotic syndrome? Most children with typical nephrotic syndrome are treated with an oral medication, a steroid called prednisone. Prednisone reduces the inflammation in the kidney and, therefore, reduces the loss of protein from the blood into the urine. You can expect that your child will respond to prednisone after several weeks and that he will have to take it over a two- to three-month period. Your doctor or other health care provider will teach you how to monitor your child's urine and follow a schedule of prednisone administration. They will educate you about the possible side effects and complications of nephrotic syndrome and its treatment. It is common for relapses to occur when the dose of prednisone is reduced or if your child gets a viral infection.

Prednisone is a very effective drug but when it is used in high doses for a prolonged period, some side effects are inevitable. These include weight gain, high blood pressure, mood changes, stomach upset and an increased chance of infections. Chicken pox infection can be severe if contracted while your child is on steroids. If your child is exposed to someone with chicken

WHEN TO SEEK HELP FOR YOUR CHILD WITH NEPHROTIC SYNDROME

- sudden increase in size of stomach
- fever
- difficulty breathing
- abdominal pain
- exposure to/development of chicken pox
- sudden arm/leg swelling and pain

pox or develops chicken pox himself, you must contact your doctor so that a preventive or treatment medication can be taken.

In the early stages of treatment, when fluid retention is at its greatest, your child might need to take "water pills" (diuretics). These help control uncomfortable swelling. Occasionally protein and diuretic medications are given intravenously if swelling is particularly problematic.

Nephrotic syndrome can cause complications. One is bacterial infection developing in the excess fluid that has accumulated inside the stomach. The infection shows up as increased swelling of the stomach with or without pain and fever. Another rare complication that can happen is the formation of blood clots. These can cause a swollen or painful limb.

Most children with nephrotic syndrome respond to prednisone; however, a few will require other medications that suppress the immune system. These drugs are prescribed if the protein loss does not improve with prednisone alone, if very frequent relapses occur or if the side effects of prednisone are becoming too problematic. Sometimes a kidney specialist might have to take a biopsy of the kidney if your child is not responding in a typical way.

While most children have one or several relapses of their condition, the majority of children with nephrotic syndrome will eventually outgrow their condition by adolescence or adulthood without any long-term kidney damage.

Posterior Urethral Valves

What are posterior urethral valves? The urethra is the tube that carries urine from the bladder to the outside of the body. In some male babies, small flaps of redundant tissue are present at the beginning of the urethra that can obstruct the outflow of urine because they act like one-way valves. Depending on the severity of the obstruction, the urethra, bladder, ureters and kidneys can become swollen and damaged (see Hydronephrosis, pages 249–50).

What do posterior urethral valves look like? Posterior urethral valves most likely develop in the early stages of growth inside the womb; therefore, your doctor might see signs on an ultrasound examination done during pregnancy. If the signs have not been seen on a prenatal ultrasound, you might notice that your baby has a weak urinary stream and difficulty urinating or he might have a swelling or mass in the abdomen due to an enlarged bladder. Posterior urethral valves can also be found as part of investigations done in a baby with a urinary tract infection.

How do you treat posterior urethral valves? Posterior urethral valves can have serious consequences and need to be evaluated and treated by a health care team including a pediatrician, urologist (a surgeon with expertise in conditions of the urinary tract) and a kidney specialist, or nephrologist. They will order tests to determine the severity of the obstruction. The tests include an ultrasound and x-rays of the urinary tract (called a VCUG, see page 253). Blood tests are also needed to assess how well the kidney is working at filtering the blood.

Often, your child's doctor will insert a urinary catheter to drain the bladder and help relieve the obstruction. Your child will need to be in hospital to receive an intravenous for fluid and/or antibiotic therapy.

The most common surgical correction of posterior urethral valves is called an endoscopic ablation. A urologist will remove the abnormal tissue by inserting a small flexible tube with a light and camera at the end through the urethra. The long-term effects on the kidneys depend on the degree of the obstruction and the timing of detection. Approximately 25 percent of children will have some long-term impairment of kidney function.

Vesicoureteral Reflux (Urinary Reflux)

What is vesicoureteral reflux? After urine is made in the kidneys, it flows down tubelike structures called ureters before entering the bladder where it is stored until it flows out through the urethra. Normally, the ureters are designed to prevent urine from flowing backward. Reflux occurs when this mechanism is faulty, causing urine to move from the bladder back into the ureter and sometimes all the way back up to the kidney. Reflux is common and tends to be more prevalent in children who have siblings or parents with this condition or who have malformations of the urinary tract. In young infants, it is more common in boys but, by early childhood, girls are more likely to have reflux.

It is associated with urinary tract infection: about 25 percent of children who have a urine infection will also have reflux.

How do you diagnose vesicoureteral reflux? Reflux is usually found when your doctor is investigating another urinary tract problem, either a urinary tract infection or hydronephrosis (see pages 128–30 and 249–50). Reflux is associated with an increased incidence of urinary tract infections. Young infants with urinary tract infections are usually taken to their doctor because of fever and fussiness. Older children might complain of tummy pain, discomfort when peeing or a change in the urine's appearance or smell.

Reflux is most commonly diagnosed and assessed with a **voiding cystourethrogram** (VCUG), which is a specific x-ray test of the urinary tract. This test involves placing a catheter through the urethra into the bladder through which dye is injected. X-ray pictures are taken as the bladder is filled and then emptied to check if urine backs up through the ureters (reflux) and, if so, how far and whether the urinary tract is swollen. Reflux is graded in terms of its severity on the VCUG with grade 1 being the most mild and grade 5 the most severe. Most children with reflux have it on the mild end of the spectrum (grades 1 to 3). More severe reflux and repeated infections can be associated with kidney damage leading to kidney scarring, high blood pressure and poor growth.

How do you treat vesicoureteral reflux? Mild reflux is most commonly outgrown by the age of 5. Generally, physicians prescribe antibiotics to prevent infections that might scar the kidneys until your child has outgrown the reflux. Using antibiotics to prevent infection is an issue that

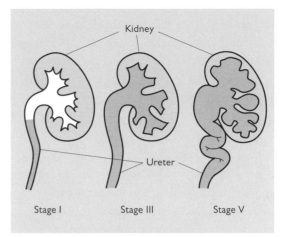

Kidney

Ureter

Stage I   Stage III   Stage V

THE STAGES OF VESICOURETERAL REFLUX
Voiding cystourethrogram (VCUG) showing grades of severity of urinary reflux back into the ureter and kidney.

is continually evaluated. Studies are being done to determine whether all children with mild reflux benefit from taking regular antibiotics. Because increasing numbers of antibiotic-resistant infections are emerging, it is important that you and his doctor regularly review your child's need for daily antibiotics and the particular antibiotic taken.

Children with higher degrees of reflux (grades 4 and 5) might also require surgery by a pediatric urologist. The decision whether to operate on a child with severe reflux is individual. Factors that are considered include the child's age (even severe reflux can improve with time), general health, frequency of infection and tolerance of them, and effectiveness of preventative antibiotics.

Balanitis and Balanoposthitis (Infected Glans/Penis)

What are balanitis and balanoposthitis? Balanitis is an infection of the foreskin and balanoposthitis an infection of the foreskin and glans, or end of the penis. These conditions can occur in children with phimosis (see pages 255–56) and might be related to difficulty cleaning under the foreskin. Balanitis can also occur as a reaction to chemicals, for example, in detergents or soaps, or contact with irritating materials.

What does balanitis look like? Discomfort, itch, redness, mild swelling and discharge can be seen with balanitis or balanoposthitis. Many, but not all, children have phimosis related to these infections.

How do I treat balanitis? Warm soaks in the bathtub, gentle cleaning and local antibiotic cream or ointment are usually sufficient. Regular local hygiene with gentle retraction of the foreskin and cleaning with soap and water, followed by a lubricant such as petroleum jelly is important to prevent recurrences. You should avoid giving your child bubble baths or using scented soaps, both of which might predispose him to these conditions. If the balanitis has been caused by irritation, your child should wear cotton underwear and you must ensure that all the detergent is rinsed out after washing his clothes. If the symptoms don't settle within a couple of days, it is advisable to take him to his doctor. He might need to take oral antibiotics. If a boy has recurrent, bothersome episodes, you might be advised to have him circumcised by a pediatric urologist or general surgeon.

Hypospadias

What is hypospadias? Hypospadias is a common malformation affecting almost 1 percent of boys. It is a congenital (present from birth) condition in which the opening of the urinary tract

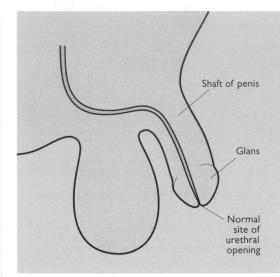

NORMAL URETHRAL OPENING

is not located at the tip of the penis but, rather, on the underside of the penis. It is usually recognized as part of the examination of the newborn baby boy. Hypospadias can be minor where the opening is located very close to the tip, or severe in which case the opening may actually be close to the base of the penis. In hypospadias, the lower half of the foreskin might be absent with the upper half forming a hood over the end of the penis. A condition that is often associated with hypospadias is called chordee and refers to the bending of the penis on erection. This will also require attention.

Why is hypospadias a concern? Hypospadias generally does not cause problems relating to the urinary tract, but hypospadias can make peeing with a direct stream while standing difficult for your child to achieve. As a boy gets older, this difference can be stigmatizing and socially cumbersome. In addition, if he has chordee and it is significant, it can have an impact on sexual function and satisfaction. For these reasons, significant hypospadias and

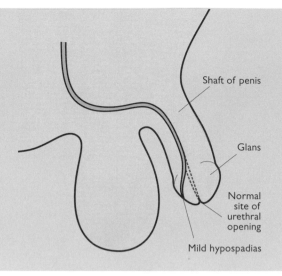

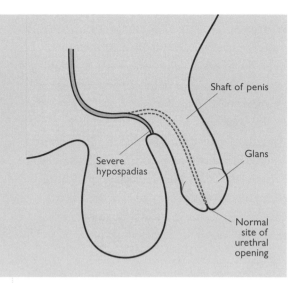

MILD HYPOSPADIAS

In mild hypospadias, the urethra opens on the underside of the penis, but close to the tip.

SEVERE HYPOSPADIAS

In severe hypospadias, the urethra opens at the base of the penis.

chordee are generally repaired. Surgical correction might not be necessary for very minor degrees of hypospadias.

How do you treat hypospadias? The type of surgical procedure depends on the degree of hypospadias. Infants with hypospadias should not be circumcised prior to any surgery because the foreskin is often used for part of the repair. Mild hypospadias is often corrected during a short outpatient procedure. More extensive hypospadias and chordee repairs require more complex procedures and time in hospital. In severe forms of hypospadias, the child's chromosomes might also be checked to exclude any genetic abnormality.

Phimosis

What is phimosis? In uncircumcised boys, the glans, or head of the penis, has a covering of skin called the foreskin. In young boys, especially those under 2, the foreskin is normally difficult to pull back but gradually becomes retractable with time in most children by between 4 and 7. Phimosis occurs when a tight layer of tissue exists around the head of the penis preventing retraction and often producing symptoms. Phimosis is most often painless.

What does phimosis look like? True phimosis, as opposed to a normal nonretractile foreskin, can cause your child difficulty when urinating, such as difficulty initiating peeing, pain when he pees, or ballooning of the foreskin during peeing. Phimosis will lead to difficulty cleaning under the foreskin, which can lead to a higher incidence of infections in this area that can cause local pain, redness, swelling and discharge. Phimosis can also develop from repeated infections (see Balanitis, pages 253–54).

It can sometimes be difficult to tell a normally nonretractile foreskin from phimosis.

With a nonretractile foreskin, gentle retraction leads to pouting (like a fish's mouth) of the tip of the foreskin while attempting to gently retract a phimotic foreskin leads to a cone-shaped foreskin with a pinpoint opening.

Paraphimosis occurs when the ring of phimosis tissue is pulled back behind the glans of the penis. This causes very painful swelling and you have to take your child to a doctor quickly. If the paraphimosis cannot be corrected, your child might need a surgical procedure to release the constriction.

How do you treat phimosis? A nonretractile foreskin is normal in young children and does not require treatment. You should not try to vigorously retract a normal but nonretractile foreskin. If your child has symptoms related to a true phimosis, he will need treatment. Your doctor might prescribe a topical steroid ointment to be applied to the tip of the penis. If your child still has persistent or recurrent symptoms related to a phimosis, you might be advised to have him circumcised by a pediatric urologist or general surgeon.

Paraphimosis. If your child's retracted foreskin has become stuck (paraphimosis) you should take him to the nearest emergency room immediately.

Undescended Testicle

What is an undescended testicle? The testes normally develop inside the fetus' abdomen while the baby is in the womb. They then descend into the scrotum during the last trimester of pregnancy. When the testicle fails to migrate into the scrotum, the condition is called an undescended testicle. Approximately 30 percent

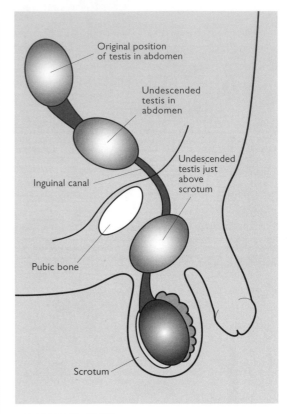

UNDESCENDED TESTIS
The testes normally move down the inguinal canal into the scrotum before birth. A testis that fails to descend may stop anywhere, from high in the abdomen to just above the scrotum.

of premature male infants have a testicle that has not come down into the scrotum, while about 3 percent of boys born after a full-term pregnancy have an undescended testicle.

Most undescended testicles discovered at birth will come down into the scrotum over the first several months of life, but about 1 in 150 boys has a testicle that remains undescended. This condition must be differentiated from a "retractile testicle," which is a normally situated testis that can appear undescended because of a protective reflex, the cremasteric, that causes the testis to pull up from the scrotum. Retractile testes can be manipulated down into the scrotum and are entirely normal.

Most undescended testicles are felt higher up in the groin area, and both sides can be affected in 10 percent to 20 percent of cases. Rarely, neither testicle can be felt and an ultrasound is done to check for the presence of the testicles in the abdomen.

Why is an undescended testicle a concern? The potential problems caused by an undescended testicle include reduced sperm production and fertility, increased risk of testicular cancer, twisting of the testis (testicular torsion) that causes the loss of its blood supply, and the adverse psychological effects of a "different" appearance. Changes inside the testicle and their adverse effects on sperm development can be seen as early as 6 months of age. The risk of developing a tumor of the testicle is up to 10 times greater in males who have an undescended testis. This risk does not change with bringing the testis down into the scrotum, but it makes examination and detection of any tumor mass easier.

How do you treat an undescended testicle? If an undescended testicle has not come down into the scrotum by the time your son is about 6 months of age, it is unlikely to descend spontaneously. The testis can usually be brought down into the scrotum with a simple outpatient surgical procedure, called an orchiopexy, which is usually performed between 9 and 15 months of age. Hormonal treatment has been used but is generally not very successful. Eighty-five percent of boys who are treated for an undescended testicle present on one side are fertile, while about 65 percent of boys with undescended testicles on both sides are fertile.

Varicocele

What is a varicocele? Each testicle is suspended in the scrotum by a spermatic cord through which blood vessels flow to and from the testicle. The veins within the spermatic cord have valves to keep blood flowing in one direction back to the body. If these valves are defective or pressure in the veins is too great, the veins swell with blood causing a varicocele. Varicoceles are very common and usually begin to appear during puberty. They affect 15 percent to 20 percent of teenaged boys to varying degrees.

What does a varicocele look like? A varicocele usually causes a painless lump above the testicle that feels like a "bag of worms." Sometimes your son will have a dull ache or feeling of heaviness in the scrotum that might increase with exercise. A varicocele is usually not very painful and often gets smaller when he lays flat. Most varicoceles occur on the left side but 10 percent can have them on both sides. They rarely involve the right side alone.

How do I treat a varicocele? Many varicoceles are not bothersome and don't require treatment. If your son has mild discomfort, simple measures like more snug-fitting underwear can be helpful. The two major reasons to have a varicocele surgically repaired are if it is very large and uncomfortable or if it causes adverse effects on sperm development and fertility. The testicle needs to be at a slightly lower temperature than the rest of the body for adequate growth and sperm development. Because a varicocele contains warm blood pooled within the veins, the temperature of the testicle can increase. Your son's doctor will measure testicular growth and, if it is being affected, he might recommend surgical repair. A urologist will perform a varicocele repair, a minor procedure, on an outpatient basis.

Varicoceles in young boys or those only involving the right side are unusual. In these cases a more detailed physical examination and ultrasound test is often done to exclude the presence of a mass pushing on and obstructing the veins.

Labial Adhesions

What are labial adhesions? Prior to puberty, a girl's external genitalia, or labia, are not exposed to very much estrogen. Because of this, they remain thin and more susceptible to irritation. Labial adhesions occur when the labia minora (the inner and thinner labia) become irritated and stick together. Thus, the same factors that cause vulvitis (see next section) can also produce labial adhesions.

What do labial adhesions look like? The inner labia become stuck together in the midline. Sometimes, labial adhesions are mistaken for a hymen that does not have a normal opening, but when your child has labial adhesions it is difficult to see her urethra (opening through which urine is passed). Irritation of the vulva with associated redness, itching and scratch marks might be present as well.

How do I treat labial adhesions? Often, no specific treatment is needed beyond attention to hygiene, avoiding irritants and regular airing of the area between diaper changes. If more than three-quarters of the labia minora are stuck to each other, your baby's doctor might prescribe a topical estrogen cream to be applied to the area

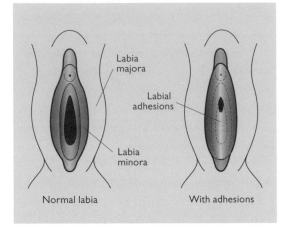

LABIAL ADHESION

Ordinarily, the inner labia surrounding the entrance to the vagina are separated. In rare cases, they stick together to block the opening, partially or completely.

of attachment. You will need to use a zinc barrier cream or petroleum jelly once separation occurs to prevent recurrences.

Prepubertal Vulvitis

What is prepubertal vulvitis? Redness, discomfort and itching of the external genitalia are common in young girls. This condition is termed vulvitis. It occurs because prior to puberty girls normally lack estrogen. As a result, the lining of the genitalia tends to be thin, relatively unprotected and prone to irritation from feces and other irritants. Irritation can lead to redness, scratch marks, pain when urinating and discomfort. A vaginal discharge is generally absent. Masturbation is a normal behavior in young girls that can irritate the vulva and should be differentiated from primary vulvitis. Confusion can also occur when they have irritation around the anus, for example, from pinworms.

What causes prepubertal vulvitis? Vulvitis is most often caused by suboptimal hygiene. Young girls who have only recently mastered the toilet are not the best of wipers. Chemical irritation by scented or treated soaps and bubble baths can also produce vulvitis. Also, bacteria that are normally present in the child's throat, particularly streptococcus, can be transferred to the vulva and produce inflammation. A vaginal discharge usually does not occur with vulvitis alone and indicates inflammation of the vagina that can occur with a bacterial infection or the presence of a foreign object. When significant vaginal discharge, rather than simple vulvitis, is present in a child before puberty, you should consider the possibility of sexual abuse. While yeast infection occurs in very young infants, this infection is uncommon in older girls prior to puberty. Yeast generally attaches to genitalia exposed to more estrogen.

How do I treat prepubertal vulvitis? Most vulvitis can be treated with a zinc barrier cream along with oatmeal baths that help to soothe the inflamed area. You need to pay attention to your child's hygiene. Avoid using irritating soaps and bubble baths. If her genitalia are more inflamed, her doctor might prescribe a local steroid ointment. Severe pain and redness can be a sign of a bacterial infection from streptococcus that also causes strep throat. Her doctor might take swabs from the vaginal area to look for these bacteria and, if positive, then prescribe oral antibiotics.

MANAGING VULVITIS

- Practice regular hygiene.
- Avoid tight synthetic underwear.
- Avoid bubble baths and heavily scented soaps.
- Take oatmeal baths.
- Use a barrier cream.
- See your child's doctor if vagina is very inflamed or significant discharge is present.

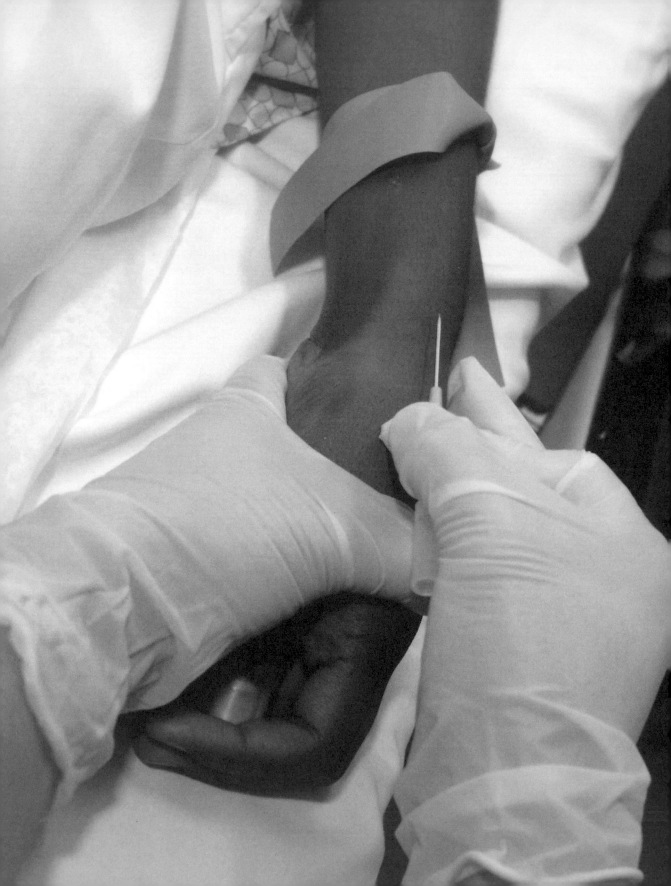

Blood Diseases and Immune Disorders

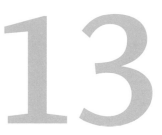

Anemia: An Overview

What is anemia? Anemia occurs when the amount of hemoglobin in a person's blood is too low. Hemoglobin is the molecule in the blood's red cells that helps deliver oxygen to the body. The red blood cells (RBCs) normally circulate for about 120 days before becoming defective and being removed from the circulation.

What causes anemia? There are three main situations that can lead to anemia:

- inadequate production of red blood cells,
- increased destruction of red blood cells,
- increased blood loss from the body.

ANEMIA CAUSED BY INADEQUATE RBC PRODUCTION

Physiological anemia of the newborn. Infants are born with higher levels of hemoglobin and more RBCs for a given volume of blood than older children and adults. After birth, the baby's hemoglobin level normally drops to a low point at about 2 months of age, a condition known as physiologic anemia of infancy. After this occurs, the infant's body gets the signal to increase RBC production. This temporary and expected drop in the blood count is considered normal and no treatment is needed.

Iron deficiency anemia. Anemia also occurs when the body lacks the materials needed to manufacture enough healthy red blood cells. The best example of this situation is iron deficiency anemia. Iron is essential for the production of hemoglobin in red blood cells. If your child is not getting enough iron in her diet, she could get iron deficiency anemia, the most common cause of anemia in children. Iron deficiency anemia can affect children at any age, but it is most commonly seen in children under 2 years of age and in adolescent girls who have started menstruating.

Megaloblastic anemia. Your child's anemia can also be caused by deficiency in folic acid and vitamin B12, both of which are necessary for normal blood production. Children will develop a type of anemia called megaloblastic anemia if one or both of these substances is deficient. People who eat little or no meat, vegetarians or vegans, may not have enough vitamin B12 in their diets. A folate deficiency can develop from eating too few folate-containing foods, such as vegetables, or in infants who drink only goat's milk. Some intestinal diseases such as **celiac disease** (gluten-sensitive enteropathy) can result in deficiencies of both vitamin B_{12} and folate. These forms of anemia are rarely found in babies and young children.

Aplastic anemia. In healthy individuals, blood cells are normally produced in the bone marrow. These mature cells are initially generated from more primitive cells, called stem cells. Aplastic anemia occurs when the bone marrow is unable to produce sufficient numbers of blood cells because of a problem in the maturation of these stem cells. Some aplastic anemias affect only red blood cells and are therefore called red cell aplasia. A few of these are inherited, such as Diamond-Blackfan and Fanconi's anemia, both of which can also be associated with other physical abnormalities, particularly of the upper limbs. More often, aplastic anemia is caused by a viral infection. Sometimes, otherwise healthy children develop a mild anemia for about one month following viral infections. In some children who have an underlying blood disorder, such as sickle-cell disease or thalassemia major, infection with a virus called parvovirus B19 can cause severe anemia. This is known as an **aplastic crisis.** The bone marrow production of RBCs slows down and cannot compensate for the breakdown of cells created by the underlying disease. Aplastic anemia can also result from exposure to certain toxic chemicals, radiation or medications, such as antibiotics, antiseizure drugs or cancer medications. Some childhood cancers cause an anemia due to decreased RBC production. For example, in leukemia, abnormal cells can crowd out the normal bone marrow needed to produce blood cells.

TEC. Another less common form of anemia resulting in the absence of all the more immature forms of RBCs (or red blood cell precursors) in the bone marrow is transient erythroblasto-penia of childhood (TEC). This is a slowly developing anemia of early childhood, usually in toddlers 18 to 26 months old, that is characterized by the gradual onset of pallor. As the word "transient" suggests, all patients with TEC recover completely without any treatment and with no long-term ill effects. The cause of TEC is unknown, although researchers have proposed a number of viral and immunologic causes.

Chronic diseases. Many chronic diseases in other organs can also result in an anemia due to poor RBC production. For example, in advanced kidney disease, hypothyroidism, Addison's disease (deficiency of the adrenal gland) and pituitary gland diseases, the body does not produce adequate hormones necessary for red blood cell production. Lead poisoning can also cause anemia by interfering with the production of heme, the iron-containing portion of the hemoglobin molecule.

ANEMIA CAUSED BY DESTRUCTION OF RED BLOOD CELLS (HEMOLYTIC ANEMIA)

Hemolysis occurs when the red blood cells are destroyed prematurely by some abnormal process. If the bone marrow can't keep up with the body's demand for replacement RBCs, a hemolytic anemia will result. This can happen for a variety of reasons. It can occur spontaneously or can be triggered by stressors such as infections, drugs, snake or spider venom, or certain foods. Toxins from advanced liver or kidney disease can also shorten the life of red blood cells.

In a condition known as autoimmune hemolytic anemia, the immune system mistakes red blood cells for foreign invaders and begins destroying them. This can occur in the newborn period when a pregnant woman's immune system targets her baby's red blood cells, if those cells are different than the mother's. The best known example of this phenomenon is when the baby and mother differ in their Rh or ABO components.

Red blood cells contain several distinct proteins on their cell walls. Two well-known groups of these proteins are the Rh and ABO components that determine a person's blood type. For example, if you have the major Rh protein, D, you are said to be Rh-positive. If the D protein is absent, you are Rh-negative. If an Rh-negative individual is somehow exposed to Rh-positive blood, anti-D antibodies will be made. This situation can sometimes create major problems: the anti-Rh antibodies from a sensitized Rh-negative mother might cross her placenta, attach to the red blood cells of her Rh-positive fetus and ultimately damage them. As for the ABO group of red cell proteins, an individual can have A proteins, B proteins or neither, in which case, they are blood type O. Most people are A, B or O blood types.

When the mother and baby differ in the components of the RBC, this produces Rh or ABO incompatibility. The baby then develops a specific type of anemia called hemolytic disease of the newborn. Other children inherit defects in the red blood cells that can involve the RBC's structure or the production of hemoglobin. Common forms of inherited hemolytic anemia include sickle-cell anemia, thalassemia and G6PD Deficiency (see pages 264–65).

Vascular grafts, prosthetic heart valves, tumors, severe burns, chemical exposure, severe hypertension (high blood pressure) and clotting disorders can all damage normal red blood cells and mark them for early destruction. In rare cases, an enlarged spleen can trap red blood cells and destroy them before their circulating time is up.

ANEMIA CAUSED BY BLOOD LOSS

Blood loss can also cause anemia, whether it's because of excessive bleeding due to injury, surgery, intestinal bleeding, heavy menstrual periods or a problem with the blood's clotting mechanism. Any of these factors will also increase the body's need for iron because iron is needed to make new red blood cells.

What does anemia look like? The most common sign of anemia is pale skin, along with decreased pinkness of your child's lips, the inner lining of the eyelids and the nail beds. Other common signs of anemia can include irritability, fatigue, dizziness, lightheadedness and a rapid heartbeat. Depending on the condition causing the anemia, other signs and symptoms—jaundice (yellow-tinged skin), dark tea-colored urine, easy bruising or bleeding, and enlargement of the spleen or liver—can occur. In infants and preschool children, iron-deficiency anemia can result in developmental delays and behavioral disturbances such as problems with social interaction and attention to tasks.

How does my child's doctor test for anemia? Anemia is usually diagnosed by a simple blood test that measures hemoglobin. It is part of the complete blood count (CBC), which also assesses the size and number of the RBCs and counts the blood's white blood cells and **platelets**. To determine the specific type of anemia, your child's doctor might order other diagnostic tests. These can include an examination of the blood smear, blood iron levels (measured either directly or indirectly with a ferritin test), hemoglobin electrophoresis (to diagnose sickle-cell disease or thalassemia) and, if needed, a bone marrow aspiration to determine whether cell production is happening normally in the bone marrow and to exclude leukemia.

How do you treat anemia? Treatment for anemia depends on the cause of the condition. If your child has iron-deficiency anemia, her doctor will prescribe iron medication. She might advise dietary changes, such as reducing excess milk intake. The doctor might prescribe folic acid and vitamin B12 supplements if the anemia is due to a deficiency of these nutrients. You should be sure to follow up with your child's doctor to ensure that the anemia is being treated adequately.

Treatment for more severe or chronic forms of anemia depends on the cause. Some children might need blood transfusions. Some might need treatment with medications or removal of the spleen to prevent blood cells from being removed from the circulation or destroyed too rapidly. Others might need medications to fight infection or stimulate the bone marrow to make more blood cells. Bone marrow transplantation might be considered in severe cases of sickle-cell disease, thalassemia and aplastic anemia. This procedure involves taking bone marrow cells from a donor and injecting them into your child's vein. The donated cells then travel through the bloodstream to your child's bone marrow, where they begin producing new blood cells.

G6PD Deficiency

What is G6PD deficiency? G6PD deficiency is the lack of glucose-6-phosphate dehydrogenase, an enzyme present in red blood cells. G6PD helps the red blood cells to function normally and protects them from natural oxygen chemicals that may build up. When this enzyme is deficient, a type of anemia

known as hemolytic anemia can occur. This can occur when people deficient in G6PD have a fever; take medications such as pain medicines, certain antibioticsand drugs to treat malaria; or when they are exposed to other specific substances, such as mothballs or fava beans.

What causes G6PD deficiency? About 400 million people worldwide have G6PD deficiency, making it the most common inherited enzyme deficiency. G6PD deficiency is inherited as an x-linked, recessive condition, meaning that this condition usually occurs in boys. Although the condition has been found in most ethnic groups, it is most common in African Americans, Arabs and people of Mediterranean heritage, including Italians, Greeks and Sephardic Jews. The condition tends to be milder in African Americans and more severe in people of Mediterranean descent.

What does G6PD deficiency look like? If your child with G6PD deficiency is exposed to a medication or infection that causes oxidative stress in his blood cells, sometimes there are no symptoms at all. In more serious cases, your child can exhibit symptoms of anemia, including pallor, fatigue, rapid heartbeat, rapid breathing or shortness of breath, jaundice (yellowing of the skin and eyes), an enlarged spleen or dark, tea-colored urine. Once the trigger is removed or clears up, the symptoms of G6PD deficiency usually disappear fairly quickly, typically within a few weeks. Newborns can develop persistent and more serious jaundice as a result of G6PD.

How do you diagnose G6PD deficiency? In most cases, it is not known that a child has G6PD deficiency until his red blood cells are exposed to oxidative stress and he develops symptoms of the disorder due to the resulting anemia. If your child's doctor suspects he has G6PD deficiency, the doctor will order laboratory tests to help make the diagnosis. The tests include a CBC, a blood smear and special blood tests that directly measure G6PD activity or look for specific DNA. Additional blood tests are usually done to make sure there are no other possible causes of the anemia.

How do you treat G6PD deficiency? Treating the symptoms associated with G6PD deficiency is usually as simple as removing the trigger. In other words, treat the child's illness or infection or discontinue the use of a certain drug. However, severe anemia might require treatment in the hospital, such as supportive care with oxygen and fluids and, sometimes, a transfusion of healthy blood cells.

You should always check with the doctor or pharmacist before giving any medication. Be careful about using herbal, naturopathic or other alternative complementary therapies. It is important to avoid the foods and drugs listed below.

Antibiotics
- sulfonamides
- co-trimoxazole, combination of trimethoprim and sulfamethoxazole (Bactrim, Septra)
- dapsone
- chloramphenicol
- nitrofurantoin
- nalidixic acid

Antimalarials
- chloroquine
- hydroxychloroquine
- primaquine
- quinine

Chemicals
- mothballs (naphthalene)
- methylene blue

Foods
- fava beans, also called broad beans

Other drugs
- aspirin (acetylsalicilic acid)
- sulfasalazine
- methyldopa
- large doses of vitamin C
- hydralazine
- procainamide
- quinidine
- some anticancer drugs

Hemophilia

What is hemophilia? Hemophilia is a rare genetic bleeding disorder that prevents blood from clotting properly. Human blood contains special proteins, known and as clotting factors, that help stop bleeding. People with hemophilia are deficient in one of those factors, either factor VIII or IX and, as a result, their blood cannot clot properly. Hemophilia A, also known as factor VIII deficiency, is the cause of about 80 percent of cases. Hemophilia B, which comprises the majority of the remaining 20 percent, is a deficiency of factor IX. Patients are classified as mild, moderate or severe, based on the amount of factor present in the blood.

Hemophilia is inherited as an X-linked disorder, which means the disease occurs almost exclusively in males. About 1 in every 8,000 boys is born with hemophilia. Affected males cannot pass the gene for hemophilia to their sons but their daughters will be carriers of the disease gene. Every female who carries the gene for hemophilia has about a one in four chance of having a child who has hemophilia.

What does hemophilia look like? Some children with hemophilia bleed only occasionally, whereas others bleed more often. About 30 percent of infant males with hemophilia bleed excessively after circumcision and 1 percent to 2 percent of newborns with hemophilia can have bleeding within the skull (intracranial hemorrhage). Once babies with hemophilia begin crawling and cruising, you might notice raised bruises on the stomach, chest, buttocks and back. These are unusual places for normal children to bruise. The shins and forearms normally bruise.

The most common type of bleeding in hemophilia involves the muscles and joints. A child with hemophilia will usually refuse to move the affected joint or muscle because of pain and swelling. Recurrent joint bleeding can also lead to chronic damage. Other signs of a clotting problem are prolonged nosebleeds, excessive bleeding following a tooth extraction or surgery, or blood in the urine.

How do you diagnose hemophilia? Diagnosing the condition requires doing a complete blood count (CBC) and a set of blood tests to assess the clotting ability of your child's blood including prothrombin time (PT) or international normalized ratio (INR), activated partial thromboplastin time (PTT), factor VIII level and factor IX level.

How do you treat hemophilia? Although hemophilia is a lifelong condition with no cure, your child's hemophilia can be successfully managed with clotting factor replacement therapy. He will receive the missing factors periodically through an intravenous line. He can receive these either at a hematology clinic or at home given by a visiting nurse, by you or once your child is older and has undergone special training, he can do it himself.

The development of recombinant, that is, biologically manufactured, clotting factors has virtually eliminated the danger of transfusion-related infection, such as HIV or hepatitis viruses. Between 14 percent and 25 percent of children with severe hemophilia A develop inhibitors (antibodies to the clotting factor). Their bodies view the clotting factor as a foreign protein and develop antibodies to fight it off. This can make the hemophilia difficult to treat. A new medication called recombinant factor VII has helped many people with inhibitors. It activates another part of the coagulation process directly and bypasses the deficiencies.

Many hemophiliacs prevent bleeds by infusing clotting factors on a regular basis, usually two or three times per week. These scheduled home-based infusions have also helped reduce the joint problems that hemophilia caused in the past. Thanks to advances like these, children with hemophilia can now participate in a wide range of sports and have the freedom to live more active lives. Swimming is strongly encouraged because it exercises all the muscle groups without putting stress on the joints.

Try to prevent your infant or young child with hemophilia from injuring himself. You should put bumper pads in your child's crib, cushion furniture with sharp edges and place gates across stairs to prevent falls. As your baby with hemophilia begins to crawl and walk, he can wear special knee and elbow pads that offer protection against joint bleeds. If your house has ceramic tile or hardwood floors, you should consider installing carpet or buying rugs to soften the floor surface. A rambunctious and adventurous toddler might need to wear a helmet to protect against head injuries.

Dental cleanings can sometimes cause bleeding. For this reason, it's important that your child's dentist knows about the condition. Hemophiliacs need to be followed by a hematologist who specializes in treating blood disorders. If your child is bleeding, he may need to be hospitalized, depending on the severity. Any injury affecting the brain or any part of the central nervous system or a vital organ should be treated as an emergency and the child should be taken to the hospital immediately.

WHEN TO CALL YOUR CHILD'S DOCTOR

Certain bleeds require medical attention, including those injuries affecting:

- the central nervous system—any suspected trauma to the head, neck or back;
- the face, including the eyes and ears;
- the throat or another portion of the airway;
- the gastrointestinal tract (which might produce signs such as bright or black blood in your child's stool);
- the urinary tract (blood in the urine, which could require treatment and bed rest);
- the genital area;
- the hips or shoulders (these can be complicated bleeds because they involve the rotator joints);
- large muscle compartments, such as the thighs.

Acetaminophen is the preferred pain reliever because many other over-the-counter pain medications, such as ibuprofen or naproxen, contain aspirin or NSAIDs (non-steroidal anti-inflammatory drugs). These can affect blood **platelets** and lead to increased bleeding.

Joint hemorrhage must be treated promptly because prolonged bleeding can cause joint disorders. The accumulation of blood in the joint spaces can erode the smooth surfaces that allow limbs to bend easily. This can lead to chronic joint damage that may require surgery to remove the damaged joint tissue.

Histiocytosis

What is histiocytosis? A histiocyte is a form of white blood cell that is found in every human body. Its job is to help destroy certain foreign materials and fight infection. Langerhans cell histiocytosis (LCH) is a rare disorder that affects 1 in 200,000 children. The cause is unknown, but for some reason, patients with this disease have too many histiocytes (Langerhans cells). These cells accumulate in certain areas and create problems. Langerhans cell histiocytosis has also been known in the past as Histiocytosis-x, eosinophilic granuloma, Hand-Schuller-Christian syndrome and Letterer-Siwe disease.

What does histiocytosis look like? Only one part of the body or many different sites can be involved. Usually the disease is more serious when several sites are affected and the patient is a young infant. Possible sites of involvement include:

- skin (rash),
- bone (single or multiple lesions),
- lung, liver and spleen (enlarged),

- teeth and gums (loose or lost teeth, swollen gums),
- ear (chronic infections or discharge),
- eye (vision problems or bulging eye),
- central nervous system (excessive thirst and urination from diabetes insipidus),
- general symptoms such as fever, weakness and failure to gain weight may be present.

How do you diagnose histiocytosis? A diagnosis of LCH is usually made after your doctor has done a biopsy to allow microscopic examination of the affected tissue. To determine the extent of the disease and subsequent treatment plan, she might order several other tests. These include blood tests, x-rays of the chest and bones (skeletal survey) and CT scans. Sometimes a biopsy of the liver or bone marrow is performed.

How do you treat histiocytosis? Treatment, if any, depends upon the individual case and is planned after thorough evaluation of your child to determine where the disease is. The goal of an overall treatment plan is to use as little treatment as possible to keep the disease under control. Although this disease is not considered to be a cancer, cancer treatments have been used in people with histiocytosis. Consequently, hematologists and oncologists who treat cancer also treat children with Langerhans cell histiocytosis. Sometimes the disease will regress without any treatment at all. In others, limited surgery, small doses of radiation therapy or chemotherapy will be prescribed, depending on the extent of the disease. Radiation therapy, if used, is given in much lower doses than cancer patients receive.

Some children with histiocytosis remain symptom-free, while others may develop lifelong chronic problems. In a few cases, the disease will be fatal. Usually these are very young infants who have a rapid downhill course and do not respond to any known treatment. Whether or not the disease responds to treatment will often depend on the extent of organ involvement. The vast majority of children will survive the disease.

Hypogammaglobulinemia

What is hypogammaglobulinemia? The body normally defends itself from the threat of foreign proteins, or antigens, by producing specific antibodies to them. These antibodies, made of immunoglobulins, play a dual role in the immune response: first, they recognize the antigen as foreign and then they trigger a biological response that culminates in its elimination. There are five major types of immunoglobulins: immunoglobulin G (IgG), immunoglobulin M (IgM), immunoglobulin A (IgA), immunoglobulin D (IgD) and immunoglobulin E (IgE). These immunoglobulins are made in cells called B-lymphocytes.

Hypogammaglobulinemia is a disorder caused by low levels of immunoglobulins in the blood because of abnormalities or deficiencies in the B-lymphocytes. The resulting **antibody** deficiency means that your child is susceptible to recurrent infections with specific types of germs. The most common congenital abnormalities of B-lymphocyte production include:

- hypogammaglobulinemia (common variable immunodeficiency),
- IgA deficiency,
- x-linked agammaglobulinemia, (Bruton's agammaglobulinemia),
- transient hypogammaglobulinemia of infancy.

Selective IgA deficiency. It is the most common antibody deficiency **syndrome**, affecting about 1 out of every 700 people. Most of these individuals are healthy but recurrent infections can occur in as many as 50 percent of people with IgA deficiency. Some people only develop symptoms later in life after an uneventful childhood and early adulthood. Recurrent or chronic upper and lower respiratory tract infections are common, as is *Giardia lamblia* infection, a parasite infestation of the gastrointestinal tract. People with undetectable levels of IgA antibodies can develop severe allergic reactions if they receive blood products.

Hypogammaglobulinemia. Also called common variable immunodeficiency (CVID), it affects 1 in 50,000 people and occurs equally in boys and girls. Most children will have a reduced amount of the immunoglobulins IgG, IgA and IgM in their blood. It is an immune deficiency disorder that can be acquired or inherited. In most cases, there is no family history of immunodeficiency. However, in instances where more than one family member is affected, an **autosomal** recessive (two abnormal genes, one from each parent) mode of inheritance is suggested. In about 5 percent of cases, one or more family members is found to be IgA deficient.

X-linked (or Bruton's) agammaglobulinemia. A mother's antibodies protect her newborn for the first 6 months of life. Symptoms in x-linked agammaglobulinemia (XLA) begin at age 7 to 9 months, after a significant decline in those antibodies. The disorder affects boys only and is characterized by recurrent bacterial infections during the second half of the first year of life. Chronic ear infections (otitis media), **sinusitis** and pneumonia are the most common infections. Children with Bruton's agammaglobulinemia often have undersized or scanty tonsils and lymph nodes. Fifteen percent of patients with XLA die of infectious complications by age 20.

Transient hypogammaglobulinemia of infancy. THI is related to a delayed onset of immunoglobulin production in infants. These children recover and develop a normal antibody response when aged 2 to 3 years. During their first years, these children have a high incidence of recurrent upper respiratory infections but not pneumonias or life-threatening infections. These children do not require IVIG therapy.

What does THI look like? Patients with hypogammaglobulinemia typically begin having bacterial infections after 7 to 9 months of age, when maternal antibodies that initially crossed the placenta fall to undetectable levels. Symptoms are related to the severity of the immunodeficiency, which may include the following:

A. **Respiratory infections:**
   - paranasal sinusitis, bronchitis, chronic cough;
   - chronic otitis media (ear infection);
   - development into more serious respiratory conditions: pneumonia, chronic bronchiectasis (dilated and damaged bronchial tubes), and interstitial emphysema.
B. **Gastrointestinal disorders:** chronic diarrhea, weight loss and malabsorption of food.
C. **Autoimmune diseases:** rheumatoid arthritis, vitiligo (areas of depigmented skin), decreases in red or white blood cells and **platelets.**
D. **Malignancy:** the risk of certain malignancies is high.

E. Growth retardation in those with early-onset recurrent infections.

How do you diagnose THI? Some test results that indicate hypogammaglobulinemia include:

- low serum immunoglobulins and B-lymphocytes,
- missing specific antibodies to any vaccines the child has received,
- absence of antibodies to A or B blood group antigens (which everyone should have).

How do you treat THI? Your child's hypogamma-globulinemia will be treated with immunoglob-ulin, given every three to four weeks intravenously (IVIG) or by injection subcutaneously. She will get antimicrobial therapy (antibiotics) at the first sign of infection. If your child has chronic sinusitis or lung disease, she may need long-term treatment with broad spectrum antibiotics. If she has developed bronchiectasis, she will need physical therapy and daily postural draining of secretions and pus from the lungs and the bronchi. If she is suffering from gastrointestinal or malabsorption problems, she should be evaluated for *Giardia lamblia*, rotavirus or other infections. Most children with immunodeficiency and arthritis who have never received immunoglobulin will find that adequate treatment with immunoglobulin usually provides symptom relief.

Immunodeficiencies

What is immunodeficiency? The immune system protects the body from potentially harmful substances, called antigens, that are components of germs, toxins, cancer cells and blood or tissues from another person. Immunodeficiency refers to the group of disorders in which the normal immune response is reduced or absent.

Each immune reaction is composed of various specific responses by the blood's white cells, namely **neutrophils** and lymphocytes. Neutrophils engulf and destroy foreign material in a process called phagocytosis.

The lymphocytes are divided into two groups: T-lymphocytes and B-lymphocytes. T-lymphocytes directly attack antigens. This is called cellular immunity. B-lymphocytes produce antibodies (humoral immunity). These antibodies attach to the antigen and make phagocytes, like neutro-phils, and body chemicals, such as complement proteins, much more efficient in the destruction of the antigen.

Immunodeficiency can be traced to the failure of one or more parts of the immune system. The causes include primary immunodeficiency, caused by congenital/inherited defects, and acquired immunodeficiency caused by a disease that hinders the immune response.

One of the more convenient ways to group the primary immunodeficiencies is according to the part of the immune system that is faulty. Thus, there are:

- B-cell (antibody) deficiencies,
- T-cell deficiencies,
- combined T-cell and B-cell deficiencies,
- defective phagocytes,
- complement deficiencies.

B-cell (antibody) deficiencies. Examples of congenital immunodeficiency disorders of **antibody** production, or B-lymphocyte abnormalities, include **hypogammaglobulinemia** (see pages 268–70), a decrease of one or more specific antibodies, that usually causes repeated mild respiratory infections, and x-**linked agammaglobulinemia**

(lack of all or most antibody production), which results in frequent severe infections and is often fatal. Other B-cell deficiencies include selective IgA deficiency and less commonly IgG subclass deficiency.

T-cell deficiencies. Congenital disorders affecting the T-lymphocytes can cause increased susceptibility to viruses and fungi, resulting in repeated candida (yeast) infections. An example of this is DiGeorge syndrome.

Combined T-cell and B-cell deficiencies. Inherited severe combined immunodeficiency (SCID) affects both T-lymphocytes and B-lymphocytes. It is often fatal within the first year of life because there is no resistance to disease or infection. Other, less severe, combined deficiencies include Wiskot-Aldrich syndrome and **ataxia telangiectasia**.

Defective phagocytes. In these inherited disorders, defective phagocytes result in infections that are unusually frequent or severe, often causing deep abscesses. These infections often respond poorly to standard antibiotic therapy. Examples of this disorder are chronic granulomatous disease, Chediak-Higashi syndrome and leukocyte adhesion defect.

Complement deficiencies. Disorders of the complement system account for about 2 percent of primary immunodeficiency. Some complement deficiencies result in the same kinds of bacterial infections seen with antibody deficiencies, as well as causing immune system disorders such as systemic lupus erythematosus (SLE) (see pages 230–31). Other complement deficiencies lead to an increase of blood-borne infections such as **meningitis** (see pages 111–12).

Acquired immunodeficiency. This can be a complication of diseases such as HIV infection and AIDS (acquired immunodeficiency syndrome). Malnutrition, particularly lack of protein, and many cancers can cause immunodeficiency. It can also be caused by chemotherapy used to treat many types of cancer. This happens because the chemotherapy often reduces the number of white blood cells available to fight infection. Drugs such as corticosteroids or other immunosuppressant medications to treat autoimmune disorders or used to prevent rejection of organ transplants can also cause immunodeficiency.

What does immunodeficiency look like? Children with immunodeficiency diseases generally go to their doctors because of frequent or unusual infections that may or may not respond well to standard antibiotic therapy. The type and pattern of infection depends on which part(s) of the host defences are missing or defective because some defences are more important against some pathogens than others. Defects in phagocyte function or humoral immunity (B-cell deficiency) results in infections with common and unusual bacteria. Defects in T-cell immunity usually result in recurrent viral, fungal or protozoal (such as *Pneumocystis carinii*) infections.

Very serious inherited immunodeficiencies become apparent shortly after birth or in the first year of life. Others, usually the milder immunodeficiencies, may not show up until people reach their 20s and 30s. Persistent, recurrent infections, or severe infection by germs that do not usually cause severe infection, can be clues that an immunodeficiency disorder is present.

Other clues include:
- Infections responding poorly to treatment with antibiotics.

THE 10 WARNING SIGNS OF PRIMARY IMMUNODEFICIENCY ARE:

1. Eight or more new ear infections in one year.
2. Two or more serious sinus infections in one year
3. Two or more months on antibiotics with little effect.
4. Two or more pneumonias within one year.
5. Failure of an infant to gain weight or grow normally.
6. Recurrent or deep abscesses in the skin or organs.
7. Persistent thrush in the mouth or on the skin, after age 1.
8. Need for intravenous antibiotics to clear infections.
9. Two or more deep-seated infections such as meningitis, osteomyelitis, **cellulitis** or sepsis.
10. A family history of primary immuno-deficiency.

- Delayed or incomplete recovery from illness.
- The presence of certain types of cancers (such as Kaposi's sarcoma or non-Hodgkins lymphoma).
- Certain opportunistic infections (such as *Pneumocystis carinii* pneumonia or recurrent fungal/yeast infections).

How do you diagnose immunodeficiency? Your child's doctor might order tests to determine whether your child has an immunodeficiency disorder. Abnormal immune function is suggested by:

- low T- (thymus derived) lymphocyte count,
- low white blood cell count,
- low antibody or **immunoglobulin** levels,
- low complement levels,
- an abnormal NBT test that is used to evaluate the effectiveness of phagocytes at killing bacteria.

Your child's doctor might order other specialized tests to confirm specific immunodeficiency disorders.

How do you treat immunodeficiency? The treatment for immunodeficiency disorders includes specific medical therapies as well as protection against and treatment of diseases and infections. Intravenous immunoglobulin (IVIG) may be given to children who cannot produce adequate amounts of antibodies or immunoglobulins, such as those with hypo- or agammaglobulinemia. Certain immunodeficiencies can be treated by bone marrow transplantation, specifically, those diseases that are characterized by deficient T-lymphocytes or combined deficiencies of T-lymphocytes and B-lymphocytes. Bone marrow transplantation is most often used to treat severe combined immunodeficiency (SCID). Gamma interferon, given as a subcutaneous injection to children with chronic granulomatous disease, has been shown to decrease the numbers of serious infections. Recently, several children with x-linked severe combined immunodeficiency have undergone gene therapy (inserting normal genes into cells that contain the defective gene) with near complete restoration of both T- and B-lymphocyte function. This very exciting breakthrough proves that gene therapy can be successful. Perhaps one day, gene therapy will be the procedure of choice for the majority of immunodeficiency diseases. Acquired immunosuppression that results from medications is often reversible once the medication is stopped.

Children with primary immunodeficiency diseases, especially those with defective T-cells and x-linked agammaglobulinemia should not receive live virus vaccines, such as the oral polio, measles and chicken pox vaccines. They should avoid contact with people who have any infection or contagious disorder. You have to treat any fever or infection aggressively. This can involve use of powerful antimicrobials to treat any infection and occasionally prolonged use of antimicrobials (antibiotics, antifungal medications, etc.) and **prophylactic therapies**.

Iron Deficiency Anemia

What is iron deficiency anemia? Iron is an essential component of hemoglobin, the oxygen-carrying protein in people's blood. Iron deficiency anemia occurs when the amount of hemoglobin becomes reduced due to a lack of iron. The causes of iron deficiency are too little iron in the diet, poor absorption of iron by the body and loss of blood, including menstrual bleeding. The most common reason for iron deficiency anemia in infants and children is the inadequate supply of iron.

In the first 6 months of life, iron stores are dependent on what has occurred during pregnancy. If your child was premature or had a low birthweight, she will be particularly vulnerable to iron deficiency due to the possible low stores of iron during pregnancy. During the following 6 to 12 months, diminished iron supplies can be brought on by poor feeding practices. Children require approximately 2.0 mg of iron in their diet daily. At this age, prolonged exclusive

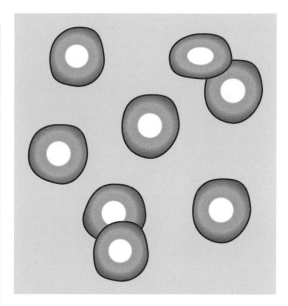

NORMAL BLOOD

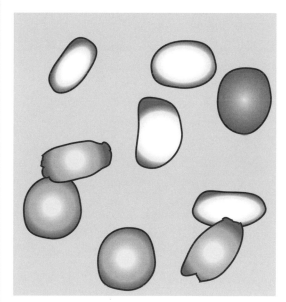

IRON DEFICIENT BLOOD

In iron deficiency, the red blood cells are smaller with reduced color when examined under a microscope.

breast-feeding, the delayed introduction of foods, lack of meat in the diet or the over-dependence on cow's milk can bring on anemia. Adolescents, especially menstruating girls, are at risk because of the growth spurts during puberty and poor eating habits.

Another cause of iron deficiency is loss of blood from the intestinal tract due to a variety of gastro-intestinal disorders, for example, inflammatory bowel disease, milk protein allergy and **celiac disease**. Although the prevalence of iron deficiency anemia has declined over the past decades, unfortunately, some children remain at increased risk, including those from low socioeconomic status, aboriginal children, infants with low birthweight, and those fed whole cow's milk during the first year of life.

What does iron deficiency anemia look like? The symptoms of iron deficiency anemia can include:

- pale skin color (pallor),
- blue-tinged or very pale sclerae (whites of eyes),
- fatigue,
- irritability,
- weakness,
- shortness of breath,
- sore tongue,
- spoon-shaped brittle nails,
- decreased appetite,
- headache,
- recurrent infections,
- unusual food cravings (called pica),
- decreased attention span, alertness and learning.

However, there may be no symptoms at all if the anemia is mild.

How do you diagnose iron deficiency anemia? Your child's doctor will order simple blood tests to make the diagnosis of iron deficiency anemia and distinguish it from other causes of anemia.

The laboratory test results that suggest iron deficiency anemia include:

- low hemoglobin and hematocrit (a test of red cell size and number) values;
- microscopically, the blood film contains small red blood cells that have reduced color in them (hypochromic);
- low serum ferritin (a sensitive measure of body iron levels);
- low serum iron.

How do I treat iron deficiency anemia? It is important to treat it because, apart from the possible symptoms described above, iron deficiency anemia has been shown to cause problems with behavior, development and cognitive function. Your child's diet is the most important way to prevent and treat mild iron deficiency. Drinking too much milk can make the anemia worse. Consuming more than a 4 cups (1 L) per day can actually cause your child to lose iron in her gut. It can also decrease her appetite for solid foods. Iron from animal, poultry and fish sources is absorbed better than iron from vegetables and cereals. Many foods are good sources of iron.

- Best sources: breast milk, formula with iron, iron-fortified cereals, liver, prune juice.
- Good sources: eggs, meat, fish, chicken, turkey, soybeans, peanut butter, dried beans, lentils, molasses, peas.
- Other sources: tuna, oatmeal, apricots, raisins, kale, prunes, greens.

If your child's diet is deficient in iron or her anemia is more severe, treatment consists of oral iron supplementation. Milk and antacids can interfere with absorption of iron and should not be taken at the same time as iron supplements. Vitamin C (ascorbic acid) can increase absorption and is essential in the production of hemoglobin. Serve a citrus fruit or juice with an iron-rich food, for example, orange juice with meat. Your child's hemoglobin should return to normal after two months of iron therapy, but iron supplements should be continued for another 6 to 12 months. This will replenish the body's iron stores, contained mostly in the bone marrow. Your child's bowel movements will often look darker while she takes iron supplements. It is important that her blood tests are rechecked about one month after starting treatment to make sure that the anemia is getting better.

PREVENTING IRON DEFICIENCY IN INFANTS AND CHILDREN

A. **Full-term, breast-fed infants:**
   1. Start a source of iron (supplemental iron at 0.45 mg/pound or 1 mg/kg per day or iron-fortified infant cereal) at age 4 months. If using supplemental iron, keep it out of reach of infants and children.
   2. After weaning from the breast, stop the iron supplement and use iron-fortified infant formula until age 12 months.
   3. Avoid cow's milk until age 12 months.

B. **Full-term, formula-fed infants:**
   1. Use iron-fortified formula until age 12 months.
   2. If feeding iron-fortified infant formula, iron-fortified cereal is not necessary but can be introduced electively at 4 to 6 months of age.
   3. Avoid cow's milk until after age 12 months.

C. **Premature infants (after discharge from hospital care):**
   1. Start supplemental iron (0.9 mg/pound or 2 mg/kg per day) or iron-fortified formula no later than age 1 month and continue to age 12 months.
   2. Preterm infants (weight under 2.2 pounds/1,000 g) fed iron-fortified formula do not need additional iron.
   3. For preterm breast-fed infants, follow the recommended guidelines under A.2 through A.3 above.

D. **Starting solid foods:**
   1. After age 4 to 6 months, use iron-fortified infant cereal and meat.
   2. Serve foods rich in ascorbic acid with meals to improve iron absorption.

You should feed your baby only iron-fortified formulas. There is no evidence to suggest that this causes increased constipation.

Idiopathic Thrombocytopenic Purpura (ITP)

What is ITP? Idiopathic thrombocytopenic purpura (ITP) is a bleeding disorder characterized by too few platelets in the bloodstream, a condition called thrombocytopenia. Platelets are small blood cells that are necessary for normal blood clotting. They work by clumping together to plug small tears in damaged vessels. The disease occurs when the immune system produces antibodies against the body's own platelets. The presence of antibodies on platelets leads to their rapid destruction in the spleen. In children, the disease often follows a viral infection that has occurred in the preceding three weeks. Usually, ITP lasts for a few weeks or months but in a minority of children it can become a chronic (long-term) disease. ITP is most common in children between the ages of 2 and 6 years.

What does ITP look like? The typical signs of ITP are those of a bleeding disorder:

- bruising,
- pinpoint bleeding spots in the skin, called **petechiae**,
- nosebleeds or bleeding gums.

Less commonly, the following signs of a clotting defect are due to ITP:

- abnormally heavy menstruation,
- gastrointestinal bleeding,
- blood in the urine, called hematuria,
- bleeding into the brain, intracranial hemorrhage (ICH), occurs in 0.1 percent to 0.5 percent of cases of **acute** ITP.

How do you diagnose ITP? The tests results used to diagnose ITP include:

- A complete blood count (CBC) that shows a low platelet count but no anemia or abnormality in the white blood cells.
- Platelet associated antibodies might be detected.
- A bone marrow aspiration and coagulation screening tests. These tests are normal in ITP and are performed only in atypical cases if other conditions that cause bleeding need to be excluded.

- A screen for other autoimmune disorders might be helpful in chronic cases, particularly in adolescent girls.

How do you treat ITP? The treatment of ITP depends on the degree of platelet reduction in the blood. Low platelets increase the risk of dangerous bleeding from trauma or spontaneous bleeding. The main reason for treating children with acute ITP is to prevent intracranial hemorrhage, a complication that occurs in fewer than 1 percent of affected children. In some children the disease often runs its course without treatment. Fifty percent of children recover in three to four weeks, 75 percent in six months, and 90 percent within 12 months. Chronic ITP is arbitrarily defined as thrombocytopenia that persists for six months or more.

Treatment should be given to children who have:

- platelet counts less than 20,000/mm^3;
- evidence of mucosal bleeding (for example, petechiae of the soft palate or inside the mouth);
- hematuria or retinal hemorrhages;
- an urgent need to raise the platelet count (for example, emergency surgery or intracranial hemorrhage).

The two main alternatives for treating your child's ITP are either intravenous **immunoglobulin** (also called immune globulin intravenous, or IVIG) or high-dose oral corticosteroids, usually prednisone. A minority of children may not respond to either therapy. In those who do respond, there is a risk of relapse in up to 25 percent of cases with either therapy. Which treatment option to use remains somewhat controversial. IVIG can be given as a single dose but this is given through an intravenous line and requires hospitalization. It might raise the platelet count more quickly and more predictably than prednisone. It avoids the potential side effects associated with high dose oral steroids but there might be transient side effects of headache, fever and nausea during the course of the infusion. Oral prednisone can be used in a high dose of 1.8 mg/pound (4 mg/kg) per day for four days and avoids potential problems with the use of a blood product such as IVIG. A less commonly used therapy is infusing anti-Rh D (**antibody** to Rh factor on red blood cells) that can also be useful in people with specific blood types.

Occasionally, ITP becomes a chronic ailment and reappears, even after remission. Your child's doctor might recommend the surgical removal of her spleen, or splenectomy, since the spleen is the major site of platelet destruction. In most instances, splenectomy is performed in children in whom thrombocytopenia has persisted for more than one year and who have serious bleeding. Most children undergoing elective splenectomy achieve a complete remission from ITP after splenectomy.

People with ITP should avoid taking aspirin, ibuprofen and warfarin because these drugs interfere with platelet function and blood clotting. Therefore, bleeding can occur with their use. Intramuscular injections are also contraindicated. Although policing your child can be a problem, you need to discourage rough play when her platelet count is low.

You will have to take your child to the doctor for regular follow-up blood counts until her platelet count has returned to 150,000/mm^3 or above. No further platelet counts are needed unless clinical signs of bruising or bleeding return.

Neutropenia

What is neutropenia? Neutropenia is an abnormally low number of neutrophils in the blood. These white blood cells serve as the major defense of the body against **acute** bacterial and certain fungal infections. Neutrophils usually constitute about 45 percent to 75 percent of all white blood cells in the bloodstream. When the neutrophil count falls below 1,000 cells per microliter of blood, the risk of infection increases somewhat; when it falls below 500 cells per microliter, the risk of infection increases greatly. Without the key defense provided by neutrophils, a child has problems controlling infections and is at risk of dying from an infection.

What causes neutropenia? Neutropenia can develop for different reasons:

- if the production of neutrophils in the bone marrow is reduced;
- if neutrophils are used up or destroyed in the bloodstream faster than the bone marrow can make new ones;
- as a hereditary disease.

Reduced production of neutrophils in the bone marrow can occur in some children with cancer; viral infections, such as influenza; bacterial infections, such as tuberculosis; or deficiencies of vitamin B12 or folic acid. Children who have received radiation therapy that involves the bone marrow can also develop neutropenia. Many drugs, including phenytoin, chloramphenicol, sulfa drugs and many drugs used in chemotherapy, as well as certain toxins (benzene and insecticides) can also impair the bone marrow's ability to produce neutrophils. Production of neutrophils in the bone marrow is also affected by **aplastic anemia**, in which the bone marrow can shut down production of all blood cells.

With some bacterial infections and some drug treatments, neutrophils are destroyed faster than they are produced. Some newborn infants and older children with an autoimmune disease can make antibodies that destroy their own neutrophils and result in neutropenia. Children with an enlarged spleen (splenomegaly) can have a low neutrophil count because the enlarged spleen traps and destroys neutrophils.

Certain rare hereditary diseases also cause the number of neutrophils to decrease. Congenital cases are generally subcategorized on the basis of associated physical findings and abnormalities in other organ systems. Kostmann syndrome (congenital **agranulocytosis**) is a severe form of congenital neutropenia and the neutrophils are severely reduced from birth. Congenital neutropenia can also be present with other symptoms, for example in Schwachman-Diamond syndrome and glycogen storage disease type 1B.

What does neutropenia look like? Neutropenia can develop suddenly over a few hours or days (acute neutropenia), or it can develop gradually and last for months or years (chronic neutropenia). The symptoms your child might have depend on the level of neutropenia. The lower the neutrophil count, the greater the risk of infection. This risk increases if low neutrophil counts persist for more than three days. Types of infection include otitis media (ear infection), tonsillitis, sore throat, mouth ulcers, gum infections and skin abscesses.

Children with Kostmann syndrome suffer from severe bacterial infections, such as infection of the umbilicus, pneumonia, skin abscesses or otitis media during their first few months of life. Therefore, most cases of congenital neutropenia are diagnosed early during infancy. In children with autoimmune neutropenia serious infections are uncommon. Children usually grow out of this disorder within two years of diagnosis.

Severe neutropenia can lead to serious problems that require prompt care and attention as your child could potentially develop a bacterial, fungal or mixed infection at any time. These infections can be life-threatening when she is persistently and severely neutropenic. It is therefore important that if your child has neutropenia and develops fever or signs or symptoms of an infection, you take her to be seen by her doctor as soon as possible so she can be treated with antibiotics to fight the infection.

How do you diagnose neutropenia? When a child has frequent or unusual infections, her doctor might suspect neutropenia and order a complete blood cell count to make the diagnosis. A low neutrophil count indicates neutropenia. In many cases, the neutropenia is expected and the cause is known, as in those receiving chemotherapy or radiation therapy. When the cause is not known, it must be determined.

Blood tests and then a bone marrow biopsy, which involves taking a small sample of the bone marrow for examination under a microscope, will generally help to decide which sort of neutropenia the child has. From the bone marrow, her doctor might also be able to determine whether the problem lies in faulty production of the cells or whether too many cells are being used or destroyed in the bloodstream. Congenital neutropenia is distinguished from autoimmune neutropenia of the newborn by its persistence after the first few weeks to months of life and by specific **antibody** tests. Chronic idiopathic neutropenia is also diagnosed by excluding infectious, malignant and autoimmune disorders.

How do you treat neutropenia? The treatment of neutropenia depends on its cause and severity. Your child's doctor will discontinue, whenever possible, any drugs that can cause neutropenia, and you will have to ensure your child avoids exposure to suspected toxins. Sometimes the bone marrow recovers by itself without treatment. Neutropenia accompanying viral infections, such as influenza, can be transient and get better by itself after the infection has cleared. Children who have mild neutropenia generally have no symptoms and may not need treatment.

If your child has severe neutropenia, she could succumb rapidly to infection because her body lacks the means to fight invading organisms. When she develops an infection, she probably will be hospitalized and immediately given strong antibiotics, even before the cause and exact location of the infection are identified. Fever, the symptom that usually indicates infection in a person who has neutropenia, is an important sign and indicates that immediate medical attention is needed.

Colony stimulating factors (CSFs), also called granulocyte colony stimulating factors (G-CSFs), filgrastim or sargramostim, is the main option of treatment for severe congenital neutropenia. CSFs are an artificial version of a natural hormone that drive the bone marrow to produce neutrophils. Many children with congenital neutropenia need CSFs every day to keep them free of dangerous infections. Some only need to boost their neutrophils when they get a severe infection. CSFs are given by an injection just under the skin using a very small needle. Corticosteroids might help if the neutropenia is caused by an autoimmune reaction.

Removing an enlarged spleen can cure the neutropenia due to an enlarged spleen trapping and destroying the neutrophils (hypersplenism). When neutropenia is caused by another disease (such as tuberculosis or leukemia or other cancers), treatment of the underlying disease might resolve the neutropenia. Bone marrow (or stem cell) transplantation might be recommended to treat certain serious causes of neutropenia, such as Kostmann syndrome, aplastic anemia or leukemia.

Sickle-Cell Disease

What is sickle-cell disease? Sickle-cell disease (SCD), or sickle-cell anemia, is a group of inherited diseases of the blood in which hemoglobin, the substance in the red blood cell responsible for carrying oxygen, is abnormal. This can cause the red cell to change from a flexible smooth shape into a rigid elongated sickle shape. These cells live for only 10 percent of the time of a normal red blood cell leading to a low total number of red blood cells (anemia).

SCD affects people whose ancestors originally lived in tropical climates, mostly those of African descent, but it can also affect people from the Middle East, the Indian subcontinent and the eastern Mediterranean regions. In North America approximately 1 in 400 African-American babies are born with sickle-cell anemia. If the child inherits the gene from only one parent then she will be a carrier and is said to have sickle-cell trait, which occurs in 1 out of every 11 African-American babies. They will not be affected from a health perspective but

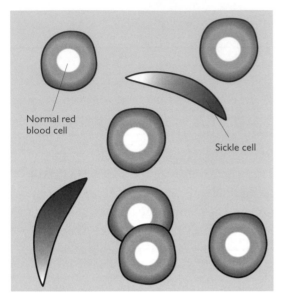

SICKLE-CELL DISEASE

Seen through a microscope, blood taken from a person affected by sickle-cell disease shows rigid, elongated sickle-shaped red blood cells.

Normal red blood cell

Sickle cell

if they marry another carrier then there is a one-in-four risk with each pregnancy of the baby having SCD.

What does sickle-cell disease look like? Symptoms do not usually start until the baby is about 6 months of age. As a result of the shortened life-span of the red blood cells, your child with sickle-cell disease will be anemic and might have pale nail beds or lips. When the red blood cells are broken down they release **bilirubin**, which is often increased in the bloodstream leading to jaundice (yellow color) of the eyes and skin.

When the red blood cells turn into the rigid sickle shape they tend to block the tiny blood vessels that are responsible for supplying oxygen to the whole body. The resulting lack of oxygen causes extremely severe pain and these episodes are known as vaso-occlusive, or painful, crises. The most common parts of the body affected

are the bones, abdomen (stomach area), chest and the penis (which produces a persistent, unwanted, painful erection). During infancy the small bones of the hands and feet are often involved causing swelling, warmth and pain. Over the course of time all parts of the body are affected to varying degrees.

In the first few years of life, your child's spleen gradually loses its function after recurrent crises and becomes severely scarred. Unfortunately the spleen is responsible for a big part of the body's defense against infections and this loss of spleen function allows bacteria (especially *Streptococcus pneumoniae*) to grow in the bloodstream, which can lead to serious infections such as **septicemia**, **meningitis**, pneumonia and osteomyelitis (bone infections).

Your child with SCD will tend to be smaller and slower to enter into puberty and to begin menstruation than her classmates. She will eventually catch up and her growth will ultimately be close to normal. Because of some damage to the kidneys, your child with SCD might have a tendency to wet her bed.

How do you treat SCD? Firstly it is important that your child's doctor make the diagnosis as quickly as possible. If both parents are known to be carriers the diagnosis can be made during pregnancy. In the United States, most states include screening for sickle-cell disease in their newborn screening by a blood sample taken shortly after birth. If your state does not screen it is advisable to have your baby checked if there is any history of sickle-cell disease in your family or if you are in a high-risk group.

Once the diagnosis is made, your child should be referred to a physician or clinic with experience in this disorder who will follow your child on a regular basis. To avoid overwhelming infection, children are started on penicillin syrup (as a **prophylactic therapy**) that is taken twice daily by mouth and is usually continued until at least the age of 5 to 6 years. In addition to the regular immunizations your child will need further protection provided by the pneumococcal and meningococcal conjugate vaccines, as well as another pneumococcal conjugate vaccine (Pneumovax) at 2 years of age. Immunizations against hepatitis and influenza are also recommended.

If the above measures are taken, the risk of a serious infection is dramatically reduced. Nevertheless, you will still be instructed to seek urgent medical attention if your child has a fever, because her immune system is still compromised. This means that those with SCD remain susceptible to life-threatening infections despite the vaccinations and daily antibiotics. You will also be shown how to feel for your child's spleen because massive enlargement of this organ can occur, causing pain on the left side of the abdomen as well as pallor and listlessness. This is known as **splenic sequestration** and is also potentially life-threatening if not urgently treated.

The most common problem encountered is the painful crisis. This might be preceded by fever, dehydration, trauma, swimming, exposure to cold and/or emotional stress, or due to unknown factors. Many of these crises can be managed at home with simple painkillers such as acetaminophen, ibuprofen or codeine in addition to some extra fluids and application of a heating pad or hot water bottle to the area. If you cannot control the pain or your child develops a fever, then you will need to seek medical attention where intravenous therapy will likely be required. If your child has to be hospitalized on a regular basis for vaso-occlusive crises there

SEE YOUR CHILD'S DOCTOR QUICKLY IF SHE HAS

- Fever,
- suddenly larger spleen,
- chest pain, trouble breathing or fast breathing,
- painful crises that don't settle with painkillers at home.

GENERAL GUIDELINES

- Complications are treatable,
- discourage "sick person" identity,
- no special diet,
- no change in discipline,
- encourage normal lifestyle (no restrictions),
- regular follow-up by medical team with immunizations and prophylactic antibiotics as recommended.

is a medication, hydroxyurea, that has shown very promising results in reducing the number of episodes in children.

Thalassemia

What is thalassemia? Thalassemia is an inherited group of blood diseases that involve decreased and defective production of hemoglobin. This molecule is present inside all red blood cells and is needed to transport oxygen throughout the body. Hemoglobin contains two different kinds of protein chains: alpha and beta. Any deficiency in these chains causes abnormalities in the formation, size and shape of red blood cells.

There are two types of thalassemia: alpha-thalassemia and beta-thalassemia. Their names describe which protein chain, alpha or beta, in the hemoglobin molecule is abnormal. Both forms of thalassemia are genetic disorders and both parents must pass the thalassemia gene to their child for her to have the disease. If only one parent passes the gene for thalassemia on to the child, then the child is said to have thalassemia trait. Thalassemia trait will not develop into the full-blown disease, has no or few symptoms and no treatment is necessary for someone who has it. However, genetic counseling is important for families that carry the thalassemia gene because someone with the trait has a 25 percent chance of having a child with the disease if his or her partner also carries the trait.

Thalassemia affects many people coming from areas around the Mediterranean (Italy, Greece and Turkey), Africa, Malaysia, China and many parts of Southeast Asia. People with different forms of thalassemia show a wide range of illness from the disease. Some people only have mild anemia with little or no effects, whereas others require frequent blood transfusions.

How do you diagnose thalassemia? The thalasse-mias can be diagnosed by a few simple blood tests: a complete blood count (CBC), including hemoglobin, and a specific test called a hemo-globin electrophoresis that is used to screen for all types of thalassemia and can be done in infancy.

ALPHA-THALASSEMIA

What does alpha-thalassemia look like? Alpha-thalassemia can range from mild to severe. Children with alpha-thalassemia trait do not have thalassemia disease. They have no signifi-cant health problems, with the exception of possibly being mildly anemic. The anemia can cause slight fatigue, and doctors might at first suspect an iron deficiency. Other cases of alpha-thalassemia resemble beta-thalassemia intermedia (see next section). Finally, the most severe form of the disorder is called alpha-thalassemia major. This type is extremely rare and is sometimes incompatible with life. Women carrying fetuses with this form of thalassemia have a high incidence of miscarriage.

How is alpha-thalassemia treated? Children with alpha-thalassemia trait require no treatment: generally, they cope well with their slight anemia. Iron supplements don't help children with thalas-semia trait. The anemia is caused by an abnormal hemoglobin protein, not a lack of iron. People with alpha-thalassemia intermedia might require occasional blood transfusions during times of physical stress, like fevers or other illnesses.

BETA-THALASSEMIA

Beta-thalassemia is the most common form of thal-assemia seen in the United States. It is grouped into three categories: beta-thalassemia minor (trait), intermedia and major (Cooley's anemia).

What does beta-thalassemia look like? Beta-thalassemia minor (trait) often goes undiagnosed because people with the condition have no real symptoms other than mild anemia. It may initially be mistaken for iron deficiency anemia because the appearance of the blood film is similar in the two conditions. No treatment is usually needed.

Children with beta-thalassemia intermedia have varying effects from the disease. They tend to have similar signs and symptoms but a milder course and better outlook than do those with thalassemia major. Mild anemia might be their only symptom or they might require blood transfusions, especially during illness, medical complications or later on during pregnancy.

Beta-thalassemia major (Cooley's anemia) is a very serious condition because of the severe anemia. The most common complaint is fatigue or shortness of breath. Some children also have mild jaundice or the liver and the spleen might be enlarged, which is sometimes painful. Another symptom of beta-thalassemia major can be bone abnormalities. Because the bone marrow is working overtime to make more red blood cells to compensate for the anemia, children can experience enlargement of their cheekbones, foreheads and other bones. They might experience bone pain or frequent nosebleeds. Gallstones are also a frequent complication of thalassemia because of abnormalities in bile production that involve the liver and the gall-bladder. Poor growth can occur as a result of low hemoglobin and reduced ability of the blood to carry oxygen to the body. Regular transfusions can help alleviate these problems. Heart failure and infection are the leading causes of death among children with untreated thalassemia major.

How do you treat thalassemia major? Thalassemia major requires regular blood transfusions in order to reduce the symptoms of severe anemia: they are necessary for survival. Without trans-fusions every few weeks, your child diagnosed with thalassemia major will usually die by age 7 due to the effects on her body of severe anemia.

Although multiple lifelong transfusions save lives, they also cause a serious side effect: an overload of iron in the body. Over time, people with thalassemia accumulate deposits of iron, especially in the liver, heart and endocrine (hormone-producing) glands. The deposits eventually cause abnormal heart rhythms or heart failure. In addition, permanent liver scarring, diabetes, and delayed growth and sexual maturation can also occur. To minimize iron deposits in the body, people affected by the disease must undergo chelation (iron-removing) therapy for up to 12 hours a day with intravenous (given through the skin directly into a vein) or subcutaneous (under the skin) doses of the iron-binding agent desferrioxamine. Before treatment of iron-chelation therapy was widely used, most children with beta-thalassemia major died before reaching adulthood. Chelation therapy is given five to seven days a week and has been proven to prevent liver and heart damage from iron overload, allow for normal growth and sexual development in children with thalassemia, and increase life span. Iron concentrations in the body are monitored every few months and are used to guide the frequency and dosing of chelation therapy.

Your child's doctor might also recommend removing her spleen because the condition can cause that organ to become extremely enlarged. Children with thalassemia also have an increased need for daily folic acid. Recently, some children have successfully undergone bone marrow transplants to treat thalassemia major; however, this is considered only in cases of severely disabling thalassemia disease.

Von Willebrand Disease

What is von Willebrand disease? Von Willebrand disease (VWD) is an inherited disorder that affects the blood's ability to clot properly. It is the most common inherited bleeding disorder, affecting as many as 1 percent or more of the population. When a blood vessel is cut or torn, platelets (small cells that float in the blood) plug the tear to stop the leak of blood. A substance in the blood known as von Willebrand factor (VWF) helps these platelets stick to damaged blood vessels. Another function of VWF is to carry the important blood clotting protein, called factor VIII, to the site of the injured blood vessel. Children with VWD have a problem with the amount or quality of one or both of these blood components.

What are the different types of VWD? Like many conditions, there are various forms of VWD. Unlike hemophilia, which affects only boys, VWD affects boys and girls equally.

- Type 1 VWD, which accounts for 70 percent to 80 percent of cases, is the mildest form of the disease. Here, the total amount of von Willebrand factor (VWF) in the blood is reduced. Although the condition can be made worse by taking aspirin and other non-steroidal anti-inflammatory drugs (NSAIDs), symptoms can be so mild that the affected person is never diagnosed. People with type 1 VWD usually do not bleed spontaneously. However, they can have significant bleeding with trauma and surgery or when they have a tooth pulled.
- In type 2 VWD (15 percent to 20 percent of VWD), the building blocks that make up the VWF (called **multimers**) are smaller than usual or break down too easily.
- In type 3 VWD, patients have severe bleeding problems and have no measurable VWF and factor VIII (the protein that helps with blood clotting).
- In the acquired type, VWD can occur in those children with Wilms' tumor, congenital heart disease, systemic lupus erythematosus and hypothyroidism.

What causes VWD? Like hemophilia, VWD is a genetic disorder that is passed from parent to child. In type 1 VWD, the child of a man or a woman with VWD has a 50 percent chance of inheriting the abnormal gene (**autosomal** dominant inheritance). In type 3 VWD, a child usually inherits the gene from both parents (autosomal recessive inheritance). In this case, the child will likely have severe symptoms, even if the parents don't have any symptoms at all. In type 2 VWD, the disease can be either autosomal dominant or recessive.

What does VWD look like? The symptoms of von Willebrand disease can include:

- bruising that is unusual in location or frequency;
- abnormal menstrual bleeding;
- bleeding in the mucous membranes, such as the gums, nose and the lining of the gastrointestinal system;
- excessive or prolonged bleeding after a tooth is pulled or tonsils are removed or prolonged oozing from cuts;
- the rare type 3 VWD can cause severe bleeding symptoms similar to severe hemophilia (for example, bleeding in joints or muscles);

- family history of a bleeding tendency, such as excess bleeding from wounds, gingival (gum) bleeding, postpartum bleeding.

How do you diagnose vwd? Because the symptoms can be mild, vwd can be difficult to diagnose and often goes undetected. Many children are diagnosed as a result of a positive family history or during routine preoperative screening.

The tests used to diagnose vwd can include:

- Factor viii level test, which measures the level of factor viii and its ability to function.
- vwf antigen test (also called factor viii antigen). This measures the amount of von Willebrand factor. The disorder is considered mild if a person has 20 percent to 40 percent of the normal amount. It is severe if the amount is less than 10 percent of normal.
- vwf activity (ristocetin cofactor activity test). It measures how well the von Willebrand factor is working.
- vwf multimers analysis. This test helps classify the type of vwd.
- Platelet function tests determine how well the platelets work and help identify the type of vwd or the presence of another disorder.
- Bleeding time, which measures the time for a puncture wound to stop bleeding. It is being done less frequently nowadays.
- pt and ptt, which are the common tests performed to screen a person's coagulation, or clotting, factors.

These tests might need to be done more than once because these levels can rise and fall over time in an individual.

How do you treat vwd? The most common treatment for excessive bleeding due to von Willebrand disease is desmopressin (DDAVP). This medication produces a temporary increase in the von Willebrand factor levels by causing release of vwf from its storage sites in the blood vessels. DDAVP can be given intravenously or intranasally (into the nose). However, it can be ineffective in some type 2 and all type 3 patients. Patients with type 3 (and some type 2) will need intravenous treatment with factor viii concentrates that contains both factor viii and von Willebrand factor. Children with type 1 may also require the use of this medication in certain situations, such as major trauma or major surgery, although they can generally be treated with DDAVP.

No evidence suggests that extensive activity restrictions are necessary for most people with mild type 1 vwd. Children with more severe forms of vwd should follow guidelines developed for those with severe hemophilia. Avoid medications with known antiplatelet effects such as aspirin, ibuprofen and naproxen. Heavy menstrual bleeding can sometimes be controlled with birth control pills. Call your child's doctor immediately if she experiences any excessive or unexplained bleeding.

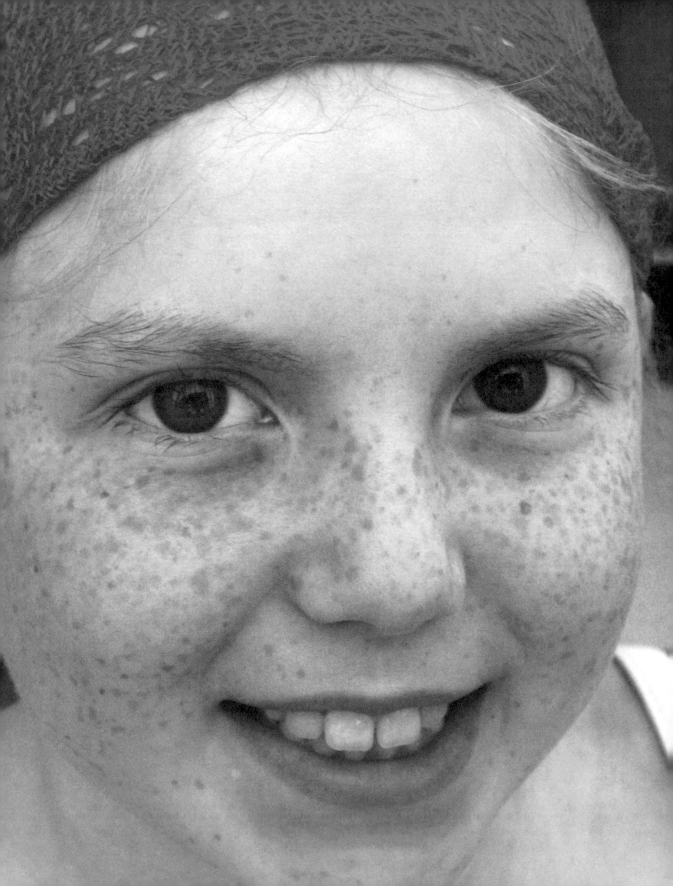

Malignancy

14

Brain Tumors

What are brain tumors? Brain tumors are cancers of the brain. Brain tumors in children are different than in adults both in terms of their location and the types of tumors seen. In children, brain tumors are most commonly found in the part of the brain called the posterior fossa, which includes the cerebellum, pons and medulla oblongata. The most common types of brain tumors in children include astrocytomas, medulloblastomas, ependymomas and germ cell tumors. The names of these different types of tumors refer to the fact that the cancerous cells arise from different types of brain cells.

Brain tumors are the second most common type of cancer in children, with leukemia (a form of blood cancer) being the most common. They are the most common type of solid tumor in children.

What do brain tumors look like? Brain tumors cause a variety of symptoms depending on where they are located and whether they are causing pressure on normal brain tissue. Brain tumors can obstruct the flow of cerebrospinal fluid in the brain, which leads to a buildup of fluid and pressure called hydrocephalus. Children with hydrocephalus will complain of headache and

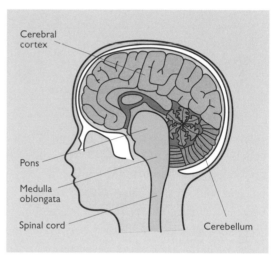

THE BRAIN

Brain tumors in children are most commonly seen in the cerebellum, pons and medulla.

vomiting, especially early in the morning. In young children, you might even notice an increase in head size, or the soft spot (fontanelle) can appear bigger or more prominent. Some children might be unable to move the eye properly (which can interfere with vision), or the face may droop on one side because the tumor is pushing on the nerves responsible for these movements.

Children with tumors in the posterior fossa often develop an unsteady gait and walk similar to someone who is drunk. If the tumor is growing slowly, the symptoms will generally develop

MALIGNANCY 287

SYMPTOMS OF BRAIN TUMORS IN CHILDREN

- headache
- vomiting
- abnormal facial movements or facial droop
- unsteady gait
- changes in personality or school performance
- weight loss
- seizure

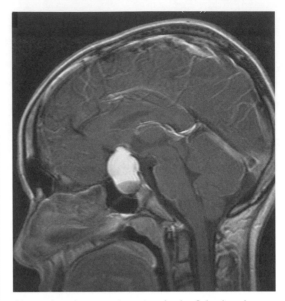

Magnetic resonance imaging (MRI) of the head.

very gradually. In these cases, there might be a change in school performance or young children might lose developmental milestones (such as walking or talking). Some children become irritable and develop a poor appetite that leads to weight loss. If the tumor occurs in the parts of the brain above the posterior fossa, the child can develop seizures, weakness on one side of the body or have changes in sensation (for example, the ability to feel touch, or tingling feelings).

How are brain tumors treated? If your child has symptoms that are consistent with a brain tumor, his doctor will begin by performing a very careful physical examination of the neurologic system. This involves performing a variety of maneuvers that test the various nerves and muscles. When intracranial pressure is raised, his doctor should notice specific changes in the appearance of the eye, called papilloedema. If, based on the physical examination, a brain tumor is suspected, he will order a CT scan or

MRI of the brain. If available, an MRI is usually the better test because it provides a better look at the posterior fossa and more detail in general. If a brain tumor is present, he might recommend a lumbar puncture to look for cancer cells in the cerebral spinal fluid that bathes the brain. This is performed by placing a tiny needle in the lower part of the spine below the bottom of the spinal cord to collect a few milliliters of cerebral spinal fluid.

The treatment for brain tumors generally consists of a combination of chemotherapy (medications used to kill the cancer cells), radiation therapy (high energy x-rays used to kill the cancer cells) and surgery to remove the tumor. The treatment will vary depending on the tumor type and location. Some children require a shunt (called a VP shunt) to drain off excessive fluid prior to removing the tumor.

The five-year survival rate associated with all brain tumors is approximately 50 percent. This will vary depending on the type of tumor. Unfortunately, many of the survivors of brain

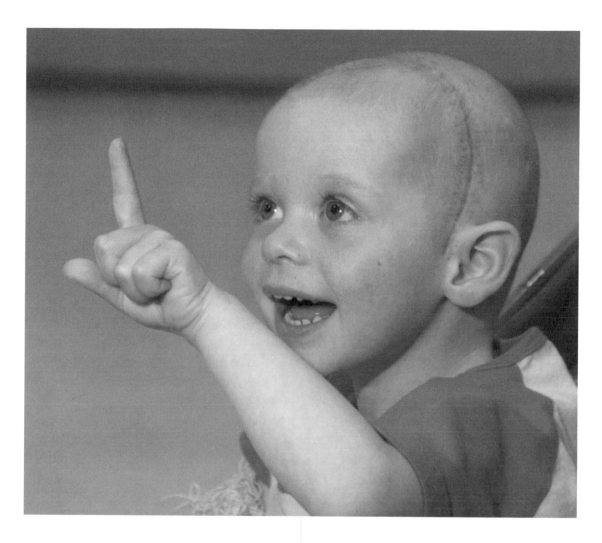

tumors must cope with residual problems related to the cancer and necessary treatment. Seizures, learning disabilities, weakness, growth and hormonal problems are common challenges that they frequently face.

Leukemia

What is leukemia? Leukemia is a cancer of the blood. It is the most common form of cancer in children. Leukemia occurs when abnormal cancerous cells (called "blasts") take over the bone marrow, which is the spongy inner part of the bone where blood cells are made. As a result, healthy blood cells cannot be normally produced.

There are three different types of blood cells normally produced in the bone marrow that all have specialized functions. The white blood cells help fight infection, the red blood cells carry oxygen and the platelets help the blood to clot. As the number of blasts increase they will "spill" out of the bone marrow into the bloodstream. They may also invade other tissues (for example, lymph nodes, liver, brain, bone or testicle).

There are two main types of leukemia. **Acute** lymphoblastic leukemia (ALL) is the most common form of leukemia in children, accounting for approximately 75 percent of cases. ALL affects a special type of mature white blood cell known as a lymphocyte. Acute myeloid leukemia (also known as acute non-lymphocytic leukemia) is a form of leukemia that affects the immature white blood cells other than the lymphocytes. It is more common in adults but still accounts for 15 percent to 20 percent of childhood leukemia. There are also chronic forms of leukemia, which are very rare in children and will not be discussed.

What does leukemia look like? The symptoms of leukemia are mainly related to the decreased number of healthy blood cells. Decreased numbers of red blood cells, a type of anemia, will result in reduced energy and pallor (pale skin). Low platelets will cause easy bruising and a skin rash that consists of small red dots, called **petechiae**. If the white blood cells are decreased your child will be more prone to infection. Some children will also have fever and poor appetite. If the leukemia has invaded his bones, your child might complain of bone pain, limp or have a swollen joint. Painless enlargement of one or both testicles can be a sign of invasion into the testicle. When a doctor examines your child, he might feel enlargement of lymph node, liver and/or spleen.

How is leukemia treated? If your child's doctor suspects he has leukemia, he will recommend a blood test called a complete blood count (CBC) to check the numbers of white blood cells, red blood cells and platelets. This will also reveal if there are any blasts present in the blood. If the

SYMPTOMS OF LEUKEMIA

- pale skin
- decreased energy
- bruising or skin rash
- unexplained fever
- poor appetite/weight loss
- bone pain

CBC is suspicious for leukemia, the bone marrow will be examined directly by aspiration (a needle sampling) and tests will be performed on this specimen to confirm the diagnosis of leukemia. This information will also be used to determine the type of leukemia. All children with confirmed leukemia will have a lumbar puncture, which is a needle placed in the lower back to remove spinal fluid. This is done to check if there are any cancer cells in the spinal fluid. Other studies might be performed based on your child's symptoms.

Once the diagnosis of leukemia is made, your child will be placed into a high- or low-risk category depending on age and the number of abnormal white blood cells. Treatment will be based on the initial risk group. Leukemia is treated with chemotherapy, a combination of oral and intravenous medications that kill cancer cells. A number of drugs are used as part of each specific treatment plan, or protocol. These protocols consist of different phases of therapy: first, to induce a remission, next to consolidate it and, finally, to maintain the remission. In total, most protocols carry on for about 120 weeks. As part of the protocol, anticancer drugs are also injected into the spinal fluid via a lumbar puncture in order to either eliminate leukemia in the spinal fluid or prevent a later relapse.

The treatment of childhood leukemia is one of modern medicine's miracles. Not long ago, the diagnosis was essentially a death sentence. Now, the majority of children with leukemia, over 70 percent of all those with ALL, will be cured of their disease.

Lymphomas

HODGKIN'S AND NON-HODGKIN'S LYMPHOMA

What is lymphoma? Lymphoma is a cancer of the lymphatic system. This system helps protect the body from infection and is one of the most important parts of the immune system. Lymphoma occurs when development of lymphocytes—a type of white blood cell used to fight infection—becomes abnormal and leads to malignant changes. These abnormal cells generally start in the lymph nodes and can then circulate throughout the entire lymphatic system. Because they are able to grow faster and live longer than normal white blood cells, they are able to flourish within the immune system.

There are two broad categories of lymphoma: Hodgkin's disease and non-Hodgkin's disease. Lymphoma is the third most common type of cancer in children, accounting for about 12 percent of pediatric malignancies.

HODGKIN'S DISEASE

What is Hodgkin's disease? Hodgkin's disease is a type of lymphoma that is more common in adolescents than younger children. Specific abnormal cells, called Reed-Sternberg cells, are seen in Hodgkin's disease and are typical for this lymphoma. Further classification of Hodgkin's disease depends on the appearance of the lymphoma under the microscope. Like most cancers, no one knows exactly what causes Hodgkin's disease although certain viruses, such as the Epstein-Barr virus (which causes infectious mononucleosis), have been associated with the disease. Children with known immunodeficiency disorders (diseases that affect the child's immune system) have an increased risk of developing Hodgkin's disease as are those who have had solid organ (for example, liver or kidney) or bone marrow transplants.

What does Hodgkin's disease look like? The first sign of Hodgkin's disease is usually a painless swelling of the lymph nodes. The most commonly affected nodes are those in the neck; those above the collarbone and in the chest are also frequently involved. When touched, the swollen lymph nodes feel firm and rubbery. They are not tender or painful and, in general, there is no redness associated with the swelling. If there are enlarged lymph nodes in the chest, your child might notice shortness of breath or chest pain. Typically, the symptoms of Hodgkin's disease develop slowly over time.

Some children develop constitutional (whole body) symptoms that include fever, profuse sweating at night (drenching the sheets) and weight loss. These are called "B" symptoms. There might also be a decrease in energy. Some children notice a nonspecific itchiness.

How do you treat Hodgkin's disease? If your child's doctor suspects your child might have Hodgkin's disease, or another form of lymphoma, he will recommend a series of tests. This usually starts with blood work to look at the white blood cells, the function of the liver and kidney, and other markers of cancer. He will order a chest x-ray to see if the lymph nodes in the chest are enlarged. A CT scan of the neck, chest and abdomen will also identify enlarged lymph nodes. In addition, the results of a lumbar puncture (needle in the back to remove spinal fluid) and bone marrow aspiration (sampling by needle) will determine if there are cancerous cells in either the spinal fluid or bone marrow. A biopsy of the enlarged lymph node generally confirms the diagnosis.

Based on the above tests, your child's oncologist (doctor specializing in the treatment of people with cancer) will assign a stage (I to IV) to your child's illness. This staging system allows doctors to determine the appropriate treatment and assists with prognosis. Treatment usually involves a combination of chemotherapy and radiation therapy. Chemotherapy uses a combination of different medications to kill the cancer cells. Radiation therapy uses high energy x-rays to kill the cancer cells. Unfortunately, these treatments also kill healthy cells, which results in side effects, such as hair loss and susceptibility to infection. The chest radiation can also injure the lungs and heart. Still, in spite of these problems, treatment has led to a very high cure rate. The survival rate for stages I and II (milder) Hodgkin's disease is over 90 percent. Even children with more advanced disease still have disease-free survival rates of 70 percent to 90 percent.

NON-HODGKIN'S LYMPHOMA

What is non-Hodgkin's lymphoma? Non-Hodgkin's lymphoma (NHL) is a term used to describe a group of lymphomas that differ from Hodgkin's disease in terms of what the cancerous cells look like, their rate of growth and how the cancer affects the body. Sixty percent of lymphomas in children are the NHL type and they tend to occur in younger children than Hodgkin's disease. The risk factors for NHL are the same as for Hodgkin's disease. There are three main types of NHL that are distinguished on the basis of their cellular make up.

What does non-Hodgkin's lymphoma look like? Children with NHL also have swelling of the lymph nodes but, in these cases, they are most commonly found in the abdomen, chest and above the collarbone. Many children will have symptoms such as abdominal pain, nausea, vomiting or changes in bowel habits. These symptoms are secondary to the lymph nodes in the abdomen, which can stick together to form a mass. Just as in Hodgkin's disease, lymph nodes in the chest can lead to shortness of breath, chest pain or swelling of the face and neck. NHL can also spread beyond the lymphatic system to involve bone, bone marrow, brain and spinal cord, skin and testicles.

Unlike Hodgkin's disease, NHL grows rapidly. Generally, the symptoms are only present for a short period of time and the majority of children will have widespread disease by the time they are diagnosed. Children with NHL are less likely to have the constitutional symptoms of fever, weight loss and night sweats than those with Hodgkin's.

How do you treat non-Hodgkin's lymphoma?
The tests performed to make a diagnosis of
non-Hodgkin's lymphoma are the same as those
used to make the diagnosis of Hodgkin's disease. NHL in children will also be staged to help
guide treatment and prognosis. Chemotherapy
is also used to treat NHL. However, different
medications, which are directed specifically
at treating NHL, are used. The survival rate for
NHL is 70 percent to 90 percent, depending on
the stage of the disease.

Neuroblastoma

What is neuroblastoma? Neuroblastoma is a
cancer that arises from the primitive nerve
cells that go on to form part of the sympathetic
nervous system and the adrenal glands (organs
that sit above the kidney and are responsible
for secreting a number of hormones). Neuroblastomas begin in the adrenal gland in 45
percent to 50 percent of cases. Otherwise, they
are found along the nerves of the sympathetic
nervous system, most commonly in the
abdomen/pelvis, chest or neck. The tumor
might extend into the neighboring organs or
lymph nodes. It can also spread to more distant locations such as bone, bone marrow
(the spongy inner part of the bone that makes
blood cells), liver or skin.

Neuroblastoma is the most common solid
tumor in children found outside of the brain. It
accounts for approximately 8 percent to 10 percent of all childhood cancers. The majority of
children with neuroblastoma are diagnosed
before the age of 5 years and it is the most common form of cancer in infants.

What does neuroblastoma look like? Most commonly your child's doctor will feel a mass in the
abdomen, arising from either the adrenal gland
or sympathetic nervous system. This mass feels
hard and smooth if touched and is not tender.
It may less commonly start with a painless mass
in the neck. If the mass is in the chest your
child might complain of shortness of breath or
chest pain. Neuroblastoma has often spread
to distant organs by the time it is diagnosed.
Some children develop dark circles and swelling
around the eyes that resemble raccoon eyes. If it
has spread to the bone, your child might limp or
complain of bone pain. Some children have a
fever, weight loss and/or decreased energy. In
infants it can spread to the skin causing small
bluish lumps that have been described as looking like a blueberry muffin. Neuroblastomas
secrete hormones that infrequently cause symptoms such as diarrhea or high blood pressure.
Rarely, children will be taken to the doctor
because of unusual jumpy eye movements,
uncoordinated gait or jerky movements.

How do you treat neuroblastoma? If a doctor feels
an abdominal mass, he will usually start with
an ultrasound of the abdomen to determine if it
is a tumor and where it is located. If neuroblastoma is suspected, he will order a CT scan or
MRI of the neck, chest and abdomen/pelvis. He
will arrange for you to collect a 24-hour urine
sample to look for the hormones secreted by
neuroblastomas. He will also order a bone marrow aspiration (needle sample) and lumbar
puncture (needle placed into the lower back to
obtain spinal fluid) to see if the neuroblastoma
has spread to either the bone marrow or spinal
fluid. A bone scan, which is a special type of

x-ray that uses a nuclear medicine dye, is used to look for spread to the bones. Another type of nuclear medicine x-ray, the MIBG scan, is good at finding areas of distant spread and will usually be ordered. A biopsy of the mass is done to confirm the diagnosis and if the tumor is confined to one area it might be removed at the same time.

Based on the findings of the tests, physicians will assign a stage (I to IV) to the neuroblastoma that is used to guide treatment and prognosis. In most cases, therapy will consist of a combination of chemotherapy (medications that kill cancer cells) and surgery. Radiation (special type of x-ray used to kill the cancer cells) therapy is often used. If the neuroblastoma has spread to the bone marrow, a bone marrow transplant might be recommended.

The prognosis depends on the stage of the neuroblastoma at the time of diagnosis. It varies from a 90 percent five-year survival in children with mild (stage I) disease to a 10 percent to 20 percent five-year survival in those children over a year of age with advanced (stage IV) disease.

Retinoblastoma

What is retinoblastoma? The retina is the part of the eye that is situated at the back of the eyeball and is responsible for converting light into nerve impulses that travel to the back of the brain where they are interpreted into a visual perception. Retinoblastoma is cancer of the retina. It can affect one or both eyes.

Retinoblastoma occurs in about 1 in 16,000 children. It is usually diagnosed before your child reaches 2 years of age, although, when both eyes are involved, which occurs about 25 percent of the time, it is usually diagnosed

before the first birthday. A retinoblastoma gene that predisposes a child to the development of retinoblastoma has been identified. About 40 percent of retinoblastomas, especially those involving both eyes, are hereditary.

What does retinoblastoma look like? Retinoblastoma is usually diagnosed when the "red eye" that is usually observed when a light is flashed into the pupil is not actually red, as expected, but white instead. This might be seen during a routine eye exam or you might notice that in a photograph only one eye is red. Your child might have decreased vision or his eye may "turn in" (**strabismus**). Larger tumors can be accompanied by an irregularity of the pupil, blood in the eye (hyphema), bulging of the eye or eye pain. Rarely, retinoblastoma can spread to the bone.

How do you treat retinoblastoma? If your child's doctor suspects he has retinoblastoma, he should be referred immediately to an eye specialist (ophthalmologist) for a complete eye assessment. The doctor will order a CT scan or MRI of the eyes and brain to evaluate the extent of the tumor.

The treatment for retinoblastoma depends on whether one or both eyes are affected. If only one eye is affected and the tumor is small enough that vision can be preserved in that eye, radiation, laser coagulation or cryotherapy (freezing) may be used to try to destroy the tumor. If the tumor is larger and vision is already lost in that eye, the eye is generally removed (enucleated). If both eyes are affected, every attempt will be made to preserve some vision in at least one eye by attempting cryotherapy or radiation prior to resorting to enucleation. Chemotherapy is only used if there is tumor remaining after the eye is removed or if the cancer has spread (metastatic disease).

The overall survival rate for retinoblastoma is greater than 90 percent. However, in the inherited type of retinoblastoma, there is a significant risk that secondary tumors, particularly bone cancer, will develop when your child grows up.

Wilms' Tumor

What is Wilms' tumor? Wilms' tumor is a cancer of the kidney. Kidney cancer in children is relatively rare, but Wilms' is the most common form. The annual incidence of Wilms' tumor is about eight children per one million. It is usually diagnosed in the toddler years (around 3 to 3 ½).

What does Wilms' tumor look like? A child with Wilms' tumor usually has an abdominal mass. Quite often there are no associated symptoms. In fact, the tumor is often noticed accidentally for the first time while you are bathing or changing your child. Some children have abdominal pain, fever, high blood pressure or blood in the urine. Wilms' tumor can spread to the lung (most commonly), liver, bones and brain.

Wilms' tumor generally occurs in otherwise healthy children. Approximately 10 percent of children with Wilms' tumor have other birth defects such as aniridia (an abnormality of the iris or "colored part" of the eye), subtle enlargement of one side of the body or urinary tract abnormalities. In some cases, the genes that cause this combination of problems are known and a blood test can look for them.

How do you treat Wilms' tumor? If your child's doctor suspects a Wilms' tumor, the first test performed is usually an ultrasound of the abdomen. A CT scan of the chest, abdomen and pelvis generally follow. The CT scans are generally sufficient to make the diagnosis. The results are then used to "stage" or grade the spread of the tumor. This staging system is used to guide treatment and prognosis. In general, no further testing is needed. An isolated biopsy of the tumor is not performed as it may cause the tumor to "spill" into the abdominal cavity causing spread of the disease.

Once the diagnosis is made, your child's doctor will plan the surgery to remove the kidney containing the tumor. A sample of neighboring lymph nodes is taken at the same time. Chemotherapy (medications used to kill cancer cells) and/or radiation (a special type of x-ray that kills cancer cells) usually follow surgery in order to completely eradicate the cancer cells.

The overall five-year survival rate for Wilms' tumor is 70 percent to 85 percent. The prognosis depends on the staging, or amount of spread, at time of diagnosis. When successfully treated, children who had a Wilms' tumor removed can expect to live a high quality of life.

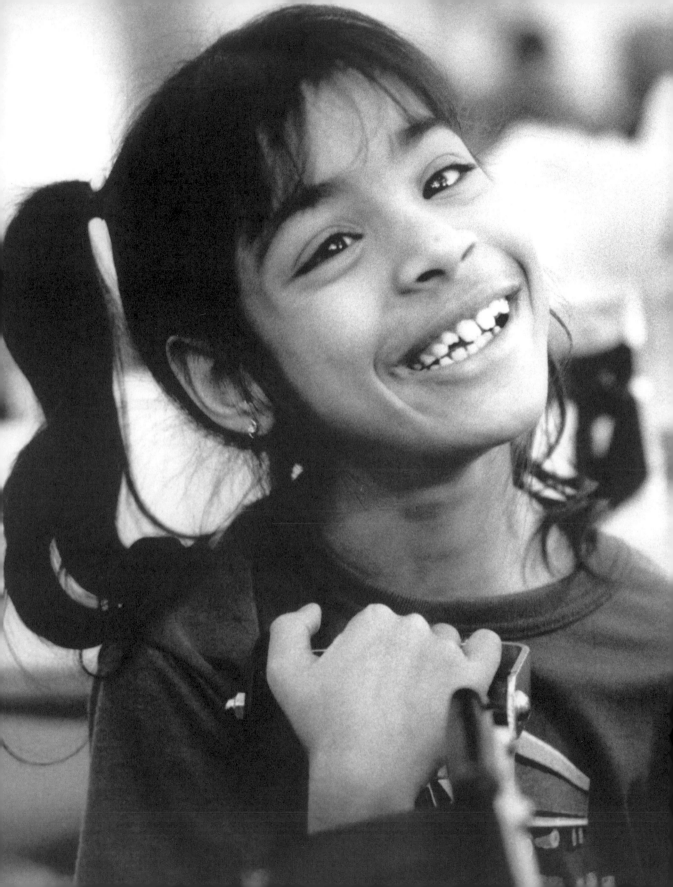

Neurological and Muscle Problems

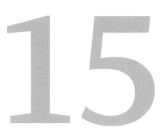

Cerebral Palsy

What is cerebral palsy? Cerebral palsy (CP) is a term used to describe a group of disorders featuring problems with movement and altered muscle tone and control. "Cerebral" means brain and "palsy" refers to disorders of movement or posture. CP is the result of earlier brain damage. This injury to the brain can occur during pregnancy (prenatal), delivery (perinatal) or immediately following birth (postnatal). Occasionally, it can follow a later injury, such as near-drowning or a motor vehicle accident. There are many potential causes of cerebral palsy. For example, some of the prenatal and perinatal causes include abnormal development of the brain, congenital infections, genetic abnormalities, prematurity and decreased oxygen to the brain (asphyxia). Some of the postnatal causes include severe jaundice, infections such as **meningitis** or brain injury secondary to accident or child abuse. The prevalence of CP is estimated to be between 2 and 5 per 1,000 babies born in North America.

There are a number of different types of CP. Of these, spastic cerebral palsy is by far the most common form. Children with spastic CP seem to have tight or stiff muscles that results

in them having difficulty moving. This spasticity might affect only a few muscles or the whole body. Spastic diplegia refers to involvement of the legs with minimal involvement of the arms. This form is most common in babies who were born prematurely. Spastic hemiplegia refers to involvement of both the arm and leg on one side of the body, as you might see in someone who has had a stroke. Often, the arm is more involved than the leg. Spastic quadriplegia is the most severe form of CP and refers to involvement of all four limbs. In these cases there is usually more widespread damage to the brain and, as a result, there is a much poorer prognosis. This sometimes results from a period of oxygen starvation to the brain.

Athetoid cerebral palsy is associated with involuntary and uncontrolled movements. Children with athetoid CP have many involuntary writhing movements and seem to be constantly in motion. Ataxic cerebral palsy features a disturbed sense of balance and depth perception. These children are usually unsteady and have poor coordination. Mixed cerebral palsy is the term used when there is a combination of any of the above types in the same child.

Cerebral palsy is thought of as a nonprogressive disorder in the sense that the brain damage does not get worse over time. However, what the children look like and are able to do changes with time because the normal brain around the damaged area continues to develop. Some children show improvement in their motor control while the muscles of others who initially were floppy (low tone) can increasingly stiffen, which results in their joints becoming fixed in one position (contractures) or other orthopedic problems.

What does cerebral palsy look like? The hallmark of CP is a delay in getting to the gross motor (rolling, sitting or walking) and/or fine motor (reaching and grabbing for objects) milestones. These developmental delays are seen in combination with physical signs such as decreased or increased muscle tone (floppy or stiff muscles) and abnormal muscle movements. Although some of these signs might be evident in the first year of life, the diagnosis is often difficult to make until 12 to 18 months of age. This is because the infant's brain is still growing and developing. In the first year of life all children vary widely in the timing of these milestones.

The degree of disability of children with CP also varies widely. Some children have only mildly impaired gait or awkward hand movements while others have severely limited muscle control, so they have to use a wheelchair to get around. Children with more severe disability need assistance with all their activities of daily living including dressing, feeding and toileting.

Children with CP also have varied mental, or cognitive, abilities. Many of these youngsters have a normal intelligence despite their physical disabilities. It is important not to underestimate your child with cerebral palsy. Some children will have difficulty expressing themselves, largely because they can't completely control the muscles involved in speech. Despite this,

your child likely will be able to communicate verbally. Children with severe CP can use special communication boards containing pictures, computers or predictable eye movements (for example, looking up for "yes") to communicate.

Unfortunately, when brain damage is more severe, your child will have significant cognitive impairment: it can appear that she never develops a meaningful form of communication. CP can also be accompanied by hearing or visual impairments that interfere with the ability to learn and communicate.

Many children with CP have feeding problems caused by the difficulty in controlling and coordinating the muscles involved in sucking and swallowing food. In fact, feeding difficulty can provide an early clue to a possible diagnosis of CP. If your child chokes and the liquid or food goes down the windpipe (trachea) instead of the esophagus, she can actually develop pneumonia and breathing difficulties from food going down the wrong way (aspiration). If she is not able to take enough calories, because of slow feeding and choking, she might not grow adequately.

Some children with CP will have seizures. These often start early in the newborn period and can be quite difficult to control. A variety of medications can be used to control the seizures.

Those with CP are also at risk for developing a number of musculoskeletal problems. The muscle stiffness can ultimately lead to the joints becoming fixed in one position, called contractures. Therapists will attempt to stretch the muscles in order to prevent this from happening. The muscles become so tight in many spastic children that their hips can be pulled either partially (subluxation) or completely (dislocation) out of the joint. This can cause your child pain and discomfort. If her hip is dislocated, she might require surgery to fix it. Children with severe CP can develop scoliosis, (curvature of the spine, see pages 220–21) that might also need surgical correction.

How do you treat cerebral palsy? Your child's doctor might suspect CP after speaking with you regarding your child's medical history and development, and then examining her. There is no single test that will tell the doctor whether your child has CP or not. Reaching the diagnosis is like constructing a jigsaw puzzle with all the clues acting as pieces of the puzzle. It is often true that not enough pieces of the puzzle are available in your child's early months to make the diagnosis.

Your child's doctor will be looking for changes in usual muscle tone, such as spasticity (high tone) or floppiness (low tone). Your baby may appear too jittery. Her reflexes, such as the knee jerk, are generally increased. Your child's doctor might recommend further testing to look for the underlying cause and to rule out any other conditions. She might order a CT scan or MRI to look for abnormalities in the structure of the brain. She could order blood tests to rule out chemical abnormalities in the blood. If your child's doctor suspects seizures, she might recommend a tracing of the electrical activity in the brain called an electroencephalogram (EEG) to look for evidence of seizure activity. She will also assess your child's hearing and vision.

If your child is diagnosed with CP, she will be referred to various therapists. Physical therapists will work on the muscles, both to improve strength and prevent contractures. You will probably be taught exercises to do at home. Occupational therapists will work on hand control and hand-eye coordination. They will also help with finding equipment, such as wheelchairs, leg braces and communication devices, to assist your child to gain as much independence as possible. Occupational or speech therapists assess feeding and look for signs of aspiration. They can give you advice regarding feeding techniques and positioning. In some cases, it could be unsafe to feed your child by mouth and a feeding tube (called a gastrostomy tube) will be recommended. This permits adequate nutrition to be given. It promotes proper growth and avoids aspiration into the lungs.

Speech therapy can also be helpful. Teamwork, involving health care professionals, teachers and the family is key.

Some children require medication to help decrease their spasticity and thus improve their motor control. Your child might take medications, such as diazepam or baclofen, to relax her muscles. In very severe cases, a pump might be inserted into the abdominal cavity to deliver medication (baclofen) directly to the cerebrospinal fluid. Another medication, called botulism toxin, might be injected into the nerves of the spastic muscles in order to decrease the tone. This will result in temporary relaxation of the muscles that lasts for four to six weeks.

Your health care team might recommend orthopedic surgery for a variety of problems including scoliosis, hip dislocations and occasionally for tight joints, such as the ankles, knees and hips.

Parenting is never easy. This is especially true when your child has cerebral palsy. Yet, in this situation, your rewards can be just as great as the challenges.

Epilepsy and Seizures

What are epilepsy and seizures? Seizures are caused when the electrical activity of groups of brain cells temporarily gets out of control and, as a result, interferes with normal brain function. The effect of these electrical discharges varies depending upon which part of the brain is involved. Seizures can involve impairment or loss of consciousness, abnormal or uncontrollable motor movements, behavioral or emotional abnormalities or changes in sensation.

Isolated seizures can be the result of a variety of medical conditions. These include problems such as infection (for example, **meningitis**), accidental poisoning or drug overdose, head trauma, brain tumor, low blood sugar (hypoglycemia), or anatomical abnormalities in the brain structure. Children between 6 months of age and 5 years can have a benign form of seizure when they have a fever, called febrile convulsions (see pages 302–303). The terms epilepsy and seizure disorder are used to describe those seizures that recur in the absence of fever. In many cases the cause of the seizure is unknown. Seizure disorders occur in 4 to 6 children in 1,000.

What do seizures look like? Seizures, sometimes called convulsions, can be divided into two types, generalized and partial. Each has a unique look and each requires a different treatment.

Generalized seizures involve a number of distinct seizure types. One of the more common types is the generalized tonic clonic seizure, previously called a grand mal seizure. During this seizure, the child will suddenly lose consciousness and develop stiffening of the arms and legs. This is the tonic phase. It is followed by rhythmic jerking, the clonic phase, that generally involves the whole body. The child might urinate or defecate and is often quite sleepy following the seizure. Sometimes, the seizures involve just stiffening (tonic) or jerking (clonic) movements. Absence seizures, previously called petit mal, are characterized by a brief staring spell during which the child is unresponsive with no speech or movement. In some cases, the seizure is accompanied by flickering of the eyes. The episode will usually last 5 to 20 seconds. Myoclonic seizures are characterized by brief, symmetric jerking movements of the muscles.

Partial seizures involve only one part or side of the body. These can include abnormal limb movements, sensations or even "automatisms," which are semipurposeful actions such as lip smacking, chewing movements of the mouth, picking or pulling at clothing. During a partial seizure, the child might move her head or eyes to one side or have shaking movements on only one side of the body. Sensory partial seizures involve changes in vision, hearing or smell. Some children will complain of an "aura" prior to the seizure, which is a distinct introductory sensation, such as stomach discomfort, an unusual smell or an unpleasant feeling.

A small percentage of children with seizures have an epileptic **syndrome** such as Lennox-Gastaut or Landau-Kleffner syndromes. These syndromes are characterized by particular and recognizable patterns of seizures, age of onset and outcomes.

How do I treat a seizure? Seizures are very frightening for anyone to see. If your child is having a seizure, try to remain calm in spite of the sense of alarm and helplessness. You should not attempt to restrain her movements.

- If possible, place your child on her side.
- Do not put anything in her mouth.
- Ensure that she cannot be injured by the convulsions; for example, do not put her on a bed where she could fall off or somewhere where the jerking will produce a collision with a hard object.

- Loosen any clothing around her head or neck.
- Unless you are very familiar with your child's seizures and are comfortable with the management, call an ambulance immediately.
- If the seizure continues for more than a few minutes, the child has difficulty breathing or is turning blue, call 9-1-1 right away.

If the seizure is prolonged, doctors might need to administer medication to stop the seizure. These medicines can be given by mouth, syringed into the rectum or by an injection.

Once the seizure is over, the doctor treating your child will order a number of tests to determine the cause of the seizure. If your child has a fever, the doctor might suggest tests to determine if an infection caused the seizure. One of these tests is a **lumbar puncture**, which tests for meningitis. If meningitis is suspected, your child will be started on antibiotics. Blood tests might be ordered to rule out low blood sugar or other problems with the body's chemistry, such as low sodium or calcium. A CT scan or MRI of the brain would help look for a brain tumor, a bleed inside the head or anything else that may be putting pressure on the brain. If the doctor suspects an anatomic abnormality, an MRI will provide more detail. If you suspect your child might have eaten a poison or medication she should not have, blood or urine tests would look for evidence.

A special test called an electroencephalogram (EEG) records brainwave activity and can detect seizure activity in the brain. This is done in a similar fashion to the ECG of the heart that most people are familiar with, only this time the sticky electrodes are placed around the head instead of the chest. Between seizures, your child's brain activity can be normal and, thus, the EEG will be normal even if your child has recurrent seizures. A number of maneuvers can bring on a seizure including having your child hyperventilate or stimulating her with flickering lights. And, in some special circumstances, your child will be deprived of sleep prior to the test.

If her doctors determine that an event was definitely a seizure, with no underlying cause that can be "fixed," they will need to make a decision about treatment. There are many medications used to treat seizures. The decision to use medication must balance the risk of further seizures with the potential side effects of the medications. Treatment is not usually started following a first generalized tonic clonic seizure. That is because children who have had one generalized tonic clonic seizure, a normal physical examination, normal EEG and no family history of seizures, have a 75 percent chance of not having any further seizures. On the other hand, children who have absence seizures or myoclonic seizures have a very high risk of recurrence and, thus, medication is started at the time of diagnosis. The choice of medication will depend on the type of seizure.

The majority of children treated with antiseizure medication will require blood tests to check for potential side effects and to see if the medication is reaching the required concentration in the blood. As your child grows and gains weight, the doctor will adjust the dose of the medication. The hope is that seizures can be controlled with just one medication. Unfortunately, however, this is not always possible and an additional drug or two may be required. If your child does not have seizures for a prolonged period (usually one to two years), the decision might be made to gradually discontinue the drug. This is generally done slowly over a four- to six-month period.

Febrile Convulsions

What is a febrile convulsion? A febrile convulsion is a seizure that occurs only in the presence of fever. It is commonly believed that the convulsion occurs as part of a young brain's response to a rising temperature.

Febrile convulsions are by far the most common form of seizures in young children. They affect approximately 4 percent of North American children. Typically, the close relatives of many children with febrile convulsions will also have a history of febrile convulsions. In fact, if an older sibling has had a febrile convulsion, there is a 10 percent to 20 percent risk that younger siblings will also have febrile convulsions. Although these seizures are extremely frightening to witness, they are generally not dangerous to the child and, unless the seizure is extremely long, there is no risk of brain damage.

Most children who experience a febrile convulsion will have only one seizure within the first 24 hours of the febrile illness. However, a small percentage of children will have more than one seizure within a 24-hour period or have a prolonged seizure. Furthermore, approximately one-third of children who experience one febrile convulsion will have a recurrence with subsequent febrile illnesses. This is more likely if the initial convulsion was prolonged (longer than 10 to 15 minutes), occurred in a younger infant or involved only one side of the body. These recurrences are most likely to occur within the first year following a febrile convulsion. Fortunately, the great majority of children with febrile seizures, over 95 percent, will never develop epilepsy nor do they seem at greater risk for neurological problems.

Children with febrile seizures generally develop normally, meaning they will reach their developmental milestones (walking, talking, etc.) at the prescribed time. Children with developmental delays, on the other hand, are at an increased risk of having epilepsy. Although children with delays might experience their first seizure during fever, these are not considered classic febrile convulsions.

What do febrile convulsions look like? Febrile convulsions generally occur early in the course of a febrile illness, often before parents have recognized the presence of any fever. During these seizures, your child will suddenly lose consciousness and her extremities will stiffen. This is followed by rhythmic jerking of the extremities and generally involves the whole body. Your child might lose bowel or bladder control and is often quite sleepy following the seizure. The majority of febrile convulsions last less than 15 minutes and, in fact, most are even shorter, lasting only a few minutes.

Other seizure types occur less commonly. These include staring with only stiffness or limpness of the body or jerking movements that are not preceded by stiffening. Some febrile convulsions involve stiffening or jerking of only one side of the body. These are called partial febrile convulsions and require more careful investigation by a physician in order to ensure there is no other cause for the seizure.

How do I treat febrile convulsions? Unfortunately, there is no evidence to suggest that lowering the temperature during a fever will prevent a febrile seizure. However, most physicians still recommend treating fever with antifever medications (antipyretics) such as acetaminophen or ibuprofen. This will help lower the fever and, more importantly, will make your child more comfortable. Tepid sponge baths, using water warm enough to avoid shivering, might also help when combined with antipyretics. In the vast majority of cases, doctors do not recommend administering antiseizure medications to prevent recurrence.

Febrile convulsions are very frightening to see and you might fear for your child's life during the seizure. If your child is having a febrile convulsion, remain calm and ensure that your child is in a safe place.

Following a febrile convulsion, a physician should assess your child. This is primarily to determine the cause of the fever and to ensure there are no signs of serious infection, which would require further treatment. For example, some children with **meningitis** will have fever and seizures. If the doctor is concerned that your child might have meningitis, she will recommend a **lumbar puncture** to check for infection and will start intravenous antibiotics, if necessary. Most often the fever is secondary to a viral illness and does not require antibiotics or it may be due to an infection, such as an ear infection, that can be treated with oral antibiotics. It is not necessary to keep your child in hospital after a typical febrile convulsion.

Once a febrile convulsion has occurred, many parents express concern about administering routine immunizations because some children develop a fever after such vaccinations. Fever tends to be more common following the administration of the DTaP (diphtheria, **tetanus** and **pertussis**) vaccines. The risk of fever and thus febrile convulsion is greatest in the 48 hours following the vaccine. Happily, the incidence of fever has been much reduced by the newer (**acellular**) form of the vaccine. Fever is also less common following the measles, mumps and rubella (MMR) vaccine, but when it does occur it is delayed until 7 to 10 days after the vaccination. The risk of fever

WHAT DO I DO IF MY CHILD IS HAVING A FEBRILE CONVULSION?

- Try to stay calm.
- Place the child on her side.
- Position the child so she cannot be injured by the convulsions.
- Do not place anything in the child's mouth.
- If seizure lasts for greater than five minutes, go to a medical facility, by ambulance whenever possible (call 9-1-1).

and febrile convulsion after the vaccination must be weighed against the benefits of immunization. Physicians generally recommend proceeding with immunizations as normal.

Guillain-Barre Syndrome

What is Guillain-Barre syndrome? Guillain-Barre syndrome (GBS) is a neurological condition that occurs when the body's own immune system attacks myelin (the protective covering of nerves) outside the brain and spinal cord. As a result, the damaged nerves cannot properly send their signals back to the brain, which produces a gradual muscle paralysis. GBS affects people of all ages and both sexes. It is not hereditary and the cause is unknown. GBS often follows a nonspecific viral infection of either the respiratory or gastrointestinal system. It has also been associated with stomach flu caused by a bacteria called *Campylobacter jejuni*.

SYMPTOMS OF GUILLAIN-BARRE SYNDROME

- Weakness that starts in the legs and moves up the body,
- abnormal tingling sensations,
- muscle pain,
- swallowing difficulties,
- breathing difficulties.

What does Guillain-Barre syndrome look like?
GBS generally begins with weakness or tingling sensations in the legs. This weakness gradually moves up the body to include the trunk, arms and finally the facial muscles. It usually starts gradually and then progresses upward over the next two to four weeks. In some cases, however, the process is more sudden and is then often associated with muscle pain or tenderness if the muscle is touched. If there is significant involvement of the facial muscles the child can have difficulty swallowing, or food can go down the wrong way into her lungs. In about half of affected children, the muscles controlling breathing become weakened to the point that the child can no longer breathe independently. In these cases, a respirator is required to assist breathing. Some children will experience either urinary incontinence (loss of control) or retention (the inability to urinate spontaneously).

The majority of children who develop GBS will completely recover. The length of illness is unpredictable and many children will have a long stay in hospital. A small minority are left with some weakness.

How do you diagnose Guillain-Barre syndrome?
The diagnosis of GBS is made by combining what the doctor finds on a physical examination with laboratory tests. In addition to muscle weakness, the deep tendon reflexes (for example, knee jerk) become absent. Doctors might perform a **lumbar puncture** to see if there are increased levels of protein. And they might also do an electrical test of both nerve and muscle function.

How do you treat Guillain-Barre syndrome?
Children with GBS are usually admitted to hospital in the early stages of the disease. This allows their breathing and other body functions to be monitored and often takes place in an intensive care unit. Some children require nasal feeding tubes and urinary catheters. If the disease gets worse quickly, there are several therapies that can be tried. Plasmapheresis (a blood cleansing technique similar to dialysis), intravenous immunoglobulin (IVIG) and/or steroids can help shorten the course of the disease.

Hypotonia (Low Tone, Floppy Baby)

What is hypotonia? Hypotonia is a term used to describe infants or children with lower than normal muscle tone. In other words, the child seems floppy and often has decreased control of muscle movements. When picked up, the infant almost feels like a rag doll. In some cases there is no serious underlying cause. This is called benign congenital hypotonia. The infant improves and will grow out of the relative limpness, leaving only slight muscle weakness or extra joint mobility. Hypotonia can also be caused by damage or dysfunction

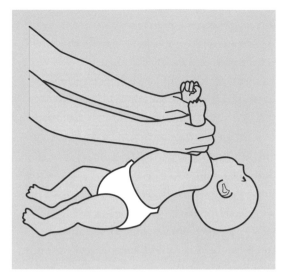

DECREASED MUSCLE TONE

A baby with low muscle tone will be slow to develop head control.

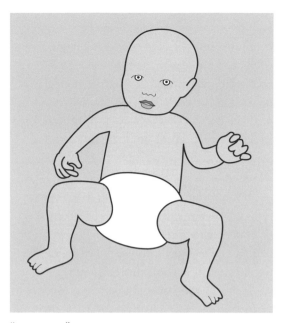

"FROG LEGS"

Hypotonic (floppy) babies lie in a "frog leg" position with arms and legs splayed out.

of the brain, spinal cord, peripheral nerves and muscles. Metabolic disorders—inherited disorders resulting in a deficiency or excessive amount of chemicals essential to body functioning—can also lead to hypotonia.

What does hypotonia look like? Sometimes your baby will not have been very active while still in the womb. An infant with hypotonia has a very characteristic appearance, regardless of the underlying cause. When lying on her back, the baby will take on a "frog leg" position with the arms and legs splayed out flat. If she is picked up under the armpits, it feels as if she will slip through your hands if you don't hold on tight. She is slow to develop control of her head.

Your baby will not move much spontaneously. This lack of movement leads to flattening of the back of the skull and loss of hair in that area. The child with hypotonia is often delayed in

reaching gross motor milestones, such as rolling, sitting or walking. In severe cases, she might never reach these milestones.

Newborn infants with hypotonia may have been born with skeletal abnormalities that consist of stiff joints or deformities, called arthrogryposis. The most common of these deformities are club foot (see pages 213–14) and hip dislocation (see Developmental Dysplasia of the Hip, pages 216–18). Those infants with a genetic disorder may have unusual facial features.

Infants with hypotonia often have feeding difficulties that can start as soon as they are born. They suck weakly or have difficulties swallowing. As a result, many gain weight poorly. These infants can also have difficulty breathing if the hypotonia is also associated with muscle weakness. As a result they can have more respiratory infections than other infants.

How do you treat hypotonia? Your baby with hypotonia might have to undergo a number of tests in an attempt to identify the underlying cause of the low tone. A pediatrician, pediatric neurologist or pediatric geneticist might assess her. The doctors will determine if the hypotonia is secondary to a problem with the central or peripheral nervous system as this will dictate which tests are performed.

If the doctor suspects a central nervous system cause, your baby will likely have a CT scan or MRI of the brain. Blood tests will look for genetic and metabolic disorders. She might also have tests that examine hearing and vision.

If the doctor suspects a peripheral nervous system problem, an **electromyogram** (EMG) and nerve conduction tests will look at the function of the muscles and nerves. Blood tests look for genetic confirmation of disorders such as **spinal muscular atrophy**, a degenerative disease of the motor nerve cells in the spinal cord that begins in utero. Sometimes the diagnosis will require a biopsy sample of muscle or nerve.

If your child is having difficulty eating and is not gaining weight, your child's doctor might recommend a special tube through the nose or directly into the stomach to assist with feeding. Physiotherapists and pediatric occupational therapists will probably also be involved as part of the team whose goal is to help your child maximize her potential.

Muscular Dystrophy

What is muscular dystrophy? Muscular dystrophy (MD) refers to a group of diseases that are characterized by weakness and a slow, progressive breakdown of muscles. Muscular dystrophy affects the skeletal muscles, which are those muscles primarily attached to bone that are responsible for moving the skeleton. The most common form is called Duchenne muscular dystrophy (DMD). Becker muscular dystrophy (BMD) is similar to DMD but milder. Other forms of muscular dystrophy include congenital muscular dystrophy, facioscapulohumeral muscular dystrophy, limb-girdle dystrophy and myotonic muscular dystrophy. These forms are also characterized by muscle weakness but the symptoms vary and they are much less common. Many types can be detected by specific, but not routine, testing of the fetus in the womb.

Duchenne muscular dystrophy is an inherited genetic disease that is carried on the X sex chromosome. Females have two X chromosomes and no Y chromosome, while males have one X and one Y sex chromosome. The second normal X chromosome in females protects them from the disease but they can carry the genetic muscular dystrophy material that can be passed on to their own children. Since males have only one X chromosome, they do develop the disease: there is no normal second X chromosome to protect them. DMD affects approximately 1 in every 3,500 males.

What does Duchenne muscular dystrophy look like? Boys with DMD generally appear healthy in the first couple of years of life and the majority will achieve their motor milestones (sitting, walking) at the normal time. Between 2 and 6 years of age, the weakness characteristic of DMD becomes evident. The first signs include development of a "waddling" gait and difficulty getting up from the floor or climbing stairs. These boys are unable to jump and have frequent falls. The muscles, especially in the calf, may become enlarged (**pseudohypertrophy**). Many boys will walk on their toes. Weakness of the shoulders and arms appears later as the disease progresses. By the teenage years, most boys lose the ability to walk and must use a wheelchair. Once confined to a wheelchair a series of new complications occur. The large joints like the knees, hips, feet, wrists and elbows lose mobility and become fixed in one position. This is called a contracture of the joint. Many boys develop a curvature of the spine called scoliosis or are hunchbacked (**kyphosis**). The muscles that control chewing and swallowing as well as bowel and bladder control are not affected. In addition to the muscle weakness, approximately one-third of boys will also have learning difficulties. Ultimately, the muscles controlling the heart and breathing weaken. Tragically, most boys with DMD will die from heart or breathing problems in their 20s or 30s.

Becker muscular dystrophy has the same symptoms as Duchenne muscular dystrophy, but these usually start later and are less severe. Most boys will walk until the late teenage years. In some cases, the heart muscle becomes more severely involved than the skeletal muscles. Males with BMD generally survive until late adulthood.

How do you diagnose and treat Becker muscular dystrophy and Duchenne muscular dystrophy? If DMD or BMD is suspected, a blood test might be done looking for an enzyme called creatine phosphokinase (CK). This enzyme is released from damaged muscle. If elevated, your son's doctor will likely recommend a muscle biopsy to look for features consistent with DMD or BMD. Your child's doctor will make a diagnosis based on the results of the muscle biopsy.

Unfortunately, there is no definitive cure for DMD or BMD at this time. However, there are a number of supportive treatments that can help improve your child's quality of life. He will have physiotherapy daily to stretch his muscles and attempt to prevent contractures. Braces that support better positioning of the muscles are also helpful. If scoliosis becomes a significant problem, your child's doctor might recommend surgery to straighten the spine. Steroid medication has been beneficial in slowing the progression of muscle weakness and increasing strength. This might also prolong your child's period of walking. These benefits must be balanced against the side effects of steroids.

Therapists will assist him with seating and getting around with techniques and aids, such as walkers and wheelchairs. As respiratory function deteriorates, many boys will need assistance with their breathing. A tube might be inserted through your child's neck directly into the airway (tracheotomy) and then attached to a ventilator to improve his breathing.

Neural Tube Defects including Spina Bifida

What are neural tube defects? Neural tube defects (NTD) occur when there is incomplete development of the brain or spinal cord and their protective coverings. These congenital abnormalities are not uncommon and are considered among the most serious forms of birth defects.

There are three main types of NTD. Spina bifida is the most common of the NTDs and affects approximately 1 in 1,000 infants. Spina bifida results from the incomplete closure of the spine early in pregnancy with the result that the protective covering, called the **meninges**,

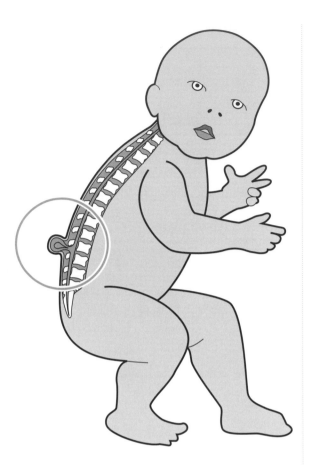

SPINA BIFIDA

Spina bifida refers to incomplete closure of the spine with the protrusion of the meninges (protective covering) or of the spinal cord itself.

or the spinal cord itself protrudes through the skin. A very mild form called spina bifida occulta occurs when there is a small opening in the vertebrae of the spine without any protrusion of the spinal cord or covering. Children with spina bifida occulta are healthy and do not have any symptoms. Anencephaly occurs when there is almost total underdevelopment of the brain: the skull might even be absent. Babies with anencephaly die within the first hours to days of life. Encephalocele results when there is a hole in the skull caused by incomplete bone closure, which allows brain tissue to protrude through it. Depending on the size and location of this defect, it might be possible to correct it surgically.

Since the 1980s, it has been recognized that maternal intake of folic acid decreases the incidence of NTDs. You will need to start taking folic acid before becoming pregnant and continue taking it for the first several months of pregnancy. This is because NTD occurs within the first weeks of pregnancy, often before the woman knows she is pregnant. The recommended dose is 0.4 mg/day.

What does spina bifida look like? Spina bifida varies depending on the location of the defect and what is protruding: the meninges and/or the spinal cord. In the majority of cases, damage to the spinal cord produces some degree of paralysis and loss of sensation. In its least severe form, the child is able to walk but has difficulties with bowel and bladder control. Other children require braces and crutches to assist with walking. In its most severe form, children with spina bifida are dependent on a wheelchair to get around.

Many children with spina bifida also develop a condition called hydrocephalus. This essentially is an excess accumulation of spinal fluid in and around the brain. A special ventriculoperitoneal (VP) shunt can be inserted to divert the extra fluid from the ventricles in the brain to the abdominal cavity. Children with spina bifida often have learning difficulties and require special assistance at school. In addition, there is an association between spina bifida and allergy to latex (rubber).

How do you treat spina bifida? The majority of children with spina bifida will require surgery within the first few days of life to close the opening in the spine. Your baby will have a CT scan or MRI of the brain to look for hydrocephalus. If present, your child might require a VP shunt.

Your child's doctor will also assess the degree of bladder and bowel control. This can even be done on a newborn by assessing how well she empties her bladder. Many children will require regular catheterization, whereby a tube is placed through the urethra into the bladder, to assist with urination. Many also have difficulty getting control of their bowels, which can be very embarrassing, especially as they get older. Medications such as suppositories and enemas can help to prevent accidents. In some cases, a special tube (called a **cecostomy tube**) can be placed into the bowel to assist with emptying the bowels.

Your child will go to a rehabilitation center where physical and occupational therapists can assist her with muscle strength exercises and help with all the necessary equipment, such as braces and wheelchairs. They often attend special classroom settings that can meet their special learning and physical needs. Some of these children with severe illness will die young; others might have a normal lifespan.

Stroke

What is a stroke? A stroke occurs when there is a sudden disruption of the blood supply to the brain. As a result, there is damage to the brain cells, which usually leads to a problem with neurological functions such as movement and speech. The difficulties experienced by the child will depend on which area of the brain is affected, and the extent of the injury.

There are two major types of stroke. The first is called an **ischemic stroke** and occurs when there is a blockage of blood supplying an area of the brain. This blockage is usually caused by a clot, or thrombus, that forms in the brain. The clot can also travel to the brain from another location, such as the heart, in which case it is called an embolism. The second type of stroke is called a **hemorrhagic stroke**. This occurs when there is bleeding from the blood vessels into the brain.

Although strokes are much less common in children than adults, they do occur. Each year, strokes afflict about 1 child in every 20,000. The causes of stroke are very different in children from those found in adults. Ischemic strokes can be caused by a variety of disorders. At least half of the children have an underlying medical condition, such as sickle-cell anemia or a heart problem. Other causes include an increased tendency to form blood clots or abnormalities of the blood vessels supplying the brain. Unfortunately, these problems are usually not discovered until after the stroke has occurred. Infection, such as **meningitis**, can also cause ischemic stroke. In some cases, despite extensive investigation, the cause is never identified. The most common cause of hemorrhagic stroke in young children is a malformation of the blood vessels in the brain called an **arteriovenous malformation** (AVM). Older children can have a dilatation of the vessels in the brain called an aneurysm, which can bleed.

What does a stroke look like? The signs that a child has had a stroke will depend on the area of the brain affected. The most common sign is weakness of one side of the body, called hemiplegia. She might also have weakness of the facial muscles, changes in vision or difficulty swallowing that can lead to drooling. Some children have difficulty with balance and coordination. Older children might complain of headache but otherwise strokes are not painful. It might not be recognized that your baby has had a stroke until months later, most commonly at 3 to 4 months of age when they should be developing purposeful hand movements. In more severe cases, the infant may have seizures and a decreased level of consciousness.

Children who have had a stroke tend to have a better recovery than adults. However, they can be left with residual difficulties in movement, speech, behavior or learning. Fortunately, in most cases these difficulties are mild.

How do you diagnose stroke? If your child's doctor suspects she has had a stroke, he will perform a variety of tests to confirm that a stroke has occurred, its site and the probable cause. This is important because the treatment will vary depending on the factors that produced the stroke. The first test performed is generally a CT scan or MRI of the brain. This helps to determine the area of brain involved and whether there has been hemorrhage or ischemia. Depending on the type of stroke, a number of blood tests will be performed to look for infection, clotting problems or chemical abnormalities. An ultrasound of the heart (echocardiogram) may also be performed to see if a clot traveling from the heart to the brain caused the stroke. An angiogram, which gives detailed information about the blood vessels in the brain, may be performed if the MRI does not give enough information.

How do you treat stroke? There are a number of treatment options following a stroke that vary depending on the cause of the stroke. If the stroke is secondary to a blood clot, your child's doctor might give her intravenous medication to shrink it. She might be started on anticoagulants, or "blood thinners," which prevent the clot from spreading. Children with underlying clotting problems can stay on blood thinners—aspirin, heparin or warfarin—for prolonged periods to prevent further stroke. If your child has had a hemorrhagic stroke, she might require surgery to remove the blood from the brain. Regardless of the cause of stroke, all children will receive rehabilitation therapy in the form of physiotherapy, occupational therapy and speech therapy.

Torticollis (Wry Neck)

What is torticollis? Torticollis means a twisted or "wry" neck. The head of children with torticollis is tilted to one side, the back of the head is rotated toward the shoulder and the chin is elevated and rotated in the opposite direction.

Torticollis can be either congenital (from birth) or acquired. The most common form is congenital muscular torticollis resulting from either an unusual position in the uterus, for example breech positioning, or a traumatic delivery. Acquired torticollis is usually secondary to infection, trauma or tumor and occurs more commonly in older children.

What does torticollis look like? Your child's congenital muscular torticollis is sometimes noticed at birth but usually is seen in the first

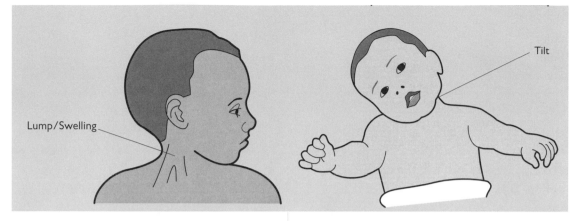

Tilt

TORTICOLLIS
In torticollis, the head is tilted to one size and a lump can often be felt in the neck muscle.

couple of weeks of life. If your baby has this condition, she will tilt her head to one side and often have a lump that can be felt in the neck muscle. This lump feels firm to touch but is not tender. She will favor holding the head to one side. As a result, if the torticollis is not treated, she can develop an asymmetrical flattening of the head, called plagiocephaly. Congenital torticollis can be associated with congenital dislocation of the hips (see Developmental Dysplasia of the Hip, pages 216–18).

Acquired torticollis occurs later in infancy or childhood. If it is secondary to infection, your child might have fever, enlargement of lymph nodes (which are often red and warm to touch) or breathing difficulties. Some signs of torticollis secondary to tumors are headache, vomiting, unusual gait or frequent falls.

How do you treat torticollis? Your child will be treated with passive stretching exercises of the neck. Initially these are performed by a physiotherapist who might teach you. Additionally, you will be encouraged to change your baby's position in the crib and place toys in a location that encourages her to look to the opposite

or "bad" side. With stretching exercises and changes in positioning, the torticollis will usually get better gradually. If the torticollis persists beyond one year, surgery may be necessary, but this is quite rare.

Treatment of acquired torticollis depends on the cause. If the torticollis has just begun, you will need to take your baby to her doctor for evaluation and the doctor will determine if further tests and treatment are needed.

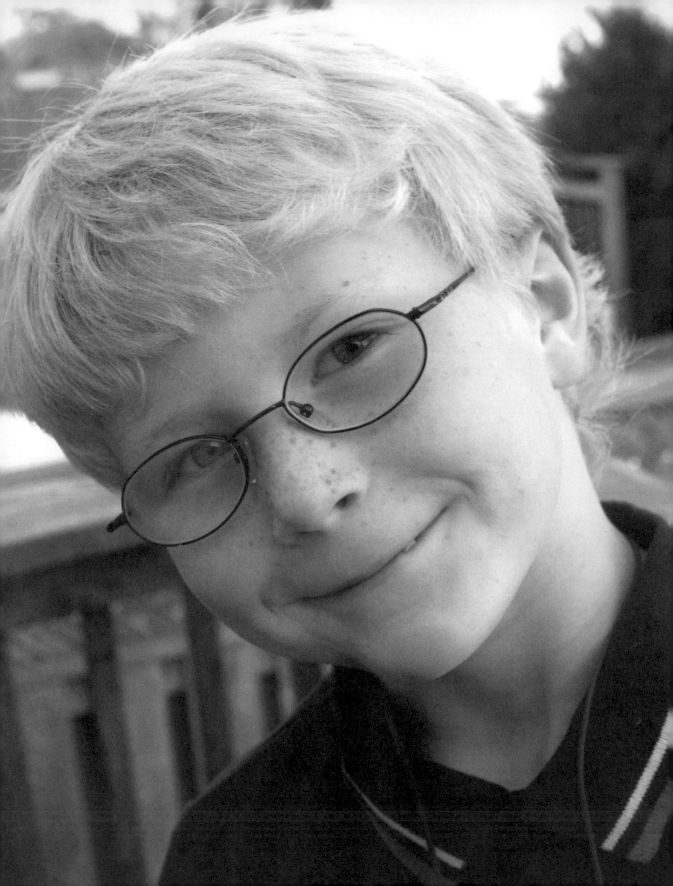

Eye Problems

Cataracts

What are cataracts? A cataract is a clouding within the normally transparent lens of the eye. Depending on their size and location, cataracts can lead to visual disturbances. People with cataracts sometimes describe their blurry vision as trying to see through a waterfall. In fact, the word, cataract, also means a waterfall.

Cataracts are common as people age. An estimated 25 percent of people over 80 years old ultimately develop cataracts; but they are rare in children. When children have cataracts, there are often other serious health problems. Some children are born with cataracts, which are called congenital cataracts. Some causes of congenital cataracts include congenital infections, such as rubella; chromosomal problems, such as **Down's syndrome**; and certain metabolic disorders. Cataracts that are not present at birth are usually secondary to other problems including insulin-dependent diabetes, significant eye trauma or some medications.

What does a cataract look like? Normally, the pupil of the eye appears as a black circle in the middle of the colored part of the eye called the iris. When a photograph is taken using a flash, often the pupils appear as a red dot, or "red eye." When

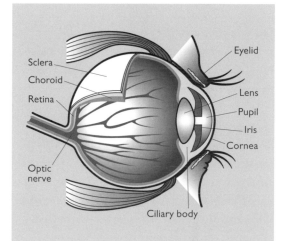

ANATOMY OF THE EYE
Light rays enter through the pupil at the front of the eye and register on the retina at the back. The light rays are converted to nerve impulses that are passed, via the optic nerve, to the brain, where they are interpreted as images.

a doctor examines the eye with an instrument called an ophthalmoscope, there should be a similar red eye appearance to the pupil, called the red reflex. However, when a cataract is present, an opacity can be seen that clouds this red reflex.

Sometimes, a cataract is so noticeable that the pupil is not a black circle but a white one. This is called "leukocoria" and it is never normal.

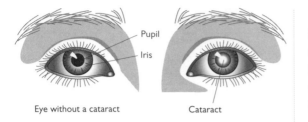

Pupil

Iris

Eye without a cataract Cataract

CATARACT

A cataract is a clouding of the normally tranparent lens. This is the part of the eye responsible for focusing light and producing clear, sharp images.

Other symptoms that could suggest the presence of a cataract include misaligned eyes, cloudy or decreased vision or abnormal eye movements.

How do you treat a cataract? Cataracts require prompt assessment after diagnosis, especially in young infants. If your young child has a cataract that obstructs his vision, it can lead to a condition called **amblyopia**, whereby the vision is impaired permanently even if the cataract is removed. Although the usual treatment for cataracts that impair vision is surgical removal, each child needs to be assessed and treated individually. It is also important that any underlying condition that produced the cataract be properly identified.

Color Blindness

What is color blindness? Colur blindness, more accurately called "color vision deficiency," occurs when specialized cells in the back wall of the eye, or retina, called photoreceptors, do not function normally. There are different forms of color vision deficiency; the inability to accurately see or distinguish shades of red and green is by far the commonest.

Approximately 5 percent to 8 percent of males and 1 percent of females have some form of color vision deficiency. In children, most instances of color vision deficiency are hereditary, which means that they are present from birth. There are various degrees of severity of color blindness and, fortunately, the condition does not worsen over time.

What does color blindness look like? Your child with a deficiency of red vision will see all shades of red as dark, while a child with a deficiency of green vision might not see any difference between the varying shades of green, brown, orange and red. Monochrome vision, which is true color blindness, is rare. Objects appear as shades of gray, much like an old movie.

Color vision deficiency can usually be diagnosed with specialized visual charts.

How do I treat color blindness? There is no treatment, but your child can learn to adapt and compensate for the inability to see certain colors. For example, instead of noting the actual color of a traffic light, red or green, your child can learn to distinguish the signal by knowing the relative position of each color, the red light being on top. Because color blindness is an inherited condition, there is no known prevention for this condition.

Eye Infections

CONJUNCTIVITIS ("PINK EYE")

What is conjunctivitis? The conjunctiva is a thin, transparent protective membrane that covers the eyeball, both over the front of the eye as well as inside the eyelids. The term "conjunctivitis" means inflammation of the conjunctiva and can occur in one or both eyes. Conjunctivitis can be caused by infections, both viral and bacterial, allergies, and chemicals and irritants.

What does conjunctivitis look like? Conjunctivitis tends to be annoying. Its symptoms include,

- redness of the whites of the eyes (the sclera),
- itchiness, irritation and a burning sensation,
- discharge that can be watery or thick and puslike, and
- matting of the lids together, usually after sleep.

Bacterial causes will usually result in a thick pussy discharge, whereas viral infections lead to red watery eyes. When your child has conjunctivitis caused by bacteria, he might also have an infection of the middle ear, otitis media. Some viral conjunctivitis can even produce bleeding beneath the conjunctival layer. This tends to look much worse than it really is. Allergic conjunctivitis usually occurs when your child has been exposed frequently to an **allergen**, such as pollens, and can be associated with other symptoms of **allergic rhinitis**. His eyelids might be swollen and he might have a clear discharge.

How do you treat conjunctivitis? The treatment for conjunctivitis depends on the underlying cause. In some instances, your child's doctor make take a swab of the eye to help identify the source of the condition. Bacterial infections are treated with antibiotic eye drops or ointments, while viral causes get better on their own after a week or two. When inserting eye drops, tilt your child's head backward and place the drops on the nasal side of the corner of the eye, allow-

ing the drops to leak into the eye. Pus can be removed from "sticky" eyes with a wet swab or clean cloth. Both bacterial and viral conjunctivitis are contagious. Help prevent transmission:

- Wash your hands properly.
- Do not share towels and face cloths.

Your child's doctor might recommend treating allergic causes with antihistamines, both orally or as eye drops, or even with anti-inflammatory eye drops.

What about conjunctivitis in newborns? Many newborns tend to have some discharge from their eyes. Usually, this is due to narrow tear ducts that temporarily get blocked, which can happen to newborns. (See Blocked Tear Ducts, pages 71–72) However, on occasion, the discharge can be caused by conjunctivitis. In this case, the sclera will be red and irritated, which is not what happens with narrow tear ducts.

If your newborn has conjunctivitis, it has different causes and is treated differently than in older children. Eye redness and discharge in the first few weeks of life can be caused by bacteria from the mother's birth canal if she happens to have a genital infection with either *Neisseria gonorrhea* or *Chlamydia trachomatis*. You might have one of these infections unknowingly, as they can infect but display no symptoms. For this reason, many authorities recommend screening women during pregnancy by use of genital swabs that are then tested for these infections. In most places, all newborns receive eye ointments immediately after birth to prevent these infections. These drops themselves can cause temporary eye redness, a benign condition called chemical conjunctivitis, which requires no treatment.

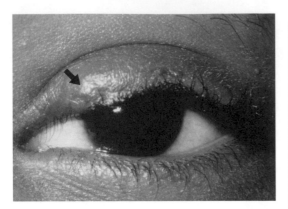

STYE

A stye appears as a red lump at the edge of the eyelid.

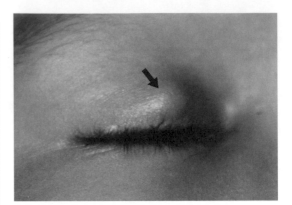

CHALAZION

A chalazion is a firm, red, tender bump within the eyelid.

COMMON EYELID PROBLEMS

What are common eyelid problems? Children can develop inflammation, redness and swelling of the eyelids and or eyelashes. Although these problems are usually harmless and get better without treatment, they can cause concern because they are so obvious. Some of the conditions, frequently given difficult names, are summarized below.

A stye, the medical term is "hordeolum," is a localized bacterial infection in a gland of the eyelid. It often appears as a red lump at the edge of the eyelid and can have a yellow head of pus around the base of the eyelash. The lump can be painful and tender to touch and might eventually drain fluid. Sties typically disappear by themselves within a few days. Warm compresses and antibiotic eye drops or ointment might help.

A chalazion is a discrete, firm, nontender bump within the eyelid and, therefore, unlike a stye, which is at the actual lid border. It is the result of an obstruction of a tear-producing gland that leads to a collection of fat, oil and other tissue, called a lipogranuloma. Time and warm compresses are often all that your child's doctor will recommend to treat a chalazion, although occasionally they will have to be excised surgically for cosmetic reasons or due to excess pressure on the eyeball.

Blepharitis is a term that refers to inflammation of the edges of the eyelids. It can be caused by irritation from skin conditions, such as seborrheic dermatitis or dandruff, viral or bacterial infections, or by an allergic reaction to cosmetics or ointment. The skin around the lashes is often red, itchy, scaly, and your child might rub the eye because of burning, causing a loss of lashes. Your child's doctor will treat the symptoms to decrease their severity. Treatment can include compresses and creams or lotions.

Dacryoadenitis is a term you probably haven't heard of. It's the medical name for an infection of the tear gland. When present, the outer portion of the upper eyelid appears swollen. The location of the swelling distinguishes dacryoadenitis from other conditions. It can be caused by a variety of common viruses, in which case there is minimal tenderness, or by several types of bacteria that are typically associated with greater tenderness. In this case, your child's doctor will prescribe oral antibiotics.

Orbital and Periorbital Cellulitis

What are orbital and periorbital cellulitis? The term cellulitis refers to an infection of the skin and its underlying tissue. Periorbital cellulitis specifically refers to an infection involving the eyelids and the soft tissues in front of the eyeball itself. Orbital cellulitis is somewhat different. It is an infection that is situated in the soft tissue directly behind the eyeball. Of the two conditions, orbital cellulitis is rarer and more serious.

Periorbital cellulitis is fairly common in young children. The cause is usually obvious. The cellulitis can spread from an infected scratch or insect bite, or from another infection, such as a stye or **conjunctivitis**. Sometimes, the inflammation has spread from a sinus infection in the maxillary sinus, which is in the cheekbone below the orbit.

Orbital cellulitis is most often the result of a direct extension of an infection located in a particular sinus, called the ethmoid sinus. This bony air sac is situated directly beside and behind the eyeball.

What do orbital and periorbital cellulitis look like? Your child with periorbital cellulitis has significant redness and swelling usually around one eye. The swelling can progress and lead to the eye being swollen completely shut. Often, the scratch, insect bite, stye or discharge is obvious. He does not look sick or "toxic" and fever is uncommon. Furthermore, he has no pain on eye movement

and his vision is not blurry. His white blood count is generally normal.

When your child has orbital cellulitis, he usually appears ill and has a fever. His eyelid is swollen and tender. There is eye pain, both when resting and particularly when he moves his eye. The eyeball may be pushed forward (proptosis). Typically he will be unable to move his eyes properly and may complain of blurred or double vision. When tested, his white blood count will be elevated and a CT scan of the orbit of the eye will show the inflammatory mass and ethmoid **sinusitis**.

How do you treat orbital and periorbital cellulitis? Periorbital cellulitis is typically a bacterial infection. Milder cases can be treated with oral antibiotics. More serious cases require treatment with intravenous therapy.

Orbital cellulitis is always a medical emergency. There is a risk of complications including loss of vision and extension of the infection into the brain causing **meningitis**, thrombosis or abscess. Treatment includes hospitalization and close monitoring, usually by CT scan, as surgical drainage can sometimes be required. Intravenous antibiotics are essential initially and follow-up oral antibiotics are usually given for two additional weeks to clear the associated sinusitis.

Glaucoma

What is glaucoma? Glaucoma is a condition in which the pressure of the fluid within the eye rises beyond normal levels. There is normally a balanced flow of fluid in and out of the eye but when there is a blockage or other impediment to drainage of this fluid, the pressure can build.

WHAT DOES GLAUCOMA LOOK LIKE?

Symptoms of glaucoma include:

- light sensitivity (photophobia),
- one eye appears larger than the other,
- cloudiness of the cornea,
- excessive tearing, and
- a tendency to squeeze the eyelid tightly (blepharospasm).

WHAT DOES REFRACTIVE ERROR LOOK LIKE?

Symptoms of refractive error include:

- squinting,
- holding objects very close in order to see them,
- eye strain,
- problems at school,
- visual complaints.

The problem with this excessive pressure is that damage can occur to important visual structures, such as the optic nerve, which leads to visual loss. Glaucoma in childhood is much less common than in adults; it is estimated to affect about 1 in 10,000 children.

Your child's doctor should examine your child who experiences one or more of these symptoms. If appropriate, he will refer your child to an ophthalmologist for further evaluation.

How do you treat glaucoma? There are many causes of childhood glaucoma. The treatment depends on the specific cause. Treatment can involve medications or various surgical procedures. The goal of treatment is to attempt to normalize the pressure within your child's eyeball.

Refractive Error (Myopia, Hyperopia, Astigmatism)

What is refractive error? Normal vision is a highly complex phenomenon that requires a series of steps to occur in near perfect alignment.

- Light from an image passes through the clear cornea at the front of the eye, through the pupil, through the eye lens, through the clear fluid that fills the eye, and onto the retina, which is a thin layer of light-sensitive nerves on the back wall of the eye.
- From the retina, the signal is passed to the optic nerve, which carries it to areas of the brain that process and perceive vision.

A refractive error occurs when the image does not fall precisely onto the retina—it might fall in front or behind it, leading to blurred vision.

Nearsightedness (myopia) occurs when the image of an object is focused in front of the retina. In this case, distant objects appear blurry and out of focus while close objects look very clear. Myopia is by far the commonest refractive error in childhood; it can affect 25 percent or more of the population, especially during and after puberty when the eye undergoes its adolescent growth phase. Myopia tends to be inherited.

Farsightedness (hyperopia) occurs when the image of an object becomes focused behind the retina. In this case, close objects appear blurred.

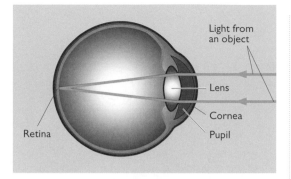

NORMAL VISION

Light from an image passes through the cornea, through the pupil, and lands on the retina.

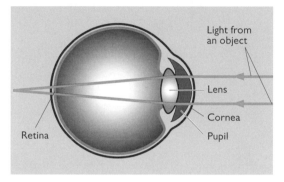

FARSIGHTEDNESS (HYPEROPIA)

Hyperopia occurs when the image is focused behind the retina, making close objects appear blurred.

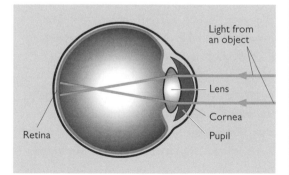

NEARSIGHTEDNESS (MYOPIA)

Myopia occurs when the image is focused in front of the retina, making distant objects appear blurred.

Hyperopia is relatively uncommon in childhood. It often runs in families.

Astigmatism occurs when irregularities in the visual system, usually involving the cornea, results in an inability to focus on all parts of an object at the same time. This causes blurring of both near and distant objects.

During routine health examinations, your child's doctor will examine the eye and visual system in different ways, depending on the child's age. If you or your doctor have any concerns about your child's ability to see clearly, your child can have further specific examinations aimed at finding out how sharp his vision is and detecting any potential problems.

Contrary to popular belief, refractive error and other visual problems are *not* caused by reading in dim light or sitting too close to the television; they are often inherited conditions related to the size and shape of the eyeball.

How do you treat refractive error? Once a specific problem is identified, the treatment usually involves corrective lenses (eyeglasses). Teenagers sometimes prefer contact lenses, but the care requirements generally make them unsuitable for younger children. As the eye grows, the refractive error can worsen before stabilization occurs when your child has completed the growth phase of puberty. This means that laser correction therapy is not an option for children.

Strabismus (Crossed Eyes, Squint)

What is strabismus? Strabismus is the medical term that describes a misalignment of the eyes, commonly called "crossed eyes" or "squint."

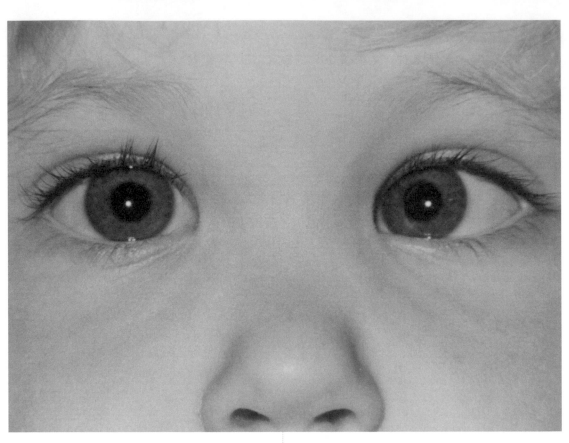

STRABISMUS

The affected eye turns inward. Note that the "reflected light" is off-center.

The condition is one of the most common pediatric eye disorders; it affects about 4 percent of all children.

There are many causes of strabismus; about half of affected children are born with the condition because the muscles attached to the eyeball, which allow its movement, are not properly balanced. Strabismus that shows up later in the toddler or childhood years is often due to farsightedness. As part of your child's natural adjustment to the farsightedness, his eye tends to turn inward.

What does strabismus look like? The affected eye(s) might appear turned inward, outward or less commonly up or down. Because the eyes aren't synchronized, your child might experience double or blurred vision causing him to cover or close the affected eye, hence the term "squint." He might sit in an odd position, twisting around to compensate for the misalignment and, thereby, to focus on a particular object.

It is important to differentiate true strabismus from a condition called "pseudostrabismus" in which the eyes appear to be out of alignment, but in actuality they are positioned normally. Your child with a broad nasal bridge or **epicanthal skin folds** over the inner corner of his eyes

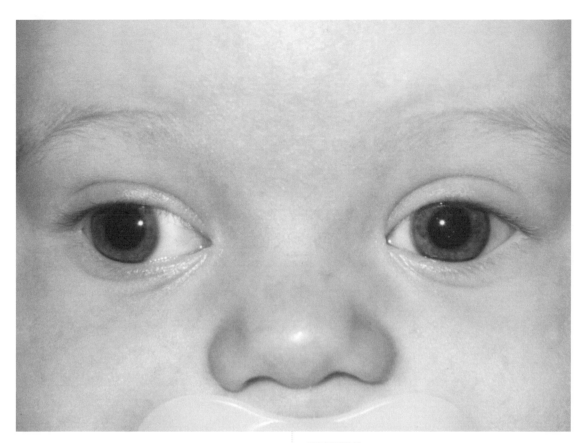

The affected eye (on the left) is turned outward.

might appear to have crossed eyes, but this is an optical illusion. His eyes are normal.

When should I worry about crossed eyes? Newborn infants often have times when their eyes are out of alignment; this is normal in the first two to four months of life. Once your child is beyond 4 months of age and continues to exhibit eye misalignment, your doctor should refer him to an ophthalmologist. Any child who has constantly crossed eyes should also be referred.

Children with strabismus are at risk of developing **amblyopia**, a condition where vision fails to develop normally. To combat blurry double vision, the brain accepts visual signals only from one eye and ignores the image from the weaker eye. Ultimately, vision in this eye will be permanently impaired because it is not being used. Amblyopia can often be prevented with prompt diagnosis and treatment of strabismus.

How do you treat strabismus? The treatment for strabismus depends on the underlying cause, but there are several types of therapy that are commonly used. These include wearing eyeglasses, wearing a patch and sometimes surgery. Glasses can correct unequal vision between the eyes or improve farsightedness. An eye patch can be used to force the child to use the weaker eye. Surgery involves realigning the eye muscles.

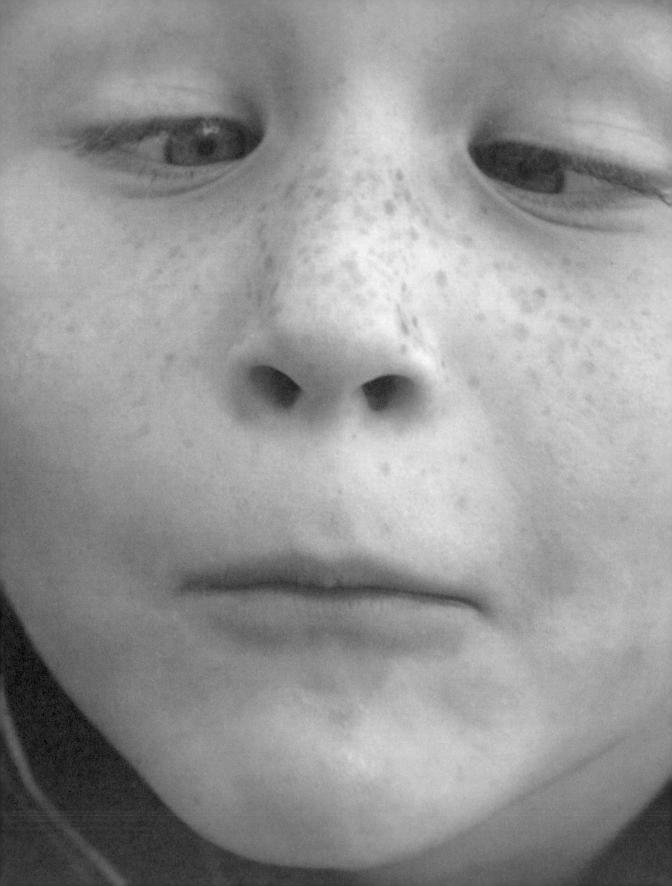

Ear, Nose and Throat Problems

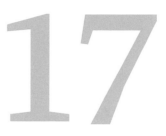

Cleft Lip and Palate

What are cleft lip and palate? A cleft is a separation in a body structure. In the developing fetus, the two sides of the upper lip and the roof of the mouth (palate) normally fuse together in the middle between the 5th and 10th week after conception. Failure to complete this closure leads to a cleft lip, a cleft palate or a combination of both. You probably were shocked to see this defect in your newborn, but these clefts are fairly common birth defects, occurring in 1 in 700 to 1 in 1,000 newborn infants.

The exact cause of clefting remains unknown, although a number of factors including genetic and environmental factors have been associated with this condition. Cleft lip and palate can occur together or separately. In some instances, clefts are associated with other medical problems, as part of a specific genetic **syndrome**.

What do cleft lip and palate look like? There is a wide spectrum in cleft lip and cleft palate. In milder forms of cleft lip, your child might have a small notch in the upper lip; in more severe forms, there can be a large opening, leading to a connection from the upper lip through the floor of the nostril including the upper gums. Some milder forms of cleft palate involve just the boneless soft palate at the back of the mouth. These might not be detected until later in life, whereas larger clefts are immediately apparent.

What are the problems associated with lip and palete clefs? Your baby with oral-facial clefts will experience a range of medical problems.

- Her feeding problems were apparent from birth, because clefts involving the lip or palate have impaired her ability to create suction while feeding. There are special devices and techniques to aid in this area; while some infants can breast-feed, this is not always possible. Specialized nipples and squeezable bottles are also available to assist with feeding.
- Middle ear infections occur much more frequently. In some cases, this can lead to hearing loss.
- Speech and language problems occur in many children; her voice might be nasal and hard to understand.
- She will have dental and orthodontic problems including dental decay and bad positioning of her teeth.

How do you treat cleft lips and palates? There is no proven prevention for cleft lips or palates. Some authorities feel that women should take

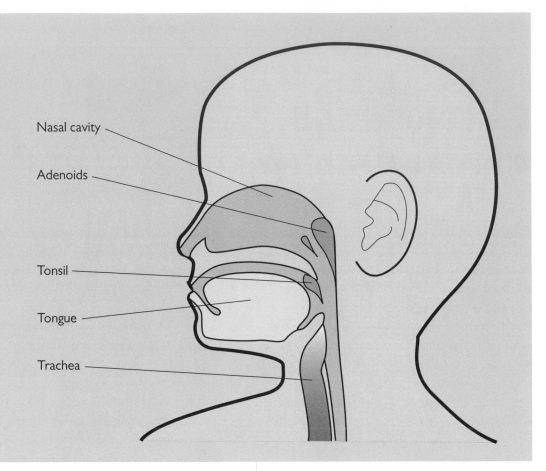

Nasal cavity

Adenoids

Tonsil

Tongue

Trachea

TONSILS AND ADENOIDS

The adenoids are at the back of the nasal cavity and cannot be seen when looking into the mouth. The tonsils are oval-shaped fleshy pouches on each side of the back of the throat.

the common B vitamin folic acid during the critical (early) part of pregnancy, which might prevent some cases of cleft lip and palate.

Despite the range of potential problems listed above, there are very good treatments available for your child. In many centers, a multidisciplinary team of health providers will provide a range of care for your child. These include medical physicians (pediatricians, geneticists), surgeons (plastic surgeons, otolaryngologists [ear, nose and throat

specialists]), dentists, nurses, speech therapists, nutritionists, occupational therapists and social workers.

Your child can have surgical treatment that will result in improved looks and speech. The timing of the surgery varies; generally the lip is repaired first. Many children require multiple surgeries over time.

Enlarged Tonsils and Adenoids

What are enlarged tonsils and adenoids? The tonsils and adenoids are part of the body's immune system, and play a role in filtering and fighting infections. Their location behind the mouth and nose is strategic, because most infections enter the body through this route. The tonsils appear as oval-shaped fleshy bumps on each side at the back of your child's throat. The adenoids cannot be seen, because they sit above and behind the soft palate, which is the back part of the roof of the mouth. After the first year of life, the tonsils and adenoids tend to grow, most likely in response to the infections and **allergens** in the environment. Normally, they shrink in late childhood and adolescence.

When should I worry about enlarged tonsils and adenoids? It is normal for young children to have relatively large tonsils and adenoids; usually there is no reason for you to be concerned. Sometimes, however, there can be symptoms caused by these large tissues. Enlarged tonsils and adenoids cause nasal obstruction that can lead to mouth breathing, snoring and possibly **obstructive sleep apnea**, during which breathing is interrupted because the airway becomes blocked (see pages 328–29.) The tonsils and adenoids can be so big that they can actually cause difficulty in swallowing. Occasionally, your child's speech can be affected, because the enlarged tissues produce a nasal voice. In some children, large adenoids can block the ventilating tube to the middle ear and lead to recurrent ear infections.

How do you treat enlarged tonsils and adenoids? There is no need to treat tonsils and adenoids simply because they are large. They will shrink over time. If your child has symptoms attributed to her large tonsils and adenoids, your child's doctor might refer her to an ear, nose and throat specialist who might recommend surgical removal (tonsillectomy and adenoidectomy).

Hearing Loss and Deafness

What is hearing loss? Hearing is a complex sense that involves the ear (comprised of the outer, middle and inner ears), the auditory nerve and the brain. The outer ear consists of the auricle, the visible funnel-shaped structure that is designed to catch sound waves, and the ear canal that leads to the eardrum. This **tympanic membrane** is a thin drumlike structure that vibrates in response to sound waves. The vibrations of the tympanic membrane are transmitted via small bones in the middle ear to the inner ear. There, a structure called the cochlea converts the vibrations to electrical

COMMUNICATION MILESTONES

By 3 months, a child *should*
- startle to loud sounds,
- smile in response to soothing sounds,
- make certain sounds (for example, "oo, ah").

By 6 months, a child *should*
- turn toward a sound,
- make several different sounds (often in reaction to a parent's sound).

By 9 months, a child *should*
- respond to her name,
- babble, often with a speechlike quality (for example, "gaga/baba"),
- understand "no."

By 12 months, a child *should*
- understand some words and simple phrases,
- communicate by using a combination of sounds and gestures.

impulses that travel through the auditory nerve to the brain. Like all of our senses, sound is "perceived" in the brain.

Hearing loss can arise from problems anywhere along this hearing pathway. Conditions affecting the outer and middle ear can impair the conduction (transmission) of sound waves and produce conductive hearing loss. Or, problems can exist in the inner ear, cochlea or auditory nerve whereby the response to sound waves is abnormal. This is called "sensorineural hearing loss."

There are numerous causes of hearing loss including:

- congenital infections, such as rubella,
- congenital malformations of any part of the ear or the part of the brain responsible for hearing,
- hereditary causes,
- infections, for example **meningitis** or **encephalitis**,
- exposure to high levels of certain medications toxic to the ear (ototoxic).

Temporary conductive hearing loss can be caused by earwax or persistent middle ear fluid collections.

Hearing loss and deafness can be present at birth (congenital deafness) or it can occur during infancy or childhood (acquired hearing loss or deafness). In many areas, newborns' hearing is screened to detect hearing loss as early as possible. Other centers will only test the hearing of babies at high risk, such as those born prematurely, those with infections known to cause hearing loss and those who have members of the family with hearing problems. The frequency of congenital hearing loss is approximately 1 or 2 per 1,000 newborns; early childhood deafness also occurs in 1 or 2 per 1,000 children.

What does hearing loss look like? Hearing loss in the first years of life can lead to delays in speech, language and cognitive development. You are usually the best judge of your child's development. If you suspect a problem, arrange for a proper hearing assessment. If your child does not meet any of the milestones in the box on page 325, she should have a hearing evaluation.

While there are several types of tests used to detect hearing loss, the common goal is early identification. Appropriate treatment can either repair the hearing problem or teach communication skills where hearing cannot be restored.

How do you treat hearing loss? When your child has been identified as having a significant hearing loss, her care will require the coordinated efforts of many professionals. From the audiologists, who perform and interpret the various types of hearing tests, to the speech and language therapists who help diagnose and treat problems, to otolaryngologists, the goal of treatment is to correct, if possible, the hearing problem, and to assist your child in her development. Depending on individual circumstances and severity, your child might be prescribed hearing aids or have a cochlear implant. These implants are sophisticated biomechanical devices that amplify sound waves and help create an impulse that the brain can interpret as sound.

If your child has conductive hearing loss due to recurring or persistent middle ear fluid her doctor might recommend inserting a ventilating tube into her eardrum.

Nosebleeds

What are nosebleeds? The medical term for a nosebleed is epistaxis. Nosebleeds, which are extremely common in childhood, usually begin in the wall between the two nostrils, called the nasal septum, an area rich in blood vessels. There are many causes for nosebleeds. One of the most common causes is digital trauma, which is a polite term for nose picking.

Often colds and allergies lead to nosebleeds. Here's why. When your child has a cold or allergy, the veins in the congested nasal passages are dilated and thin-walled. Blowing the nose or sneezing raises the pressure inside the vein to the point that it pops, like a flat tire, causing bleeding. It is much less likely, but possible, that epistaxis is the result of foreign bodies, injury, polyps or a bleeding disorder such as hemophilia.

When should I worry about my child's nosebleed? If the bleeding hasn't stopped within 20 to 30 minutes or the nosebleed is part of a head injury, you should take your child to a doctor. While nosebleeds may appear frightening, it is important to remember that they are common and often completely harmless. The real amount of blood lost is usually much less than it appears. If your child has recurrent, severe nosebleeds or your family has a history of bleeding tendencies, your child should be evaluated for a bleeding problem. In rare cases, the bleeding can be difficult to control, or be severe enough to cause low blood levels (anemia).

How do I treat nosebleed? There are many myths and misconceptions about how to stop a bleeding nose. The best way to stop a nosebleed is to

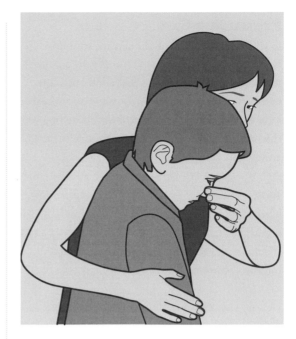

HOW TO STOP A NOSEBLEED
Pinching the nostrils stems the flow of a bloody nose.

tightly squeeze together the two sides of the soft part of the nose, just above the nostrils, below the bony part. Firm pressure for at least 10 to 15 minutes (resisting the urge to continue checking to see if the bleeding has stopped!) will usually stop the bleeding. Your child's head should be tilted forward to avoid blood trickling into the back of her throat. She should try not to sniff, pick at or blow the nose for the next few hours.

You can often prevent recurrent nosebleeds by keeping the nasal septum moistened with lubricating creams or ointments. If the environment is very dry in your home, you might use a room humidifier. In recurrent or severe cases, your child's doctor might treat the bleeding areas with cautery, a chemical burning of the bleeding site, to prevent further bleeding episodes.

Protruding Ears

What are protruding ears? Some children have unusually prominent ears that stick out. This can involve one or both ears and, in some cases, runs in the family. In the majority of instances, this is a cosmetic problem that does not affect hearing or health.

When should I worry about my child's protruding ears? While protruding ears pose no medical risks, they can have a negative impact on a child or adolescent if they cause embarrassment, anguish or low self-esteem.

How do you treat protruding ears? A common surgical procedure called otoplasty, in which the protruding ears are repositioned closer to the head, is the cosmetic procedure doctors use to improve the appearance of protruding ears.

Snoring and Obstructive Sleep Apnea

What is snoring? Snoring is the sound that we hope we aren't making in our sleep. It is created by the vibration of the soft palate when you sleep with an open mouth. Anything that causes obstruction of airflow through the nose—seasonal allergies, upper respiratory infections and enlarged adenoids—can contribute to snoring.

When should I worry about my child's snoring? Snoring is common. By some estimates it affects 10 percent of children at some point. Doctors

feel most instances of snoring are benign and get better on their own. However snoring can be associated with a condition called obstructive sleep apnea. This refers to episodes of partial or complete blockage of the upper air passages during sleep, which leads to abnormal breathing and sleep patterns. Obstructive sleep apnea can have a negative impact on your child's health:

- daytime sleepiness,
- behavioral and attention problems,
- growth problems,
- high blood pressure.

However, you should remember that not all children who snore have obstructive sleep apnea.

What does obstructive sleep apnea look like? If your child has obstructive sleep apnea, she might pause during snoring due to complete blockage of airflow, gasp, sleep restlessly and sweat.

The best tool for assessing sleep apnea is a sleep study. During this test, a technician records numerous body functions and vital signs while your child sleeps. Unfortunately, sleep studies are difficult to perform and interpret, and they are expensive. Some authorities have recommended that, if you are concerned, you should videotape your child sleeping, so that your health provider can watch and have a better assessment of the child's sleep.

How do you treat obstructive sleep apnea? Snoring itself requires no treatment. Sleep apnea is another, more complicated, story. Opinions can differ. The difficulty in accurately diagnosing obstructive sleep apnea in the first place is only one of the many controversies in this area. While many children with obstructive sleep apnea do benefit from surgery, others may not. The treatment for obstructive sleep apnea is usually surgical removal of the tonsils and adenoids in an operation called a tonsillectomy and adenoidectomy.

Swimmer's Ear (Otitis Externa)

What is swimmer's ear? Otitis externa refers to an infection that affects the ear canal, the cylindrical passage from the outside world to the eardrum. The term "swimmer's ear" relates to the observation that these infections are more common in the summer months, especially in children who spend many hours in the water. One of the factors producing otitis externa is prolonged exposure to water, which softens the skin and promotes bacterial growth. Otitis externa can also be caused by trauma caused by scratching or by well-meaning parents who use cotton swabs in an attempt to "clean" the ear.

What does otitis externa look like? Your child might complain of itching; discomfort or pain, especially with movement of the outer ear; discharge; and temporary hearing loss from blockage of the ear canal with swelling and debris. There might be a red scaly area around the opening of the ear. In more severe cases, your child's outer ear might swell and she might have a fever.

A similar pattern can also be produced by otitis media, the infection of the middle ear behind the eardrum that often accompanies colds, if the eardrum perforates.

How do you treat otitis externa? There are a number of options. Your child's doctor might clean the ear canal and/or prescribe different types of ear drops that can contain a combination of antiseptics, antibiotics and anti-inflammatory medication. If the pain is significant, your child could take acetaminophen or ibuprofen as needed. In more severe cases, your child might need to take oral or intravenous antibiotics. It is wise to keep the ear dry until the infection has healed.

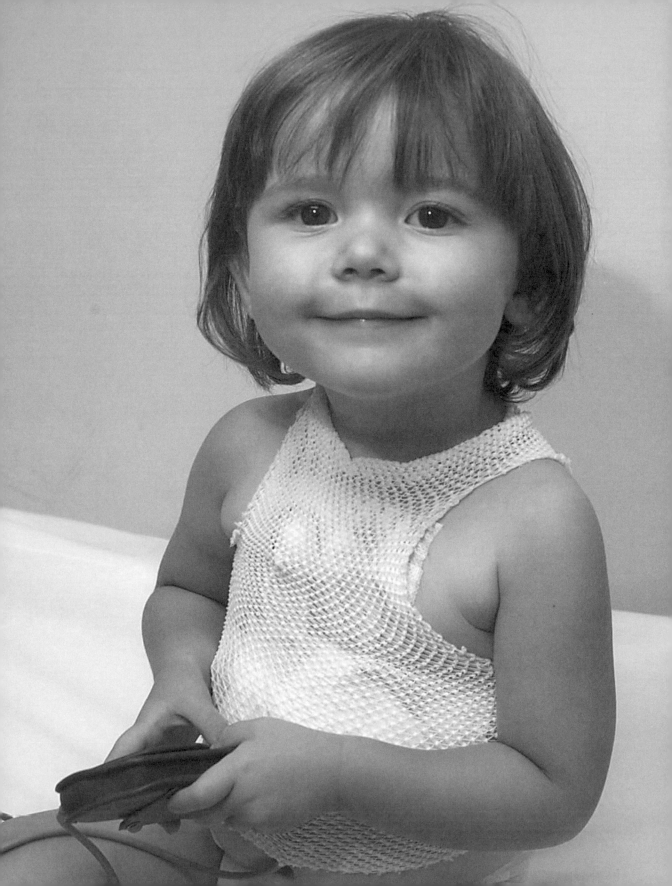

Heart and Circulatory Problems 18

All About Heart Murmurs

What are heart murmurs? The human heart is quite noisy. The various sounds that it makes are the result of blood flowing through the heart's chambers and then out of them again.

There are actually four different chambers in the heart: two on the right side, which pump blood to the lungs, and two on the left, which supply oxygenated blood to the body. The powerful chambers, one on the right and one on the left, are called ventricles. They are filled by antechambers, each called an atrium. The flow of blood is maintained in the proper direction by four heart valves, each at the outflow of a chamber.

The sounds of the heartbeat are really the sounds of the four valves closing. The mitral and tricuspid valves close at the same time. This makes the first heart sound. The pulmonary and aortic valves also close together. This produces the second heart sound.

A heart murmur is simply another type of sound that is heard with a stethoscope when blood courses through the heart. It can signify a normal variation in blood flow similar to the sound of water flowing rapidly out of a faucet. On the other hand, a murmur can also reflect abnormal flow through a defect between the

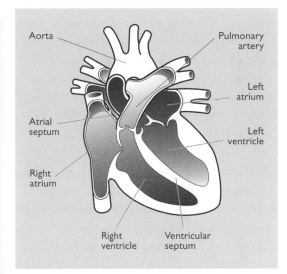

NORMAL HEART

The right ventricle pumps blood into the lungs through the pulmonary arteries. After the blood is oxygenated in the lungs, it returns to the left ventricle, which pumps it through the body via the aorta.

chambers of the heart or through an abnormal valve, similar to the hissing of air escaping from a balloon. They can occur when the two ventricles are contracting (systolic murmurs) or when the two atria contract (diastolic murmurs). The timing of the murmur, its intensity and quality can all help distinguish between innocent, harmless murmurs and those that need further investigations and treatment.

When should I be worried about my child's heart murmur? Between 50 percent and 80 percent of children will have a heart murmur heard during childhood, but less than 1 percent of children actually have a congenital heart problem. This suggests that the vast majority of murmurs are harmless or "innocent murmurs." These murmurs are heard in many children due to the flow of blood through an entirely normal heart. They are more likely to be heard when the child has a fever or exercises. Innocent murmurs tend to be fairly "soft" or gentle-sounding and cannot be felt by placing your hand over your child's heart. Such murmurs can change or become inaudible when your child changes position. As he gets older the murmur will often disappear. No investigation or treatment is required for innocent heart murmurs.

Aren't some murmurs a sign of heart disease? Yes. A minority of murmurs are indeed caused by a cardiac abnormality. They are called pathologic murmurs and can be categorized by their timing and location. Depending on the intensity of the murmur, where the murmur seems loudest and the timing of the murmur during the heart cycle, your child's doctor might suspect specific abnormalities of his heart. When the ventricles are emptying (systole), loud murmurs that do not sound like one of the innocent murmurs can often suggest a problem with one of the valves of the heart or a defect in the wall between the two ventricles. Murmurs heard when the atria are emptying and the ventricles are filling (diastole) can also suggest a valve abnormality. Continuous murmurs heard throughout diastole and systole that do not sound like innocent venous hums (the normal sound of blood flowing through the veins) can occur when blood flows across a narrowing in

the aorta (coarctation of the aorta), or when the ductus remains patent after birth (see Patent Ductus Arteriosus, page 337). Pathologic murmurs can sometimes be felt by placing the palm of your hand over the left side of the chest. They do not tend to change or disappear when your child changes position.

How do you treat murmurs? Innocent murmurs are harmless and require no treatment. If uncertainty exists as to the nature of the murmur, your child's doctor might refer him to a cardiologist. Pathologic murmurs require further investigation to diagnose the underlying abnormality. Your child will have a chest x-ray and an electrocardiogram (ECG) and blood pressure measurements in both arms and legs to help distinguish between innocent and pathologic murmurs. These tests can help assess the size of the chambers of the heart, the rhythm of the heart and the flow of blood to the lungs and to the body.

The best method to determine exactly what might be causing a heart murmur is an echocardiogram. This simple, safe ultrasound of the heart is a painless procedure that allows the physician to see the chambers and valves of the heart. It can detect any defects in the walls between the chambers, abnormalities of the valves or abnormalities of the vessels leading from the heart.

Specific treatment for pathologic murmurs depends on the underlying diagnosis (see Congenital Heart Defects, pages 334–37). While some abnormalities might not require regular medication or surgery in the short term, your child might require antibiotics before certain surgical or dental procedures to prevent bacterial infections in the heart (see Infective Endocarditis pages 343–44). Some pathologic murmurs will go away as your child grows and the valves and wall defects change. Repeat assessment by a cardiologist will help ascertain what treatment your child requires as he grows. Over 50 percent of children will have a heart murmur, yet the incidence of actual congenital heart disease is lower than 1 percent!

Arrhythmias

What are arrhythmias? Think of the heart simply as a muscular pump designed to propel blood throughout the body. The rate at which the heart pumps depends on the body's needs and is controlled by a system of electrical signals. These electric impulses travel through the heart's conducting system stimulating muscle contraction in a coordinated, efficient manner.

Arrhythmias are abnormal heart rhythms. In other words, the coordinated electrical impulses are disturbed in some way. This often produces an abnormal heart rate. This abnormally slow or fast rate can affect the efficiency of the heart's pumping to varying degrees. Children of different ages have varying ranges of normal heart rates. A heart rate for a 1-month-old varies between 100 and 180 beats per minute whereas an adolescent is more likely to vary between 50 and 100 beats per minute. Heart rates are usually slowest during sleep or deep relaxation and fastest during periods of exercise, anxiety or fever.

Arrhythmias are generally categorized as either sinus (regular) or non-sinus (abnormal). If a child has an abnormally fast heart rate for his age, it is called a tachycardia. Similarly, an abnormally slow heart rate for his age is called a bradycardia. Tachycardia and bradycardia can be either sinus or non-sinus. Sinus bradycardia is more common in older athletic children who have low resting heart rates. Although the heart is pumping more slowly than most children's,

rather than indicating disease, this sinus bradycardia is usually just a sign of an efficient pump that does not need to go as fast. Sinus tachycardia is often seen in children who are exercising, or if they are dehydrated, or have a fever or a serious infection. Non-sinus tachycardias and bradycardias are distinguished from sinus (normal) ones, by performing an electrocardiogram (ECG). Non-sinus abnormalities in rate are a sign of abnormal conduction in the heart's electrical pathways.

Many children with structurally normal hearts have arrhythmias, but some types of rhythm disturbances are more common in children with congenital heart defects or after heart surgery. Some children have a familial predisposition for arrhythmias. Arrhythmias are also more common in children with abnormal levels of certain electrolytes and minerals, which can occur in the presence of a variety of other noncardiac illnesses. Also, you should be aware that certain medications can cause arrhythmias.

What do arrhythmias look like? The signs and symptoms attributable to arrhythmias depend on the type of arrhythmia and the age of the child. Older children and adolescents can describe what they are experiencing. They might describe an awareness of their heart pounding (a palpitation), or feel it skipping a beat.

Infants might eat poorly, be lethargic, pale and sweaty, and breathe rapidly if an arrhythmia persists. Other arrhythmias are never felt and are only found on an ECG. In some cases, arrhythmias show up because the child has fainting spells, called syncope.

Often a child's pulse can feel irregular, or abnormally fast or slow. This can be confirmed when a nurse or physician listens to his heartbeat with a stethoscope. In some cases, your child's doctor might suspect he has an arrhythmia based on a family history of sudden deaths.

In the majority of cases, your child's doctor will conduct further investigations of his heart rhythm abnormality with an ECG, which helps display how electricity is conducted throughout his heart. Some cases might require prolonged ECG monitoring for 12 to 24 hours. The machine your child will wear is called a Holter monitor; it helps evaluate the effects of exercise and regular activities on heart rhythm. Your child might also have an ECG to assess the structure and function of the heart. Since some arrhythmias are associated with electrolyte or mineral abnormalities, your child's doctor will also order blood screening of calcium, potassium and magnesium.

How do you treat arrythmias? If you suspect your child's heart is beating irregularly or is either too fast or slow, get it checked out promptly. Either call your physician or go to an emergency department. The actual treatment will depend on the cause and type of arrhythmia and whether or not your child has any associated cardiac defects. Your child with sinus tachycardia or bradycardia does not require specific treatment. But his underlying illness, such as dehydration or infection, has to be treated. If your child has electrolyte and mineral abnormalities, they must be corrected.

The treatment of non-sinus arrhythmias can be separated into immediate and long-term components. Immediate treatment of any arrhythmia will depend on how stable your infant or child appears. His blood pressure and circulation will be monitored, and his doctor will assess him for heart failure.

If your child has tachycardia caused by abnormal electrical impulses arising in the atria

(supraventricular tachycardia) it might be treated by medical staff placing a bag of ice partially over the child's face for 30 seconds, which might stimulate a reflex response that slows the heart. If that fails, it is also treated with an intravenous medication and, in some cases, with cardioversion, which involves discharging an electrical shock to the heart to jolt it back into sinus rhythm. Your child might see a pediatric cardiologist who will prescribe long-term oral medications to control arrhythmias to help prevent recurrence. If your child has had cardiac surgery followed by arrhythmias, he might benefit from a pacemaker.

Some arrhythmias disappear as children grow and are not a cause for concern. However, there are some rhythm abnormalities arising in the ventricles that need more aggressive treatment, particularly if children have already had a syncopal episode. These children are at risk for sudden death. Long-term treatment is directed by a pediatric cardiologist, and can include oral medications and surgical implantation of a defibrillator device.

Congenital Heart Defects

What are congenital heart defects? Congenital heart defects are abnormalities of the structure of the heart that occur during fetal development. Less than 1 percent of babies have one. In most cases, there is no underlying cause for the problem. In some instances, infections during pregnancy or maternal medical conditions, such as diabetes, or certain medications taken during pregnancy can increase the risk of congenital heart disease. Congenital heart defects are more common if there is a family history of congenital heart disease. Some children born with heart defects have distinct genetic **syndromes** or chromosomal abnormalities, such as **Down's syndrome**. Whatever the cause, many babies born with abnormalities of other parts of their bodies have congenital heart defects as well.

The severity, treatment and prognosis of the common congenital heart defects vary widely, and each defect is best addressed individually. In all cases, the echocardiogram, essentially an ultrasound of the heart, is the best noninvasive test used to make a diagnosis. Here are some of the more important congenital heart defects.

VENTRICULAR SEPTAL DEFECT

What is a ventricular septal defect? Think of the heart as not just one pump, but two. The right pump, or ventricle, pushes blood under low pressure into the lungs while the stronger left ventricle pumps blood under higher pressure to the entire body. Separating these two pumps is a wall, or septum. A ventricular septal defect (VSD) is an opening in that septum. VSDs allow some of the blood pumped from the high pressured left ventricle to re-enter the right ventricle rather than exit out the main artery, the aorta, to the body. This recirculating of blood from the left side of the heart back to the right is inefficient and can overwork the heart. A VSD is usually character- ized as small, moderate or large, as the size of the hole determines the amount of shunting and, hence, the burden placed upon the heart. VSDs are the most common congenital heart defect, accounting for 15 percent to 20 percent of isolated congenital heart defects. This is commonly referred to as "a hole in the heart."

How do you diagnose ventricular septal defect? The signs and symptoms of a VSD are directly related to the amount of blood that shunts through the

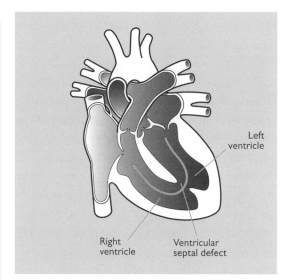

VENTRICULAR SEPTAL DEFECT
The ventrical septal defect is an opening in the wall separating the left and right ventricles.

defect from the left to right ventricle. Small VSDs generally do not cause any symptoms in infants or children since the shunt across the defect is not particularly stressful on the heart. However, a dis- tinct sound, called a murmur, might be heard when listening to the heart with a stethoscope.

More stress is placed on the heart if your child has a moderate or large VSD, since more blood shunts across the defect instead of pump- ing out to the body. The heart, therefore, has to work much harder than usual. Your child's heart murmur is so loud that it can sometimes actually be felt by his doctor's hand as well as heard through the stethoscope. Your child might have varying degrees of heart failure, which is charac- terized by faster heart rates and respiratory rates, as well as enlargement of the liver. He tends to fatigue easily and sweat excessively, especially when eating. Due to feeding difficulties, his weight gain may be less than normal. In all cases, an echocardiogram will help characterize the size, location and clinical significance of the VSD.

How do you treat VSD? If your child's VSD is small or moderately sized, the defect closes spontaneously within the first six months of life in one-third of cases. Larger VSDs will cause symptoms of heart failure by about 3 months of age. Your child's symptoms can be treated with medications that help the heart. You and your doctor will pay particular attention to nutrition in order to improve your child's growth.

If left uncorrected, large VSDs can eventually lead to damage of the blood vessels in the lungs, so your child's doctor will recommend surgically closing the defect before lung vessel damage develops. In the absence of lung vessel damage, there is no limitation to exercise. Most children have surgery to close VSDs between the ages of 6 and 12 months, or even sooner if medical management of their heart failure is unsuccessful.

Your child should receive antibiotics to prevent infective endocarditis (see pages 343–44). After surgical closure of the VSD, he should continue to receive preventative medication for infective endocarditis until his cardiologist feels it is no longer necessary.

ATRIAL SEPTAL DEFECT

What is an atrial septal defect? An atrial septal defect (ASD) is an opening in the wall, or septum, that separates the heart's two minor pumping chambers, the right and the left atrium. The defect can lead to shunting of blood from the left atrium back into the right atrium.

How do you diagnose ASD? Children with ASDs usually have no symptoms. In infants, there is often no murmur and the heart sounds are normal. In older children, a soft murmur can be heard and the second heart sound is abnormal.

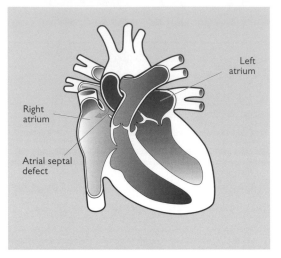

ATRIAL SEPTAL DEFECT
The atrial septal defect is an opening in the wall separating the left and right atriums.

There can be changes in your child's electrocardiogram that suggest the right side of the heart is working hard. An echocardiogram is used to diagnose and confirm the presence of an ASD, to describe its position along the septum, the size of the defect and the degree of blood flow shunting across the defect. It is rare for ASDs to produce heart failure in infants.

How do you treat ASD? Some ASDs will spontaneously close within the first four years of life. If your child still has persistent ASDs by age 4, he will usually require surgery. That is because children with untreated ASDs are at a slightly higher risk of stroke. Furthermore, ASDs that are not surgically closed in childhood can cause even greater problems in young adulthood, due to heart failure and permanent damage to the blood vessels in the lungs. ASD is also associated with abnormal heart rates, or arrhythmias, in adulthood. Your child will not have to take preventive medication for infective endocarditis and there are no exercise restrictions.

PATENT DUCTUS ARTERIOSUS (PDA)

What is patent ductus arteriosus? The ductus arteriosus is an open connection between the main artery that carries blood out of the heart to the body, called the aorta, and the pulmonary artery that connects the right ventricle with the lung. Before birth, this duct allows blood to circulate efficiently in the fetus. Normally, within hours of delivery, the ductus arteriosus will close. If the duct does remain open, or patent, after birth, blood can shunt inefficiently from the aorta through the ductus to the pulmonary artery and then back to the lungs. PDAs occur quite commonly in premature infants.

Your child with a small PDA might have a murmur but no other symptoms. Large PDAs can cause heart failure, a continuous murmur and very strong pulses felt in the baby's limbs. Your child's doctor will order an echocardiogram to assess the size of the defect and the degree of shunting.

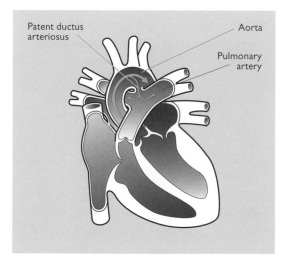

PATENT DUCTUS ARTERIOSUS

Patent ductus arteriosus occurs when the connection between the aorta and the pulmonary artery, which is normally open in the womb, fails to close after birth.

How do you treat PDA? Some PDAs will close spontaneously. Premature infants with heart failure can benefit from medication (indomethacin) that helps close the PDA. Your child might have to take antibiotics to prevent infective endocarditis. If your premature baby does not respond to medication, he will require surgery to close the PDA. In other children, the PDA usually closes by age 2. There are usually no exercise restrictions for children after closure of a PDA.

Abnormalities of the Heart Valves

What are abnormalities of the heart valves? The heart contains special valves that prevent the backflow of circulating blood. Abnormalities of any of the four valves can lead to changes in the way that blood flows through the heart. Valves that cannot open fully have stenosis, or narrowing. Generally, stenosis will obstruct some blood flow, causing the heart chamber that is pumping blood across the valve to work harder. Aortic stenosis and pulmonary stenosis are the two most frequent types. Valves that close incompletely create a valvular insufficiency or incompetence that also can stress the heart and produce heart failure.

PULMONARY STENOSIS

How do you diagnose pulmonary stenosis? Pulmonary stenosis is a narrow opening in the area at or near the pulmonary valve that causes a decreased blood flow to the lungs. Many children with mild stenosis have no symptoms and the only sign is a **systolic murmur.** If the obstruction is more significant,

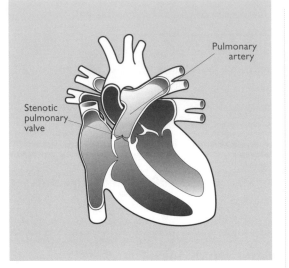

PULMONARY STENOSIS

Pulmonary stenosis occurs when there is a narrow opening in or near the pulmonary valve, causing decreased blood flow to the lungs.

children might get tired when they exercise. In more severe stenosis, children can develop signs of heart failure.

How do you treat pulmonary stenosis? Pulmonary stenosis requires treatment only if the obstruction is severe. The stenosis can often be improved with a procedure called a **balloon valvuloplasty**. Your child's cardiologist performs this minimally invasive procedure. He will use a catheter that contains a balloon to dilate the narrow area. Some valves, however, cannot be treated with valvuloplasty and must be repaired surgically. The timing of surgery depends on your child's symptoms and degree of stenosis. Your child will need to take antibiotics to prevent infective endocarditis.

AORTIC STENOSIS

What is aortic stenosis? Aortic stenosis involves an obstruction at or near the aortic valve and is more common in males. Many children have no symptoms but a doctor can hear a systolic murmur and, sometimes, also a "clicking" sound. However, infants with severe obstruction have weaker pulses in their limbs and can develop heart failure in the first few months of life. Older children with more significant obstruction can have chest pain or fainting and difficulty with exercise. An echocardiogram can estimate the degree of obstruction for both types of stenosis.

How do you treat aortic stenosis? Your child with moderate or severe aortic stenosis cannot participate in strenuous exercise or activities. He will need intervention to relieve the obstruction, which is either a balloon valvuloplasty or surgery. In addition, you will have to ensure that you take him for regular follow-up after surgery because he might experience further valvular damage and could require a valve replacement later in life. Children with aortic stenosis should take antibiotics to prevent infective endocarditis.

COARCTATION OF THE AORTA

What is coarctation of the aorta? This defect is a narrowing or obstruction of the aorta, which is the large artery that carries blood from the left ventricle to the entire body. Coarctation of the aorta is often associated with other cardiac abnormalities, particularly of the aortic valve.

How do you diagnose coarctation of the aorta?
Because the blood cannot pass effectively through the aorta, an infant with coarctation will have difficulty breathing, be pale, and feed and gain weight poorly. The lower half of some infants' bodies can appear blue and blood pressure and pulses are decreased in their legs. They can have heart failure within the first few months of life. Some infants develop life-threatening shock and kidney failure.

In a few babies with coarctation of the aorta, smaller arteries bypass the obstruction and successfully deliver blood to the lower part of the aorta. This group of infants is more likely to have either no symptoms or very mild pain and weakness in the legs after exercise because the bypass system cannot supply enough oxygen to the lower half of the body. However, these infants or children do have a systolic murmur, elevated blood pressure in the arms and abnormally lower blood pressure in the legs. Often, the pulses in the legs feel weaker, too.

The diagnosis of coarctation of the aorta is confirmed by a variety of cardiac tests and procedures, including chest x-ray, electrocardiogram (ECG), echocardiography and cardiac catheterization.

How do you treat coarctation of the aorta? For critically ill newborns, a medication called prostaglandin can be given intravenously to help the ductus arteriosus remain open as a temporary bypass. This allows oxygen to reach the lower body. Children often need intensive treatment with oxygen, medications and assistance with breathing. They need surgery urgently. When heart failure develops later or if your child is not

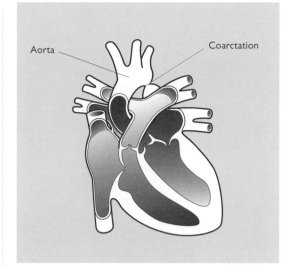

COARCTATION OF THE AORTA
Coarctation of the aorta is a narrowing or obstruction of the aorta.

sick, surgery will still be performed but it is less of an emergency. Your child might need repeat procedures (either balloon angioplasty or further surgery) if the narrowing recurs. He will have to take preventative medication against infective endocarditis. All children with coarctation of the aorta will need regular monitoring of blood pressure in all limbs into adulthood.

Cyanotic Congenital Heart Defects

What is cyanotic heart disease? Cyanotic heart disease is a term used to describe heart defects that lead to mixing of oxygen-poor blood and oxygen-rich blood. While there are many complex and rare congenital heart defects that can cause cyanosis, tetralogy of Fallot is the most common. Other conditions not described

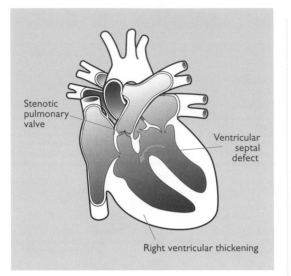

Stenotic
pulmonary
valve

Ventricular
septal
defect

Right ventricular thickening

TETRALOGY OF FALLOT

Tetralogy of Fallot is a combination of VSD, pulmonary stenosis, right ventricular thickening and an abnormal position of the aorta.

here include transposition of the great arteries, pulmonary atresia and total anomalous pulmonary venous drainage.

TETRALOGY OF FALLOT

What is it? In tetralogy of Fallot, there are four distinct abnormalities of the heart: ventricular septal defect, pulmonary **stenosis**, right ventricular thickening and an abnormality of the aortic position. Blood has difficulty pumping out from the right ventricle to the lungs due to the pulmonary stenosis. Children have difficulty getting enough blood to the lungs and, consequently, the body's circulating blood lacks sufficient oxygen.

How do you diagnose tetralogy of Fallot? Some children with tetralogy of Fallot are blue, or cyanosed, at birth while others are not, depending on the degree of pulmonary stenosis. The doctor examining your newborn can often hear a murmur. Depending on the severity of the defect, your child can have breathing difficulty; not tolerate exercise; and his lips, fingers and toes will have a bluish hue. Some children can have the sudden onset of **hypoxic spells**, cyanotic (blue) episodes or "tet" spells as well, which are associated with fast breathing, irritability and crying. Your child's doctor will order an echocardiogram to help determine the degree of obstruction near the pulmonary valve.

How do you treat tetralogy of Fallot? Hypoxic spells are serious. You need to know how to recognize the signs of hypoxic spells, when to seek medical care and how to place your child in knee-chest position in order to attempt to stop the spell. Your child might require oral medication to prevent hypoxic spells.

Children with tetralogy of Fallot require surgery. The type and timing of surgery will depend on the specific findings of the echocardiogram, and your child's overall health. He will probably have to take preventative antibiotics against infective endocarditis for the rest of his life. Some children have exercise restrictions both before and after surgery.

Hypertension (High Blood Pressure)

What is hypertension? The heart acts as a central pump, propelling blood throughout the entire body. As blood is pumped out of the heart through the arteries, oxygen and other nutrients are delivered to all of our organs. In order to efficiently supply these tissues, there must be sufficient blood pressure within the arteries.

This pressure is not constant but comes in pulses. Initially, blood pressure rises as the heart contracts, pushing out a volume of blood from its left ventricle. Then, as this pumping chamber refills, pressure is maintained by the elasticity of the arteries and the resistance to flow in the body's organs.

Usually, blood pressure is described by two measurements:

- Systolic pressure is the peak pressure generated by the heart as it pumps blood out to the body.
- Diastolic pressure occurs when the arterial pressure is at its lowest ebb.

Blood pressure is most easily measured using a cuff that inflates over the arm (or leg) and is recorded in millimeters of mercury (mm Hg). In older children, the systolic and diastolic measurements are recorded together—for example, 90/60, where the systolic pressure is 90 mm Hg and the diastolic pressure is 60 mm Hg. Optimally, your child should be sitting and relaxed. If your child is uncooperative, upset or apprehensive his blood pressure can temporarily elevate. Sometimes, automated machines or instruments that record the sound of the pulse with a sensor (a Doppler) might be used to measure blood pressure.

Hypertension, or high blood pressure, is defined as an elevation of either the systolic or diastolic pressure, or both. In children, the expected values for blood pressure vary, depending on the age, sex and height of the child. There is no single perfect blood pressure; rather there exists an acceptable range of normal for both systolic and diastolic blood pressures. For every age and size and both sexes, there are children who have below-average, average or above-average blood pressures. One method of comparing a child's blood pressure to the normal range is via a blood pressure chart that defines the value as a percentile. Because blood pressure can fluctuate considerably, hypertension is diagnosed when a child has had three separate systolic or diastolic blood pressure measurements that are all above the 95th percentile for height and age.

What are the signs of high blood pressure? Hypertension is often not apparent. There are rarely any signs that you can look for or symptoms that even older children can tell you about. Therefore, blood pressure monitoring is an important part of the annual pediatric health examination and should be measured by your child's doctor from the age of 3 years onward.

The blood pressure of children who are known to have underlying conditions such as a heart murmur, kidney disease, recurrent urinary tract infections, thyroid disease or **obesity**, should be measured earlier in life. If your child is receiving a prolonged course of steroids or other medications known to cause hypertension, blood pressure monitoring should be part of your child's health assessment.

In rare cases, usually when the blood pressure is extremely elevated above the normal range, hypertension is symptomatic: children can experience headaches, seizures or changes in their level of consciousness.

What causes hypertension? High blood pressure can occur either without an obvious cause (primary hypertension) or secondary to certain diseases (secondary hypertension). Primary hypertension, also known as essential hypertension, is usually inherited and can be seen in obese children and adolescents. The blood pressure is usually only mildly elevated and there is often a family history of hypertension.

TYPES OF HYPERTENSION

PRIMARY HYPERTENSION
- more common in adolescents
- they are often obese
- usually family history of hypertension
- treat with lifestyle changes +/– meds

SECONDARY HYPERTENSION
- more common in infants and children
- no family history of hypertension
- requires investigations to diagnose underlying condition
- treat underlying condition +/– lifestyle and meds

This is the most common form of hypertension in adolescents and adults.

Several medical conditions can produce secondary hypertension. Kidney disease or narrowing of the renal arteries, inflammatory conditions in the arteries, various hormonal imbalances, narrowing (coarctation) of the aorta and some neurological disorders can all cause secondary hypertension. Other less common causes of secondary hypertension include lead or mercury exposure, excessive ingestion of licorice and overuse of some cough and cold medications. Infants and young children are more likely to have secondary hypertension: there is usually an identifiable disease that produces their high blood pressure. Furthermore, a cause will often be found in adolescents with extremely elevated systolic or diastolic blood pressures.

What tests will be performed once hypertension is diagnosed? All younger children and some adolescents will benefit from some investigation to help determine the cause of the hypertension. The blood pressure of younger children with hypertension should be measured in both arms and both legs. Blood tests and urine tests to assess kidney function, and an ultrasound of the kidneys and their blood vessels are the most common tests that are routinely performed. An electrocardiogram and echocardiogram of the heart will help exclude coarctation of the aorta as a cause, and determine if the hypertension has begun to place a strain on the heart. In some cases, more extensive hormone levels or renal scans are necessary to determine the cause of hypertension.

How do you treat hypertension? Untreated elevated blood pressure in childhood and adolescence can eventually lead to heart disease, stroke, damage to the blood vessels in the eye and kidney failure. Children with secondary hypertension may need specific treatment (surgery or medication) aimed at the underlying problem. There are several lifestyle modifications that can help reduce high blood pressure in children and adolescents:

- weight control,
- prevention of obesity,
- physical activity,
- sodium (salt) restriction.

Teens who lose weight and increase physical activity leading to improved cardiovascular conditioning can lower their blood pressure.

Reducing the amount of salt in their diet can lower blood pressure as well.

Various medications called antihypertensives are available for children. If your child has elevated blood pressure that has not responded to lifestyle modifications, or in whom the blood pressure is well above the 95th percentile, he might require antihypertensive therapy. Some children and adolescents require long-term treatment with antihypertensives while others are able to discontinue therapy once their blood pressure normalizes.

Infective Endocarditis (IE)

What is infective endocarditis? The inner lining of the heart is a smooth surface that allows blood to flow through freely without forming clots. This smooth surface also prevents bacteria traveling within the bloodstream from lodging and remaining within the heart. However, irregular surfaces within the heart or heart valves can allow bacteria to infect the heart and blood clots to form within the heart. Certain bacteria or fungi are known to cause infective endocarditis (IE) more than others because of their ability to adhere to irregular surfaces, to multiply and to form clumps (vegetations).

Infective endocarditis is a serious infection within the heart's valves or chambers that most often occurs in children with certain kinds of congenital heart disease. It can also occur in children who have large intravenous catheters sitting in the heart (central lines). Less than 10 percent of all cases of IE occur in children who have normal hearts and no central lines.

While not all children with heart disease are at greater risk for IE, some children with abnormal flow through heart valves or defects between the heart chambers are known to be at high risk. Potential for development of IE occurs during periods when bacteria are likely to enter the bloodstream, such as during certain medical and dental procedures and operations, particularly when some degree of bleeding is anticipated.

What does infective endocarditis look like? Your child will invariably have a fever, and can have general weakness, fatigue, muscle and joint aches. He might develop blood in the urine, painful bumps or red/purple lesions on the pads of the fingers or toes, red or purple dots on the skin, red or purple lines under fingernails or toenails, red-rimmed white spots in the retina of the eye or enlargement of the spleen. In rare cases, cerebral hemorrhage (bleeding in the brain) or stroke can occur as a result of IE. In those instances, your child might have seizures or weakness on one side of his body.

He can also have a new heart murmur or a change in the sound or intensity of an old heart murmur. In order for your child's doctor to make the diagnosis, he will have had two specimens of blood taken and they will show evidence of blood infection with bacteria that is known to cause IE. An echocardiogram (an ultrasound of the heart) should also show evidence of a vegetation or a new abnormality of a heart valve.

How do you treat infective endocarditis? Prevention of IE is an important aspect of the medical care of children who have congenital heart disease. You should always inform your child's health care providers of any known underlying heart condition, and ask whether preventive antibiotics are required prior to any new medical or dental procedure or surgery. Most often, one dose of oral or intravenous antibiotic prior to the procedure is adequate to decrease the chance of IE in children at risk.

Treatment of IE involves a long course of intravenous (IV) antibiotics (several weeks to months). The type of antibiotic will depend on the type of bacteria isolated in the blood culture. Often, your child will be discharged from the hospital on home IV antibiotic therapy. Repeat echocardiograms and blood culture samples are used to ensure that the infection is being completely treated.

In some cases, your child might require heart surgery to help clear the infection. This depends on the type of bacteria causing the infection, the location of the infection within the heart and the underlying condition of the heart muscle and valves.

For information on how you can help prevent infective endocarditis in your child go to: www.americanheart.org.

Rheumatic Fever

What is rheumatic fever? Rheumatic fever is a condition that occurs in children primarily between the ages of 5 and 18 after untreated infections caused by certain types of group A streptococcus bacteria. Certain children can be more prone to an immune reaction to the bacteria that develops after a group A strep infection, such as a throat infection or tonsillitis. Rheumatic fever is also more common in crowded environments, as well as in cold and humid climates or in high altitude areas. It is therefore more common in certain countries, but can occur in any part of the world.

Rheumatic fever is caused by an immune system reaction to the bacteria. In trying to eradicate the infection, the immune system will attack anything in the body that resembles the bacteria. Unfortunately, certain parts of the body share common protein structures (antigens) with group A streptococcus, and the immune system cannot distinguish between foreign bacteria and these naturally occurring antigens. If your child does not receive appropriate antibiotics to kill the bacteria, rheumatic fever can occur.

Rheumatic fever has decreased in frequency over the last 100 years with improvement in living conditions and hygiene, and the introduction of antibiotics. However, sporadic cases occur in both urban and rural areas and in children with varying socioeconomic backgrounds.

What does rheumatic fever look like? Children with rheumatic fever can develop a variety of symptoms but invariably have fever and are weak and pale. Other possible symptoms include joint pain and swelling, which is seen in 80 percent of patients. This pain and swelling can switch from one joint to another, and often involves more than five joints such as knees, ankles, elbows, wrists and shoulders. The arthritis usually gets better with treatment.

The heart is seriously affected by the immune response of rheumatic fever. Inflammation of the heart valves, the heart muscle itself or the sac around the heart can cause a fast heart rate, a new murmur, enlargement of the heart, rhythm disturbances, chest pain and difficulty breathing. The mitral and aortic valves are the most common affected areas in the heart. The valves can become ineffective and not close completely, thereby placing strain on the heart. Valvular changes often do not go away and can worsen as children grow into adulthood.

Mood swings can accompany chorea, which is a term describing abnormal involuntary movement of the face and limbs that often causes the handwriting to deteriorate. Chorea is

CRITERIA USED TO DIAGNOSE RHEUMATIC FEVER

MAJOR CRITERIA
- cardiac inflammation
- joint swelling/pain
- chorea
- classic rash
- classic nodules

MINOR CRITERIA
- fever
- painful joints (no swelling)
- previous rheumatic fever
- low hemoglobin
- abnormal blood tests suggesting inflammation
- abnormal ECG findings

more common in adolescent girls and usually resolves after several weeks or months.

Painless firm nodules under the skin of the knees, elbows, wrists and feet are seen less commonly but can be associated with heart involvement. A typical rash that has a red border and a clear center can sometimes be seen over the abdomen, chest, arms and thighs. This non-itchy rash only lasts a few days. Nosebleeds can also frequently be seen.

Evidence of a previous group A strep infection is an important factor in making the diagnosis. This is often gathered with a throat swab, or one of the blood antistreptococcal **antibody** tests. Cardiac investigations include a chest x-ray, an ECG and an echocardiogram.

How do you treat rheumatic fever? The most important treatment involves preventing rheumatic fever at the outset by ensuring that your take your child with tonsillitis and group A strep infections to his doctor for a diagnostic throat swab and prescription of appropriate antibiotics. Once rheumatic fever occurs, treatment involves eradicating the bacteria and preventing further exposure to the bacteria. Regular treatment of group A strep infections

usually involves a course of antibiotics such as penicillin.

Once your child has had rheumatic fever, he is at risk for repeated episodes when exposed to group A strep bacteria. Ongoing preventative medication can help prevent recurrence of symptoms. This can be achieved with regular daily oral antibiotics until the age of 21 or at least five years after the last episode of rheumatic fever. Alternatively, regular intramuscular penicillin injections every few weeks can be administered.

Arthritis often responds well to anti-inflammatory medications. If your child's heart has been affected, he will require treatment with oral steroids to decrease the inflammatory damage to the heart. However, some damage to the heart might remain and your child will require ongoing evaluation and monitoring by a cardiologist. Sometimes he might require medication or surgery in adolescence or adulthood. Your child will need antibiotic prophylaxis for infective endocarditis (see pages 343–44) prior to surgery or dental work.

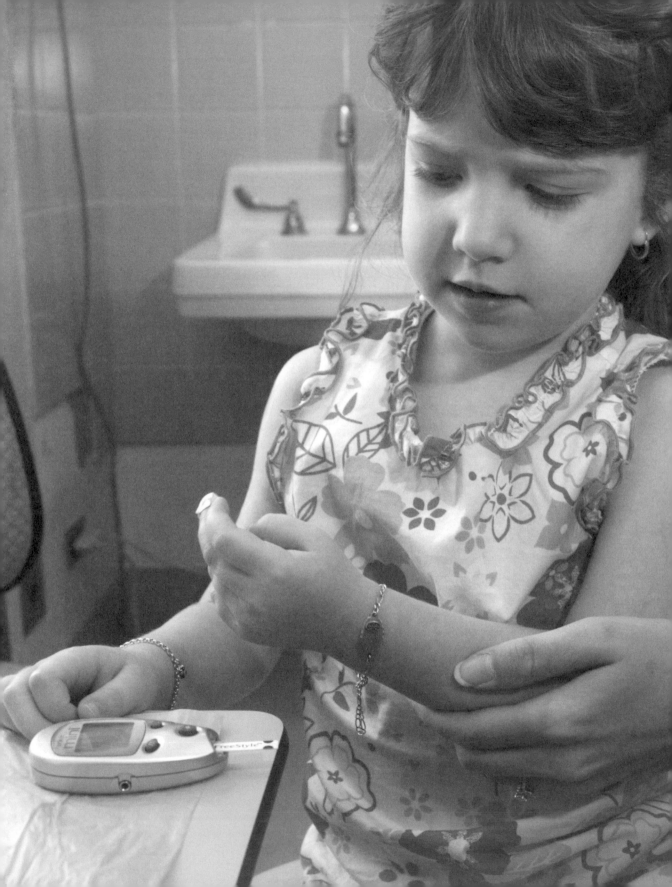

Endocrine Disease 19

Addison's Disease

What is Addison's disease? Addison's disease is a rare illness that results from permanent failure of the outer layer of the adrenal glands. The adrenal glands are two small organs that rest on top of each of the kidneys. The outer section of each adrenal gland, called the cortex, makes three important types of hormones. Glucocorticoids, such as cortisol, help to keep the blood sugar and blood pressure in the normal range. This steroid hormone also helps regulate the body's response to stress. The adrenal cortex also produces mineralocorticoids, such as aldosterone, that assist in regulating blood pressure and the salts found in the blood, particularly sodium and potassium. These two hormones are essential to sustain life. Lastly the cortex releases sex hormones, called androgens, that aid in the production of underarm and pubic hair. In Addison's disease the middle part of the adrenal gland, called the medulla, which makes adrenaline, continues to function adequately.

The most common cause of damage to the adrenal glands in Addison's disease is autoimmunity. For an unknown reason, the body makes antibodies that attack and destroy the cortex of the gland. Tuberculosis infection used to be the most common cause of Addison's disease. In

most cases, Addison's disease is not inherited, but other autoimmune endocrine diseases may run in the family.

What does Addison's disease look like? Children with Addison's disease have symptoms caused by the missing hormones. These can include:

* salt craving,
* tiredness,
* loss of appetite,
* weakness,
* weight loss,
* dizziness,
* vomiting,
* dark skin tanning when exposed to the sun,
* darkening of the skin in non-sun-exposed areas such as the knuckles, elbows, nipples and gums.

Since the symptoms usually start gradually and are nonspecific and the disease is uncommon, it often takes a long time before the diagnosis of Addison's disease is made, after many trips to the doctor. The disease is often not recognized until a stressful event (for example, a viral illness) causes the child to get sicker. This is known as an Addisonian crisis or **acute** adrenal insufficiency. This is a

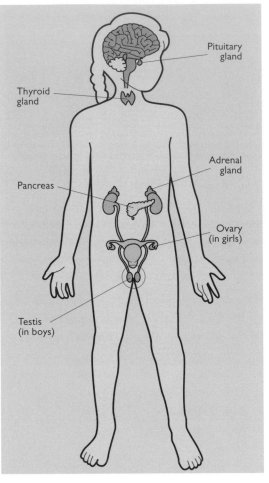

THE ENDOCRINE SYSTEM

The endocrine glands manufacture hormones, the body's chemical messengers. Hormones are distributed to all parts of the body by the blood and help to regulate internal processes, such as growth. Some glands, such as the testis and ovary, are inactive until puberty.

Labels on figure:
- Pituitary gland
- Thyroid gland
- Pancreas
- Adrenal gland
- Ovary (in girls)
- Testis (in boys)

potentially life-threatening situation with severe vomiting and diarrhea, dehydration, low blood pressure and loss of consciousness.

How do you treat Addison's disease? Your child with Addison's disease will have to take medications daily by mouth for the rest of her life to replace the hormones normally produced by the adrenal gland. Most people with Addison's disease are prescribed a combination of two pills to replace the missing cortisol and aldosterone. Even though your child is taking steroids, she is only replacing what the body should be making for itself. It sometimes requires adjusting of the doses to reach the right balance for each individual, as everyone is a little bit different. With the correct amount of medication, people with Addison's disease can lead normal, full lives. At times of stress, such as surgery or illness, your child might have to take extra steroid medication and doubling or tripling the usual daily dosage is often recommended. The body needs steroids to survive, so if medications cannot be taken by mouth they need to be injected. Your child will have to carry an injection kit and wear a medical alert bracelet in case of emergency. Monitoring for other autoimmune disorders that may coexist, such as Graves' disease or Hashimoto's disease, is important.

Congenital Adrenal Hyperplasia

What is congenital adrenal hyperplasia? Congenital adrenal hyperplasia (CAH) is a group of conditions in which the production of certain adrenal hormones is altered because of defective production pathways.

The adrenal glands are two small organs that rest on top of the kidneys. The outer layer, or cortex of the adrenals, produce hormones called glucocorticoids. An example is cortisol, which helps the body respond to stress. The adrenal cortex also produces mineralocorticoids like aldosterone that assist in regulating blood pressure and controlling the body's sodium and potassium levels. These two types of hormones are essential to sustain life. Lastly, the adrenal cortex releases androgens, which are male sex hormones that aid in the production of underarm and pubic hair in both genders, although less in females.

The production of glucocorticoids, mineralocorticoids and androgens are the result of a chain of interconnected chemical reactions that are controlled by specific proteins, called enzymes. Inherited deficiencies of the various enzymes lead to CAH. The most common missing enzyme is called 21-hydroxylase. The 21-hydroxylase enzyme is necessary for the production of glucocorticoids and mineralocorticoids. In 21-hydroxylase deficiency, the adrenal gland is unable to produce adequate amounts of cortisol and aldosterone. In an attempt to compensate, the adrenal gland becomes enlarged, hence the name adrenal hyperplasia. As a result of this enlargement excess androgens are produced. The results can be dramatic.

What does CAH look like? The symptoms of the disease depend on the specific enzyme defect. Children with 21-hydroxylase deficiency may have a severe or mild form. Males and females are affected equally, but the signs of CAH are different in each.

In the severe form, female fetuses are exposed to excess male sex hormones during early pregnancy, when the genitals are being formed. As a consequence, they get masculinized. The clitoris becomes enlarged, and the lips of the vagina seal together, making it look like a scrotum. The female chromosomes and all the internal organs, such as the uterus, remain normal. This condition often causes initial confusion regarding the sex of the newborn baby.

Extra androgens do not present a problem for the male fetus. Boys will have early puberty. In mild cases, females can also have early pubic or underarm hair, rapid growth, acne, male pattern hair growth (hirsutism) and absent menstrual periods.

If there is a lack of mineral corticoids, both sexes can have a "salt-wasting" crisis in the first few weeks of life. This is associated with vomiting, poor weight gain and a low blood sodium level. Because of cortisol deficiency, they may also have low blood sugar or an adrenal crisis (see Addison's Disease, pages 347–48).

Other, more rare types of CAH are associated with too much aldosterone. This results in high blood pressure. And, in some forms, too little androgen is made so that the male external sex organs are underdeveloped.

How do you test for CAH? The abnormal hormone levels can be detected in the blood. In some states in the U.S., newborns are screened for 21-hydroxylase deficiency. Initially, the serum levels of sodium and potassium are affected in the untreated infant.

How do you treat CAH? There is no cure, but there is effective treatment. Your child can take oral steroids, both glucocorticoids and mineralocorticoids, to replace the missing hormones. She will have to take them for the rest of her life and have ongoing monitoring of her growth and puberty. She might have to have surgery to repair the ambiguous genitalia.

You should be aware that there is a 25 percent chance of recurrence of CAH in each future pregnancy. You can have special testing during pregnancy to see if a fetus is affected with the disease. Virilization can be reduced or prevented by taking steroids starting in early pregnancy.

Diabetes Mellitus

What is diabetes mellitus? Diabetes is the disease that occurs when the hormone involved in controlling sugar metabolism, insulin, is deficient. Normally, the pancreas, a gland situated in the abdomen nestled beside the stomach, produces insulin.

There are two types of diabetes mellitus:

- Type 1 diabetes, formerly known as insulin-dependent or juvenile-onset diabetes mellitus, is caused by a failure of the pancreas to secrete insulin.
- Type 2 diabetes, which used to be called either non-insulin-dependent or adult-onset diabetes mellitus, is caused by "insulin resistance." In this case, unlike in type 1, insulin is still produced, but it may not be in a large enough quantity to meet the body's demands, or in some cases the body is not able to respond to it appropriately.

What does insulin do? Insulin has many functions in the body, but its most important role involves blood sugar regulation. When we eat certain foods, sugar is absorbed from the stomach and enters the bloodstream. Insulin allows sugar that is in the blood to move into the cells of the body where it can be used as energy. When insulin levels are low, as in diabetes, sugar builds up in the bloodstream. There is lots of sugar around, but the cells in the body are unable to use the sugar they need to survive.

What causes diabetes? Nobody knows for sure. It is not caused by eating too much sugar, and you cannot catch it from someone else. The body's own immune system seems to attack the cells in the pancreas (the islets of Langerhans) that make insulin and damages them.

There are many factors that together affect a person's risk of getting diabetes. As with many autoimmune conditions, it happens as a result of inherited factors in combination with an environmental trigger. The genes alone cannot be blamed. It has to do with being the wrong person in the wrong place at the wrong time. Your child is at a higher risk of becoming diabetic if she has close relatives with the disease. Even in relatives who are identified as at risk by measuring the insulin antibodies in their blood, there is no known way to prevent the disease. Current studies are looking at this.

Who gets diabetes? Diabetes is not rare. It affects 1 in 400 North American children. In fact, diabetes is the most common endocrine disorder. You probably know someone who has it. It affects children of all ages. Type 2 diabetes used to be seen only in older people but it is becoming more common in children because of the high prevalence of **obesity**. It is also more common if there is a family history of type 2 diabetes, and in certain ethnic backgrounds such as in African-American, Hispanic and North American native populations.

What does diabetes look like? Symptoms of type 1 diabetes mellitus include being very thirsty, very hungry and peeing a lot. Your child who was toilet trained might start wetting the bed at night. Other symptoms include stomach pain, blurred vision, weight loss, tiredness and sweet-smelling breath. If the symptoms go on long enough without being recognized, or an illness with fever occurs, a condition called diabetic ketoacidosis (DKA) can develop. Children with DKA have vomiting, abdominal pain, dehydration, heavy breathing or are even in a coma. It is a serious, potentially life-threatening situation.

Approximately 60 percent of children with type 2 diabetes have no symptoms or they might have all the same symptoms as those with type 1 diabetes. If you suspect that your child has diabetes, take her to her doctor right away.

How do you test for diabetes? A blood test can be done to measure your child's blood sugar level, which will be high if she has diabetes. The extra blood sugar spills over into the urine. When a doctor checks her urine with a special dipstick there will be sugar in it. Under normal circumstances, there is no sugar in your urine.

How do you treat diabetes? There is still no cure for diabetes although there are many new therapies, such as pancreas and islet transplantation, that are being studied. Diabetes is a lifelong condition. Your child's type 1 diabetes can be well controlled using insulin given under the skin, either by needle or by a special pump. Your child can learn to give the injections herself, with adult supervision. She will need to monitor her blood sugar several times a day by taking samples of blood by a tiny prick. The blood sugar is then measured with a small handheld machine, called a glucose meter. The dose of insulin needs to be adjusted on a daily basis, based on the blood sugar measurement at any given time and your child's diet, activity level and state of health. Your child will have to eat a balanced diet and match her food intake with appropriate changes in insulin. The specific regime of insulin will vary based on many factors such as your child's age and family lifestyle. This means that the dose and type of insulin

(short, intermediate or long acting), number of shots and route of administration will change as she grows older.

Your child's type 2 diabetes might be treated with diet and exercise alone, or in combination with pills or insulin. Regular monitoring of blood sugars with a glucose meter is also recommended.

Your child's diabetes will require regular follow-up and monitoring of the disease. Most centers have a team or diabetes education center where you and your child will learn together what to do. A team of health care professionals will be involved with her care. Your child's doctor will check for other autoimmune diseases, for example thyroid problems, that can develop with higher frequency. There are many organizations such as the Juvenile Diabetes Research Foundation that can offer support and information for families.

Why is it important to have the disease under good control? There are many long-term complications of uncontrolled type 1 and type 2 diabetes including:

- blindness,
- nerve damage,
- kidney failure,
- high blood pressure,
- heart disease and stroke.

We know now from studying a large group of diabetic patients over many years that, by keeping the blood sugar as close to normal as possible, these complications can be markedly reduced. Once your child enters her teenage years, she should be counseled about compliance with her medication and how smoking and obesity can worsen the complications of the disease. Adolescent girls with diabetes have twice the risk of eating disorders, and this too can lead to bad control of their disease when doses of insulin are skipped in order to not eat and thereby lose weight.

If her blood sugar repeatedly goes too low, that is also not good. It can cause sweating, light-headedness, fainting and even seizures. Repeated episodes of low blood sugar can affect intelligence in preschool children. You should have an emergency kit at home and at school to give sugar solutions or an injection of glucagon in the case of severe low blood sugar. The diabetes educators can help you to teach your child's other care-givers, teachers and coaches about how to look for high and low blood sugars and what to do.

Growth Hormone Deficiency

What is growth hormone deficiency? Growth hormone deficiency (GHD) is a rare illness that is one of the causes of short stature. Just as the name implies, GHD is due to a partial or total lack of growth hormone in the body. Growth hormone is made by the pituitary gland, a pea-sized gland that sits at the base of the brain and regulates

many hormones in the body. Growth hormone stimulates growth through complex chemical interactions in the body. Other pituitary hormones such as thyroid stimulating hormone (TSH) and adrenocorticotropic hormone (ACTH) can affect growth too.

What causes growth hormone deficiency? GHD can be congenital or acquired. In either case it might occur alone, or as part of damage to the pituitary gland where any of the other pituitary hormones can also be affected. There are many different causes of permanent injury to the pituitary including lack of oxygen at birth, head trauma, radiation damage in cancer patients, severe infections, such as **meningitis**, and benign tumors, such as craniopharyngiomas. There are some rare inherited problems that can cause congenital GHD. Often the cause of growth hormone deficiency cannot be found.

What does growth hormone deficiency look like? The rate of growth in a child with GHD will be slow. In congenital GHD, the child will often be a normal length at birth and will grow normally until age two or three years. This is because, in infancy, hormones such as insulin play a big role in stimulating growth, but after this time growth hormone becomes the major factor. When that happens, the growth rate slows down. Your child's height might be below the third percentile on the growth curve when the doctor plots it, whereas her weight will continue to plot in the normal or average range. As opposed to the abnormal body proportions that are seen in dwarfism, in GHD the body proportions are normal (the limbs are in proportion to the trunk). Children with congenital GHD have typical features including a high-pitched voice, a babyish face, a plump build and a smallish penis. They may have encountered problems such as low blood sugar or prolonged jaundice around the time of birth. A physical exam might show signs of other pituitary hormone deficiencies such as delayed onset of puberty. GHD does not affect intelligence.

How do I know my child is too short? It is important to collect as many accurate growth measurements as possible. Your child's doctor will take these measurements and plot them on an appropriate graph, called a growth chart. There are separate graphs for boys and girls of different ages. (You can find growth charts on page 134.) The growth chart displays a pattern of growth over time. The growth velocity is an important clue as to whether there is a growth problem or not. There are normal values for the tempo of growth. We grow at different rates at different times in our life, with big spurts in the first year of life and during the teenage years. Your child's doctor and you will be concerned if your child:

- plots way below the bottom curve on the growth chart,
- is inappropriately short when compared to the parents' heights,
- is older than 2 years and used to plot on a much higher percentile curve but has dropped down, or
- has a slow growth velocity (for example, less than 2 inches/5 cm a year in childhood).

How do you test for growth hormone deficiency? Your child's doctor will order a bone age test, which is simply an x-ray of the left hand and wrist, to look at the level of maturation of her bones. The bone age is a general marker of growth status. In GHD the bone age will be delayed; for example, a 5-year-old child will appear to have the bones of a 3-year-old. Delayed bone age is not specific for GHD as it can be seen in other conditions, such as constitutional growth delay. So, your child's doctor might also order blood tests to look at other pituitary hormones (for example, thyroid hormones). Other blood tests that investigate short stature can include:

- chromosome analysis to rule out **Turner syndrome** in girls,
- kidney function,
- a complete blood count, and
- an erythrocyte sedimentation rate (ESR), to measure inflammation in the body (see Short Stature, pages 146–47).

Growth hormone testing will be done when other causes of short stature have been ruled out. Normally, growth hormone gets released from the pituitary in "bursts." Therefore, random blood samples are not helpful in diagnosing GHD. Growth hormone testing involves trying to stimulate the pituitary gland to secrete growth hormone by supplying intravenous medicines (for example, insulin) or by exercising, which normally causes growth hormone release. If your child has GHD, her body's response will be blunted or absent after these stimulations. GHD needs to be proven on more than one test before a child is eligible for treatment with replacement growth hormone. If GHD is confirmed, your child's doctor will also order MRI images of the brain to get a close look at her pituitary gland.

How do you treat growth hormone deficiency? Your child will be treated with synthetic growth hormone given by injection six or seven days a week until she has finished growing. Treatment usually takes years, and growth occurs slowly over months— not overnight! You and your older child can learn to administer the needles yourselves. If other hormones are missing they can also be replaced by medication. All hormones need to be in the right balance for proper growth to take place. If treatment is started early, your child with GHD should achieve her full growth potential. In some countries, children who are short but do not have GHD are treated with synthetic GH at higher doses. In general, these children do not achieve the same height increase as those with GHD, and there is some controversy about how helpful this treatment is for those without true GHD.

You need to be aware that your child who is much shorter than her peers might get teased and suffer physical and emotional stress. Some people treat short children as if they were younger, just because they are smaller. She might need support around these issues.

Hyperthyroidism

What is hyperthyroidism? Hyperthyroidism is a condition that occurs due to elevated levels of thyroid hormone, which is produced by the thyroid gland, a butterfly-shaped gland found in the neck. Like most endocrine glands, the thyroid is under the control of the master gland in the brain, the pituitary. The pituitary gland makes thyroid stimulating hormone (TSH) that stimulates the thyroid to produce thyroid hormone, called thyroxine. In babies thyroxine is critical for normal brain development and in older children it works all over the body to control our growth and metabolism.

What causes hyperthyroidism? There are many causes of hyperthyroidism. Graves' disease is the most common cause in children. In this autoimmune condition, the body makes an **antibody** similar in effect to TSH that causes overstimulation of the thyroid gland. Graves' often shows up in the teenage years, to girls more often than boys, and there could be other family members with thyroid problems or other autoimmune conditions such as diabetes mellitus. Babies born to mothers who have Graves' disease can have temporary hyperthyroidism due to the mother's antibodies crossing the placenta. Hyperthyroidism can also be caused by a lump or nodule in the gland that starts secreting lots of thyroid hormone. (Thyroid cancer is very rare in children.) Children can also get a viral infection of the thyroid called thyroiditis that causes the gland to be painful and release extra hormone.

What does hyperthyroidism look like? Symptoms of hyperthyroidism often develop gradually and are the result of a hyperactive metabolism. Symptoms include:

- sweatiness,
- feeling hot,
- fast heartbeat or palpitations,
- increased appetite,
- weight loss,
- fatigue,
- trouble sleeping,
- diarrhea,
- irregular menstrual periods,
- a fast growth rate,
- muscle weakness,
- difficulty concentrating,
- hyperactivity,
- deteriorating school performance, and
- shakiness.

Some people with hyperthyroidism get bulging eyes (proptosis) or a swelling in the neck (goiter) due to the enlarged thyroid.

How do you diagnose hyperthyroidism? Sometimes your child's doctor might feel a goiter. She will order blood tests to measure thyroid hormones and antithyroid antibodies. She might also order ultrasound and thyroid scans to assess thyroid nodules.

How do you treat hyperthyroidism? There are different treatment options. Your child's doctor might order antithyroid medicines, such as propylthiouracil or methimazole, to stop hormone production within the thyroid gland. Medications known as beta-blockers can be taken temporarily to control the unpleasant symptoms, such as palpitations. Some children will only need to take the antithyroid medications for a few years because, in some cases, the condition improves and the medications can be gradually stopped.

Your child's hyperthyroidism can be cured quickly in one of two ways. She might take a small amount of radioactive iodine by mouth in order to burn out the thyroid gland. This treatment is often used if your child experiences side effects from taking antithyroid medications. Alternately, the gland can be surgically removed. This is rarely necessary. In most cases these treatments cause the thyroid to stop functioning completely and lifelong thyroid hormone replacement by mouth becomes necessary.

The eye problems most often clear up with the treatment of the disease. Your child will have to have thyroid blood tests over time. Treatment of this disease is usually straight-forward and successful.

Hypothyroidism

What is hypothyroidism? Hypothyroidism is a condition that results from reduced levels of thyroid hormone (thyroxine) in the blood. This hormone is produced by the thyroid, a butterfly-shaped gland that is situated in the neck. Like all endocrine glands, the thyroid gland is under the control of the pituitary gland in the brain. The pituitary makes thyroid stimulating hormone (TSH) that acts on the thyroid and stimulates it to produce thyroxine. In babies it is important for brain development, and in older children it is important for normal growth and metabolism.

What causes hypothyroidism? There are many possible causes of hypothyroidism. An under-active thyroid can be congenital or acquired. Congenital causes include a thyroid gland that never developed properly or else grew in the wrong place, lack of stimulation from an abnormal pituitary gland or inherited conditions where the gland is unable to make thyroxine.

The most common cause of acquired hypothyroidism is an autoimmune condition known as Hashimoto's disease where the body makes antibodies that attack and destroy its own thyroid gland. Other reasons include iodine deficiency, certain drugs, previous thyroid surgery, radiation to the neck and any permanent injury to the pituitary (for example, in **meningitis**, benign tumors and head trauma). Hypothyroidism is common in certain genetic conditions such as **Down's syndrome**.

What does hypothyroidism look like? Your baby's congenital hypothyroidism will show up weeks to months after birth. Symptoms can include:

- dry skin and hair,
- low body temperature,

- a large tongue with poor feeding and breathing difficulty,
- hoarse voice,
- slow heart rate,
- constipation,
- prolonged jaundice (yellow skin),
- low muscle tone,
- large soft spot on the head,
- poor growth, and
- a hernia through the belly button.

Untreated hypothyroidism at this age can quickly lead to mental retardation, or cretinism. Treatment started within the first two weeks of life leads to normal intelligence. If treatment is started later, it cannot prevent mental retardation totally but can prevent further retardation and other symptoms.

Because of the potential for brain damage if not recognized, and the ease with which hypothyroidism can be diagnosed and treated, all newborns are screened for hypothyroidism at birth. Before discharge home from hospital a sample of your baby's blood was taken by heel prick, smeared on a special card and sent to the laboratory to measure the TSH. Babies who are diagnosed with congenital hypothyroidism by newborn screening might not have developed any symptoms of hypothyroidism by the time of diagnosis.

Symptoms of acquired hypothyroidism are due to an underactive metabolism. They are nonspecific and can show up at any age—most typically, in female teenagers. Symptoms include:

- weight gain,
- growth problems,
- muscle weakness,
- dry skin and hair,
- feeling cold,

- slow heart rate,
- constipation,
- tiredness,
- puffiness, and
- swelling in the front of the neck (goiter).

If your teen's pituitary gland is the cause of her problem, there can be evidence of other hormone deficiencies or excess, for example, growth failure or early puberty.

How do you diagnose hypothyroidism? Your child's doctor might feel a goiter during a physical exam. She might order blood tests to measure antithyroid antibodies, levels of TSH and thyroid hormone. She might also order a scan to look for the thyroid gland.

How do you treat hypothyroidism? Your child can take thyroxine medication by mouth once daily to replace the missing hormone in the body without side effects. You will have to ensure that you take your child to the doctor to follow up with monitoring of growth, thyroid tests and medication adjustment as necessary.

- Congenital hypothyroidism is often clinically undetectable at first. A simple screening test can diagnose the problem and prevent mental retardation.
- Hashimoto's disease is the most common late onset form of hypothyroidism.

Polycystic Ovarian Syndrome

What is polycystic ovarian syndrome? There is controversy about the precise definition of polycystic ovarian syndrome (PCOS). Still, this condition is one of the most common endocrine diseases. Most people feel the condition is the result of a combination of excess male hormone (androgen) and abnormal menstrual periods due to failure of the ovaries to release eggs (anovulation). Cysts full of fluid and immature eggs collect in the ovaries.

What does polycystic ovarian syndrome look like? PCOS affects only females. In PCOS, there are a group of related symptoms that are found in various combinations in different people. These symptoms can include:

- pimples,
- **obesity,**
- balding of the type males tend to develop,
- excessive male-pattern hair growth in a female, such as a mustache or beard (hirsutism),
- cysts in the ovaries,
- irregular or absent menstrual periods,
- difficulty becoming pregnant.

Long-term effects include type II diabetes, cancer of the uterus and, possibly, premature heart disease.

Previously it was thought that PCOS was seen only in older women, but it is now recognized that symptoms often start in the teenage years. Menstrual periods may never develop, or they start but then go away, or are associated with persistent irregular bleeding. It is difficult to diagnose PCOS in children because, during puberty, symptoms such as irregular periods and acne are common. Regular monthly periods often do not develop for the first 12 to 18 months after the initial period. Your child's doctor will be concerned if your child's periods have not begun by age 16.

What causes polycystic ovarian syndrome? No one knows for sure. PCOS is likely due to a combination of inherited and environmental factors. High levels of insulin, which are often linked to increased body weight, seem to be a factor in PCOS.

How do you diagnose polycystic ovarian syndrome? There is no one test that makes the diagnosis of PCOS. Your daughter's diagnosis will mostly depend on the combination of symptoms that send her to the doctor. Blood tests can be done to measure male hormone levels. Her doctor should order tests of other hormone levels and chromosomes and a pregnancy test to rule out conditions that look like PCOS. A pelvic ultrasound might show numerous cysts in the ovaries. The ultrasound is also helpful to rule out other rare disorders, such as ovarian tumors, adrenal gland abnormalities and genetic diseases associated with missing ovaries, such as **Turner syndrome**. The test is not specific; having normal ovaries does not exclude PCOS, and cystic ovaries are seen in other conditions. Blood fat (lipid) levels and glucose tolerance tests should be done to monitor for complications of the disease.

How do you treat polycystic ovarian syndrome? PCOS is a chronic condition for which there is no cure. Your daughter's symptoms can be successfully managed by her taking the birth control pill and antiandrogen medications. She can have cosmetic treatment for increased hair growth, such as waxing and electrolysis. Medications to lower insulin levels might also be useful. She ought to try and maintain a healthy weight with proper diet and adequate exercise. She will need support regarding this lifelong condition in which cosmetic problems can affect self-esteem.

Problems with Puberty

What is puberty? Puberty is the period during which a child's body matures sexually into its adult form. This transformation is regulated by bursts of hormones released from the brain. The sequence of changes in puberty is very predictable, and more reliable than the specific age at which the changes occur.

In girls, breast development is the first sign of puberty, followed by the growth spurt and pubic hair development. Menarche (the onset of menstrual periods) is the final stage, at which point growth is almost complete.

In boys, enlargement of the testicles is the first sign of puberty. Then the penis enlarges and pubic hair grows. The growth spurt occurs later in puberty allowing boys to grow for a longer time than girls and achieve taller final adult height. It is common for boys to get some breast enlargement during mid-puberty. In some boys and girls, pubic hair development is the first sign of puberty.

DELAYED PUBERTY

What is delayed puberty? The physical changes that transform children into adults, in other words, puberty, normally occur over the span of a few years during adolescence. If puberty has not begun by age 13 in girls, and 14 in boys, it is considered delayed. The average age at which periods begin is approximately 12 ½. The diagnosis of delayed puberty is also made if your daughter's menstrual periods have not started by age 16, or five years after puberty begins. Periods usually start within two years after puberty begins (the development of the breast buds). In boys, delayed puberty is more common than in girls, and is usually not due to any serious diseases.

What causes delayed puberty? Delayed puberty in boys is often "constitutional." This means that there is no detectable disease or problem causing the delay. You might have a family history of late bloomers. These boys will ultimately catch up to their peers.

It is much more likely that there is an underlying reason for the delay in girls. There can be problems in a part of the brain called the hypothalamus or in the pituitary gland, which regulates many hormonal functions. Sometimes, the sex organs are not working normally. For example, in some genetic diseases, such as **Turner syndrome**, the ovaries do not form properly. Also, any chronic illness can cause pubertal delay. Examples would include inflammatory bowel disease, chronic kidney failure, cystic fibrosis, diabetes and eating disorders, such as anorexia nervosa. Untreated hypothyroidism, malnutrition and excessive exercise can also cause delayed puberty.

What does delayed puberty look like? The signs of late puberty depend on its underlying cause. Your child's doctor will take a full history and do a complete physical exam as part of her evaluation. This involves looking for signs of increased pressure in the brain, such as severe, worsening headaches associated with vomiting in the morning and double vision. An eye exam might show swelling in the back of the eye.

If the problem is due to a lack of hormone stimulation from the hypothalamus or pituitary gland, there may be evidence of other hormone deficiencies. If your child is drinking a lot and

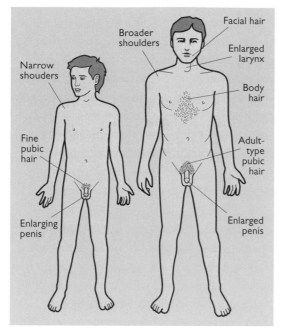

PUBERTY IN BOYS

In early puberty, the testes and scrotum start to enlarge. By the age of about 17 years, a boy's penis will have reached its maximum size, and hair will have grown under the arms and on the face, legs, chest and abdomen. The voice deepens as the larynx and vocal cords enlarge.

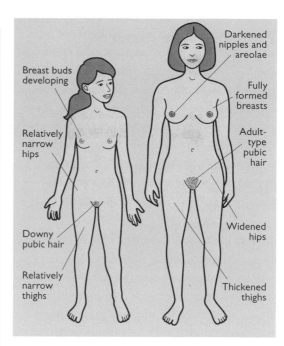

PUBERTY IN GIRLS

In girls, puberty is heralded by emerging breast buds and growth of downy pubic hair. By 15 or 16 years, a girl will have reached adult proportions, with wider hips, fat deposits in the abdomen and thighs, fully developed breasts and adult-type pubic and underarm hair.

voiding excessively because antidiuretic hormone is missing; if her growth is slow due to growth hormone deficiency; or if she is gaining weight and feeling cold then thyroid hormone is deficient. Some characteristic physical features of Turner syndrome are short stature, webbing of the neck and a low hairline at the back of the head. She might also have associated problems such as a heart murmur. In constitutional delay, other than the lack of signs of puberty, the rest of the examination is normal. Your child's doctor will assess the stage of puberty, called the "Tanner stage," by a standardized method, and measure her growth, particularly height,

weight and head circumference, in comparison to her previous values.

How do you diagnose delayed puberty? It is possible to measure sex hormone levels in the blood and the hormones made in the brain that stimulate the release of testosterone and estrogen from the testicles and ovaries, respectively. This can help to determine if the problem is in your child's sex organs, or in the stimulation center in the brain, that is, the hypothalamus and pituitary gland. If the test results point to a pituitary problem, other hormones such as thyroid hormone and growth hormone testing can be measured in the blood too. An x-ray of your child's left hand and wrist will display the level of maturity and number of bones. This bone age correlates more with the level of sexual maturity than with the chronological age. There are reference standard for children of all ages. An MRI of the brain can be done to rule out any lesions. A blood test for chromosomes to look at genetic causes, such as Turner syndrome in girls and Klinefelter syndrome in boys, should be also done.

How do you treat delayed puberty? In constitutional delay, waiting is best. With time, boys will go into normal puberty and go through all the usual changes with a normal outcome. It can be hard for the physically immature adolescent to deal with peer comparisons. If the delayed puberty is significantly affecting a boy's well-being, it is possible to "kick-start" puberty by giving him testosterone shots for a few months. When the sex hormones are missing, as they are in Turner syndrome, they can be replaced with medications such as estrogen, progesterone and testosterone. If your child has an underlying chronic illness, puberty should proceed spontaneously after treatment of the illness and improved nutrition. Any pituitary tumor in the brain, usually a craniopharyngioma, must be removed, although hormone replacement after surgery might still be necessary. Reassurance, follow-up and support are important aspects of the care.

PRECOCIOUS PUBERTY

What is precocious puberty? Puberty happens in girls before it occurs in boys. Normal puberty is starting earlier than it did in prior generations. It also starts earlier in children of certain ethnic backgrounds, for example, African-American girls. If puberty starts before 7 years of age in girls (6 years in African-American girls) and 9 years in boys, then it is called precocious puberty. Early puberty is more common in girls, and is usually not serious. In contrast, late puberty in girls is often a sign of an underlying problem. In boys the opposite is true. In both sexes, a pattern of early puberty can run in the family.

What causes precocious puberty? Early puberty can be caused by a problem in the brain (central) caused by an early triggering of the normal forces in the brain that stimulate the onset of puberty. In these cases puberty happens in the normal sequence, but starts too early. This can be due to injury to the brain caused by, for example, infections, benign or cancerous growths, and trauma. In girls commonly no cause can be found. In boys it is much more likely that an underlying problem in the brain will be identified.

Less commonly, precocious puberty can also be caused by peripheral problems, for example abnormalities in the sex organs such as tumors in the ovaries or testicles. In these "noncentral" causes the sequence of events does not happen in the usual order.

There are also incomplete forms of precocious puberty such as premature **thelarche** (early breast development). This is a normal event that commonly occurs in girls in the first two years of life and is due to an early release of estrogen from the ovary. Usually the breast development goes away without any treatment. It is very important to monitor for other signs of puberty in the rare event that the premature thelarche is really the first sign of central precocious puberty.

What does precocious puberty look like? The appearance of precocious puberty depends on the type and cause as described above. Your child's doctor will include a full history and physical exam as part of her evaluation. The doctor will rate the stage of pubertal development using a set of standards known as Tanner staging. The pace of puberty is also very important. Height (has the growth spurt happened yet?), weight and head circumference (could something abnormal be going on inside the brain leading to central precocious puberty?) need to be measured, and compared to your child's previous values. It is important to assess for progressively severe headaches, especially occurring in the morning or associated with vomiting and seizures, that can provide a clue to an underlying abnormality in the brain.

How do you test for precocious puberty? Your child's doctor will do a bone age test, which is simply an x-ray of the left hand and wrist, to look at the level of maturity of her bones. The bone age correlates more with the level of sexual maturity than her chronological (actual) age. There are reference standards for children of all ages. In precocious puberty, the bone age will be advanced, for example, an 8-year-old will appear to have the bones of a 10-year-old. The doctor can order blood tests to measure hormone levels. She can also order a magnetic resonance image (MRI) scan of the brain to rule out any lesions in the brain as the cause of the early puberty. This is especially important in boys.

Why is it important to treat precocious puberty? Precocious puberty can be caused by some serious but treatable diseases. Even though the growth spurt has started early in this condition, unfortu-nately your child's bones fuse prematurely as well and final adult height can be slightly shorter than it would otherwise have been. This is especially true if puberty starts very early. Also, there can be social consequences to an early puberty. Children may get teased or treated as if they were older because of their advanced sexual maturity.

How do you treat precocious puberty? Again, treatment depends on the cause of the problem. If there is an ovarian tumor, puberty will stop progressing after treatment of the underlying disease. If no cause is found (idiopathic precocious puberty), your child can take medications to stop the progression of puberty. These hormone-like drugs, called gonadotropin-releasing hormone analogues, are given by injection. They prevent the release of the sex hormones in the body. Your child will continue the treatment until she reaches the normal age for puberty to develop. Not all children require treatment—this is usually is a decision made by the family and the doctor together. Your child will need to be closely monitored with regular examinations, blood tests and bone age assessment.

- The sequence of events in puberty are predictable. In girls, breast development is the first sign, and in boys testicular enlargement happens first.
- Early puberty is defined as puberty before age 7 in girls (age 6 in African-American girls), and age 9 in boys.
- Early puberty is more common in girls. When it happens in boys it is important to look for underlying problems.

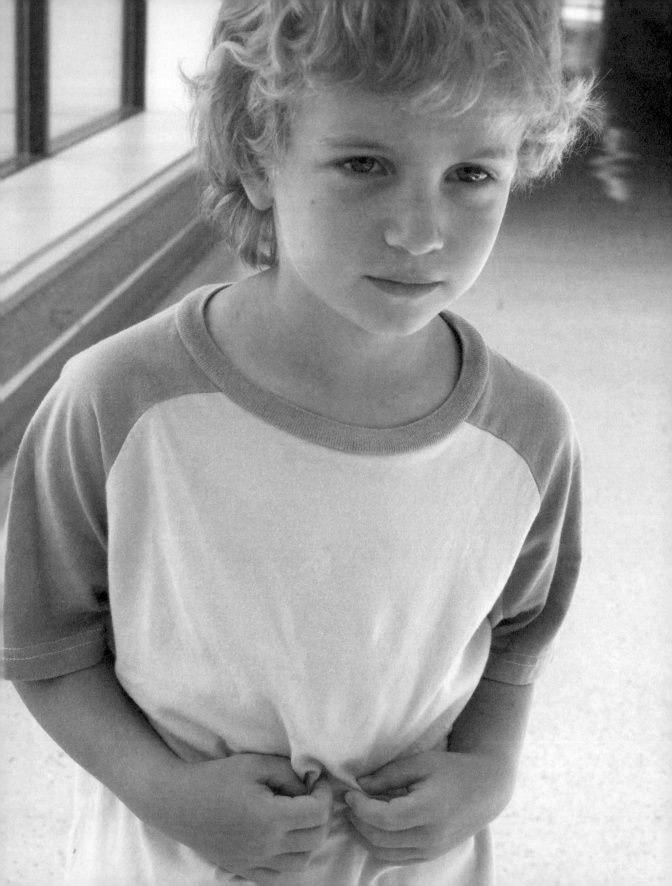

Gastrointestinal Problems

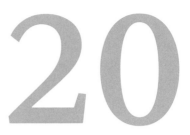

Anal Fissure

What is an anal fissure? An anal fissure is a small laceration, or tear, that can develop at the opening of the anus. It is most common in infants and is always associated with constipation. Anal fissures develop when hard stool is passed through the anal opening, causing a tear in the lining. Such fissures are one of the most common causes of bloody stools in infants.

What does an anal fissure look like? Your baby will have had a history of hard bowel movements that are difficult and painful to pass. Often, he may cry when moving his bowels due to the pain associated with the fissure, and blood might be seen covering the surface of the stool that is passed. Your older child might avoid passing stool due to the pain. This retention only worsens the underlying constipation and prevents the healing of the fissure. The tear can be easily seen when you inspect the anus. It looks like a straight red line or scab radiating from the anal opening. Sometimes an extra piece of skin (a skin tag) develops near the fissure.

How do I treat an anal fissure? The successful treatment of anal fissures depends on the successful treatment of the constipation. You can

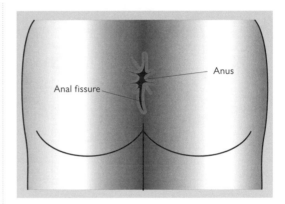

ANAL FISSURE
Anal fissures are small tears at the opening of the anus, usually associated with constipation.

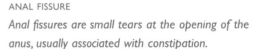

give your child stool softeners and modify his diet by adding more fluids and fiber to prevent repeated passage of hard stools. This allows the fissure to heal and prevents recurrence. You might want to lubricate the anal opening with petroleum jelly to help alleviate the pain in the initial few days until stools become softer.

Appendicitis

What is appendicitis? The appendix is a pouch of bowel that extends like a tail from part of the large intestine (the cecum). It is usually found in

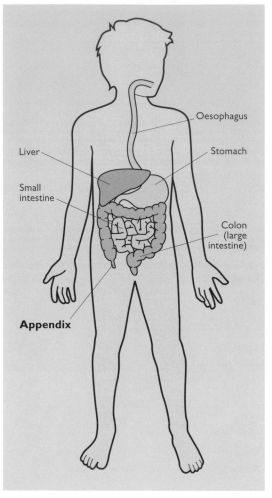

APPENDICITIS

The appendix is a pouch of bowel extending like a tail from the large intestine.

the right lower part of the abdomen. The appendix is not vital to digestion. In fact, it is quite unnecessary. However, it can cause problems. That is because the appendix can become obstructed by a hard piece of feces or swell in reaction to infection. When the appendix is inflamed like that, the term used to describe it is appendicitis. In some cases, the appendix can even burst or perforate. Appendicitis can be found at any age, but is rarely seen in children younger

than 2 years of age. The incidence of appendicitis peaks in adolescents and in young adults.

What does appendicitis look like? The classic symptoms and signs of appendicitis usually start with vague, crampy abdominal pain centered around the navel. Often, the pain is followed by a **low-grade fever**, lack of appetite, nausea and vomiting. As inflammation of the appendix progresses, the pain can change locations and become intense and sharp, most commonly in the right lower abdomen. Along with the pain, your child might not be able to tolerate any vibration or shaking of the abdomen, including coughing, car rides or movement of his bed.

The diagnosis in children is sometimes more difficult than in adults: children do not always exhibit the classic symptoms. The location and nature of the pain can vary from the classic description of appendicitis. Moreover, many of the initial symptoms mimic viral gastroenteritis, which can be quite common in children.

Your child's appendix can perforate within 48 hours of the onset of symptoms. Appendiceal rupture is more common in children than in adults, in part because the diagnosis might be delayed due to the vagueness of symptoms. In those children who have a ruptured appendix, there will be more severe signs of generalized infection, including high fever, high white blood cell count, fast heart rate and low blood pressure.

A test of your child's blood will usually show a mildly elevated white blood cell count. His doctor might order an ultrasound and CT scan to help assess his appendix for inflammation as well as for the presence of an abscess if there is suspicion of rupture.

How do I treat appendicitis? If you suspect your child has appendicitis, get medical care immediately. In the emergency room, the doctor will have an IV for fluids started and might order an ultrasound and/or CT scan to confirm the diagnosis as well as a surgical consultation. If the diagnosis of appendicitis is confirmed, your child will have to have emergency surgery in order to prevent complications from rupture.

The earlier the diagnosis is made the better; but even if your child's appendix has already ruptured, as long as it is diagnosed promptly he can still be effectively treated with intravenous antibiotics, pain medication and bowel rest for five to seven days. Some children may require drainage of collections of pus from within the abdomen. An appendectomy is performed at a later date once the inflammation has settled.

Biliary Atresia

What is biliary atresia? The bile ducts are a network of channels in and outside the liver that pick up and drain bile. This is a liquid made in the liver that gets passed through the ducts and secreted into the small intestines where it helps digest fat and certain vitamins in the food we eat. Biliary atresia (BA) is a disease in which the bile ducts outside the liver are destroyed. In BA, bile gets trapped in the liver and damages the liver cells. It also spills into the blood in the form of conjugated **bilirubin**, which produces jaundice, a yellow coloring of the skin and whites of the eyes.

What causes biliary atresia? No one knows what leads to the progressive inflammation and destruction of the bile ducts. There is some suggestion that a viral infection in a baby who is predisposed to get BA might play a role

in the process. The process starts very soon after birth. BA is not inherited, contagious or preventable.

What does biliary atresia look like? Your baby might have appeared healthy when he was born. BA shows up in the first few weeks to months after birth with jaundice. Your baby's doctor might not have diagnosed BA initially because the jaundice was initially attributed to breast milk, a common cause of jaundice in the first month of life. If your baby's jaundice lasts for more than a few weeks, it is important to search for an underlying problem such as liver disease. Other signs and symptoms of BA include:

- crankiness,
- dark urine,
- pale, clay-colored stools,
- poor growth or weight gain, and
- a swollen stomach with an enlarged liver.

Ten percent to 15 percent of children with BA will have other associated birth defects including problems in the heart, spleen, blood vessels and intestines.

How do you test for biliary atresia? Your baby's doctor will order an ultrasound of his liver to rule out some other conditions that may look like BA. The next test is usually a HIDA scan. In this test, a "radiotracer" that gets selectively taken up by the bile ducts is injected into the blood. Pictures are then taken by a nuclear medicine camera or scanner, called scintigraphy, to watch the flow of bile. In BA, the bile will not flow normally into the intestines. The most definitive diagnostic test is a liver biopsy, where a sample of the liver is taken while your baby is under anesthetic.

How do you treat biliary atresia? Early diagnosis of BA is critical. If it is detected before 2 to 3 months of age, an operation known as the Kasai procedure, or hepatoportoenterostomy, can be performed. The outcome is better the earlier it is performed. In this procedure, your baby's blocked bile ducts are removed, and his liver is connected directly to the intestines. If the Kasai procedure is unsuccessful, stops working or if your child has been diagnosed too late, a liver transplant is the only treatment option.

Most children with BA eventually will need a liver transplant. Because many advances have been made in the area of pediatric transplantation, successful treatment of children with BA is now possible.

Celiac Disease

What is celiac disease? Celiac disease is a condition where the small intestines are unable to tolerate gluten, which is a protein found in barley, wheat, rye and possibly oats. Hence, celiac disease's other name: gluten-sensitive enteropathy.

What causes celiac disease? Your baby will have inherited a predisposition to the disease. Close family members are also at risk of developing celiac disease. About 10 percent of first-degree relatives have damage without symptoms, while about 2 percent to 5 percent have celiac disease with symptoms. Exposure to gluten in the diet (which usually starts with the introduction of infant cereals) and a trigger such as a viral infection are also necessary to start the ball rolling. When these features are present, your baby's immune system makes antibodies that attack the small bowel and damage its lining. The injured intestine has a diminished capacity to digest food.

What does celiac disease look like? The symptoms can take months or years to show up; they can develop at any time from late infancy to adulthood. It is rarely seen in young babies because it takes time for the symptoms to develop after gluten is introduced into the diet. Some children may have very few or vague symptoms, and it can take a long time before your child's doctor makes the diagnosis. The signs and symptoms include:

- a poor appetite,
- crankiness,
- poor weight gain and growth,
- vomiting,
- greasy loose stools (although some children actually have constipation), and
- pallor.

Your child's doctor might also find your child has a bloated stomach and wasted buttocks. He could have mouth sores, and his teeth might be slow to come in. If he is a teenager, puberty could be late.

How do you diagnose celiac disease? Certain antibodies that are particularly associated with celiac disease can be measured in your child's blood. These are screening tests that suggest celiac disease but, which by themselves, are not diagnostic. The best test is an upper **endoscopy** with biopsies. During this procedure, conducted while your child is under anesthetic, the doctor will examine the small bowel through a small flexible tube placed in the mouth, and passed through the bowel to the small intestines. Small tissue samples are taken to analyze under the microscope for specific signs of injury.

How do you treat celiac disease? The main treatment is the lifelong strict removal of gluten from the diet. Gluten is found in foods like bread, pasta and cookies. A dietician will help you and your family learn about the special diet, teach you to read food labels and learn about hidden sources of gluten in foods (for example, in additives and preservatives). Only if your child has been diagnosed by blood tests and biopsies should he be committed to this restrictive diet. The special diet can be challenging for parents and children. There are organizations, support groups and cookbooks. You can find the Celiac Disease Foundation at www.celiac.org and the Celiac Sprue Association at www.csaceliacs.org.

The best confirmation that your child has the disease is when his symptoms clinically improve (usually over a few months) and damage to his bowel is reversed while he is on the diet. A repeat biopsy is not routinely necessary. People with celiac disease can develop other autoimmune conditions such as diabetes mellitus and hypothyroidism. They are also at higher risk for bowel cancer; although it seems that the risk is less if he follows a gluten-free diet.

Gastroesophageal Reflux (Spitting Up)

What is gastroesophageal reflux? Gastroesophageal reflux (GER) is the backward movement of stomach contents, both food and acid, into the esophagus. GER is an extremely common phenomenon: all babies spit up to some degree. This natural process

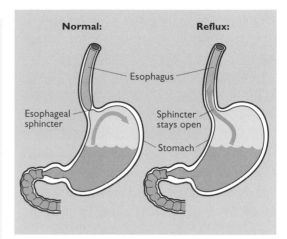

GASTROESOPHAGEAL REFLUX

Gastroesophageal reflux is the backward movement of stomach contents into the esophagus.

usually disappears by the end of the infant's first year and almost always by the second.

When reflux changes from just a messy nuisance to a real problem, it is referred to as gastroesophageal reflux disease (GERD). In this situation, the reflux happens for longer periods, or is more frequent. This leads to problems caused by esophageal irritation such as pain, irritability when eating, refusing to eat and poor weight gain.

Why does gastroesophageal reflux happen? There is a functional valve, called the lower esophageal sphincter, at the junction of the stomach and the esophagus. Normally it prevents food from coming back up the esophagus. In GER, the lower esophageal sphincter functions poorly, and relaxes inappropriately. Food can travel all the way up the esophagus, causing "spit up," or it may travel only partway, causing what adults know as heartburn or indigestion. Anything that increases pressure in the abdomen, such as coughing, can aggravate the condition.

What does gastroesophageal reflux look like? The baby with GER usually spits up effortlessly what he has eaten but sometimes it can appear forceful. The reflux is most likely to happen after a meal, but can occur at any time. It is usually the color of what he has eaten (white if milk), clear or slightly yellow-tinged. With forceful repetitive vomiting, there may even be specks of blood in what he has spat up (the emesis). Spit up due to reflux should never be dark green. This is usually a sign of a blockage somewhere lower down in the gastrointestinal tract.

Reflux is more severe in children with neurological problems, such as cerebral palsy, and chronic respiratory conditions, such as cystic fibrosis. In children with underlying problems, the reflux is less likely to disappear over time.

When GERD is the problem, your baby finds it unpleasant to feed due to the irritation in his esophagus. He will arch his back, twist his neck and stiffen and pull away when he is being fed. If the stomach contents pass all the way up and are breathed into the windpipe (the trachea), he can develop respiratory difficulties such as pneumonia, wheezing and coughing. He might even have a "spell" where he holds his breath and goes limp and blue.

GERD usually starts around 1 to 4 months of age and, like simple reflux, frequently goes away by 1 or 2 years of age. However, on occasion, GERD can occur in older children of any age. At that age, the signs are different and include dental cavities (caused by contact with stomach acid), heartburn, pain with swallowing, burping and a sour taste in the mouth. Many of these children will go on to have reflux as adults.

How do you diagnose gastroesophageal reflux? Because reflux is so common in the first few months of life, your baby's doctor will have diagnosed GER based on the typical story and the absence of any worrisome findings after doing an examination. Vomiting is an extremely common symptom that can be due to numerous causes including infectious and metabolic, neurological and surgical problems. Your child's doctor should take care that he does not overlook a more serious and unusual diagnosis.

There are tests to diagnose GERD, but none of them are ideal. The easiest test is the barium swallow (upper gastrointestinal series). For this test the baby drinks a chalky white liquid that shows up on x-rays. Pictures are then taken to show the flow of the barium. The diagnosis is consistent with GERD if the barium goes from the esophagus into the stomach, and then returns back up into the esophagus. This test is mainly good for ruling out mechanical problems such as blockages at different levels in the stomach and intestines that can also cause vomiting. The barium swallow has limitations. It only measures what is happening over a few seconds at a particular time. Just because a baby does not reflux during the test, it does not mean he does not have GERD. Furthermore, reflux is so common that just because it is seen on barium swallow does not mean that it is the cause of your baby's problems.

The pH probe is a test in which a small wire with an acid sensor at the tip is placed through the baby's nostril and is passed down the esophagus and allowed to rest at the lower end of the esophagus just before the entry into the stomach. Apart from being a little uncomfortable when the wire is passed through the nose, babies seem to tolerate this test very well. Over a 24-hour period, the frequency and duration of time that the lower esophagus is exposed to the acidic stomach contents is recorded. It is also possible to correlate the baby's symptoms, for example, coughing, arching and crying, to the periods of acid reflux.

More rarely, in serious cases your child's doctor will perform an **endoscopy** while your child is asleep under anesthetic. His doctor can look directly at the esophagus and stomach through a very small tube. Biopsies (small tissue samples) can also be taken to look at under the microscope for evidence of reflux and its complications.

How do I treat gastroesophageal reflux? The most important thing to remember is that, in most cases, your child will get better with time. While you are waiting for nature to do its work, there are a number of recommended strategies. While sleeping, your child's head should be 30 degrees upright. You can elevate the head of the crib or mattress, or keep him in an upright position after feeding. Don't keep your baby slumped in a seat or swing after he drinks because this increases the pressure over his stomach and actually causes more reflux! Reflux is known to happen less often when a baby lies prone, that is, on his stomach, than when he lies supine (on his back). Nevertheless, you should still put your baby under a year of age on his back to sleep. This is because the risk of SIDS (**sudden infant death syndrome**) generally outweighs the risks of reflux.

Changing your baby's food is also a big treatment issue. You can thicken your baby's formula with up to 1 tablespoon (15 mL) of infant cereal per 1 ounce (30 mL) of formula. This increases the calories in the meal and has been shown to reduce the amount and severity of regurgitation. You might need to widen the hole in the nipple to allow the milk to flow properly. It is not worth stopping breast-feeding in order to thicken feeds: there is no evidence to suggest that discontinuing nursing is ever helpful.

Some doctors suggest that giving smaller feeds more frequently might help. The evidence supporting this is not strong and it is sometimes not very practical, as most babies demand to be fed until they have had enough! Suffice to say that babies with GER should not be overfed.

Many parents make numerous formula changes in the hope of finding a more suitable one for their baby. Most of the time, this does not make a difference. There is some evidence that a very small group of babies vomit due to a milk allergy. This is more likely if there is a strong history of allergies in the family. In severe cases, it may be worthwhile trying a one to two week trial of a hypoallergenic formula to see if symptoms improve.

Older children should avoid foods that can make reflux worse such as citrus fruits, tomato, coffee, carbonated beverages, mint or spicy foods. If your older child is obese, you should help him lose some weight, which will also help.

There are effective medications that your baby or child can take by mouth to treat reflux. Many of the treatments do not actually prevent the reflux, but act to lessen the symptoms. Antacids can reduce the acidity of the gastric contents so that they do not burn the esophagus when they come back up. The most commonly used acid-blocking agents are either ranitidine or the newer group of proton pump inhibitors (for example, omeprazole). These can be used as early as the neonatal period if necessary and are effective in improving and sometimes resolving symptoms. Motility, or prokinetic, agents help the stomach empty more efficiently. Examples of these include metoclopramide and domperidone. Their effectiveness is a little less certain.

Rarely, in severe cases of GERD, which do not improve with maximal medical therapy, your baby's doctor might recommend surgery.

A procedure called a fundoplication can be performed. In this operation, the top of the stomach is wrapped around the bottom of the esophagus like a pleat that tightens the sphincter so that your child cannot vomit. This procedure can sometimes be performed by laparoscopy, a less invasive keyhole surgery.

Reflux can be a frustrating, anxiety-provoking and messy problem for you to deal with. It is important to try and be patient and remember that time is often the best healer. Protect your clothes and furniture with towels. Do not feed your baby when you are dressed up in your best outfit. As your child gets older, he will probably outgrow his reflux whether it is treated or not. By the time he is eating solid foods and spending more time upright, the reflux will usually have disappeared.

Hernias

What are hernias? A hernia is the bulge created whenever an organ protrudes from the wall that contains it. Most hernias happen when part of the intestine protrudes through a part of the abdominal wall. This can occur in the groin, producing an inguinal hernia; the belly button, causing an umbilical hernia; or at other less common sites.

In the womb, all fetuses have a tubular pathway that connects the abdomen with the scrotum or labia. This channel is known as the "processus vaginalis" and it usually closes off around the time of birth. However, if it remains open, a loop of bowel can get lodged in the canal. When this happens, your baby has an inguinal hernia. Most of the time, the loop of bowel can easily be pushed back into the abdomen but occasionally, the bowel can get stuck,

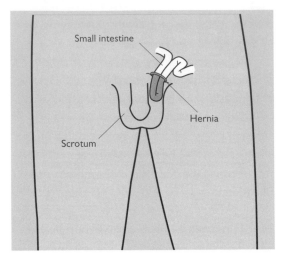

HERNIA

The tract to the scrotum lies under the skin. The hernia appears as a bulge in the groin crease or scrotum.

or "incarcerated," creating a bowel obstruction.

Umbilical hernias are a slightly different matter. Often the site where the umbilical cord originally attached to the baby's abdomen has relatively little muscle or fibrous tissue beneath the skin of the belly button. Because of this relative weakness in the abdominal wall, whenever your baby cries or otherwise raises the pressure inside the abdomen, a bulge occurs at the navel. This protrusion is called an umbilical hernia. Unlike an inguinal hernia, strangulation of the bowel does not tend to occur. Furthermore, most umbilical hernias get better on their own as the abdominal muscles develop in the first few years of life.

Inguinal and umbilical hernias are very common. Inguinal hernias occur in up to 5 percent of children; they are seen more frequently on the right side, mainly in boys and in premature babies. Umbilical hernias are more common in infants of African heritage. No one knows why hernias happen and there is no way to prevent them from occurring.

What do hernias look like? You or your baby's doctor may or may not have noticed the inguinal hernia at your baby's birth. A painless bulge can be seen in the groin crease, scrotum or lips of the vagina. It is normal for young boys to have "retractile" testicles that move in and out of the scrotum: a testicle retracted into the groin should not be confused with a hernia. Hernias can occur on one or both sides. The swelling can be intermittent and grows in size when there is increased pressure in the abdomen; for example from coughing, crying or straining. There is a risk that the intestines will move through the hole and get stuck there—incarcerated. If this happens your child might develop vomiting, pain and possibly redness in the scrotum. You should take your baby immediately to his doctor or to the emergency department of your local hospital so that a doctor can attempt manual reduction: pushing the bowel back through the hole with gentle pressure. If manual reduction is unsuccessful, this becomes a surgical emergency. The segment of bowel could die from lack of blood supply and the testicle could get permanently damaged if an operation is not performed urgently.

An umbilical hernia looks and feels like a soft, squishy swelling covered with skin. It comes out from the belly button. Remember, there is almost no risk of complication with this type of hernia.

How do you treat a hernia? Surgery is always necessary to repair an inguinal hernia to prevent possible incarceration. The timing of the hernia repair will depend on whether your baby has any complications. There is no rush to repair a painless inguinal hernia, whereas an incarcerated or strangulated hernia needs to be repaired immediately. At the time of the surgery some surgeons

WHEN SHOULD I WORRY ABOUT A HERNIA?

- pain
- vomiting
- redness
- unable to push it back

will check for and fix a hernia on the other side, which can be found 10 percent of the time. Most times your child can go home the same day as the operation. It is rare for the hernia to recur.

Umbilical hernias do not require surgery unless they are extremely big, or do not go away by age 5.

Inflammatory Bowel Disease

What is inflammatory bowel disease? Inflammatory bowel disease (IBD) is a term used to describe chronic conditions that involve inflammation of the gastrointestinal tract. Crohn's disease and ulcerative colitis are two distinct yet similar conditions that fall into this category. Inflammatory bowel disease has no clear cause. Like other inflammatory diseases, IBD can run in families. It is believed to occur in individuals with a predisposition who experience some type of environmental trigger that leads to intestinal inflammation. The intestine's immune system cannot adequately control the inflammation, causing it to wax and wane throughout life. While both ulcerative colitis and Crohn's disease can be diagnosed in children as young as 4 or 5 years of age, it is most often seen in preteens, teens and young adults.

The inflammation of ulcerative colitis is limited to the colon (large bowel) and involves only its inside layer. Some individuals can suffer from inflammation involving the entire colon, while others might only have rectal inflammation. Generally, the rectum and the lowest parts of the colon are the most affected. There is tremendous variability with respect to severity and response to medication. Individuals with ulcerative colitis may experience inflammation in the eyes, joints and skin.

Crohn's disease can involve any part of the gastrointestinal tract from a child's mouth to anus, not just the colon. This inflammation typically involves all the layers of the intestinal wall (not just the inner layer, as in ulcerative colitis) and is usually patchy in distribution, with healthy areas of intestine interspersed with inflamed areas. Involvement of the small bowel can prevent normal absorption of nutrients leading to nutritional deficiencies and growth problems. There is also an increased incidence of lactose intolerance in individuals with Crohn's disease. Your child with Crohn's disease can also have inflamed skin, eyes and joints that may precede any obvious involvement of the gastrointestinal tract. The degree of symptoms can vary from individual to individual, and often flare-ups and remissions are experienced.

What does inflammatory bowel disease look like?

Ulcerative colitis
- Bloody, mucuslike stools. Often, stools are loose and a lot of blood can be lost.
- Symptoms can begin and progress quickly.
- Abdominal pain, poor appetite, joint symptoms, eye inflammation, weight loss are also common but fever, vomiting and skin lesions are less frequent.

- In severe cases, your child could develop a serious condition called "toxic megacolon," which is a dilatation of the colon that predisposes it to perforation and subsequently severe abdominal infection.
- Multiple flare-ups and remissions.

Crohn's disease
- A history of chronic abdominal pain, poor appetite, weight loss or poor growth, and diarrhea.
- There may also be blood in the stool, nausea and vomiting, fatigue, abscesses or ulcers near the anus, mouth ulcers, fever, painful or swollen joints, eye inflammation and rare skin rashes that are specifically associated with IBD.
- Delayed puberty in preadolescents and adolescents.
- If colon involvement is significant, your child can have an urgent feeling (that he must have a bowel movement immediately or he'll have an accident) prior to bowel movements, or pain with bowel movements.
- Thickening of the intestinal wall might narrow the inside of the intestine to the point that the bowel becomes obstructed.

How do you diagnose inflammatory bowel disease?
Two tests are helpful in evaluating the gastrointestinal tract for signs of inflammation: barium x-rays and **endoscopy**.

Barium x-rays use barium to outline the lining of the intestines. Your child will be given a barium enema that will pass through the rectum and colon and swallow a barium drink that is followed through the esophagus, stomach and small bowel in what is called an upper GI series.

Upper and lower endoscopy are more invasive tests and require your child to be sedated or under general anesthetic as well as having special preparation of his bowel. Upper endoscopy involves insertion of a long flexible telescope into the esophagus, stomach and duodenum (first part of the small bowel). Your child's doctor or a specialist can see the lining of the tract and take biopsies (small samples of tissue). Detailed information about the inflammation at a cellular level is provided by examination of the biopsies under a microscope. Similarly, through lower endoscopy the rectum, colon and often a small part of the terminal ileum (end part of the small bowel) can be seen. Both barium studies and endoscopy are important in confirming the diagnosis of Crohn's disease. In ulcerative colitis, lower endoscopy (colonoscopy) is the best way of making the diagnosis. The barium enema is a useful adjunct test.

Many children with Crohn's disease develop anemia from increased blood loss and poor absorption of iron, vitamin B12 and folic acid. Your child's blood tests can show signs of inflammation as well as anemia. Sometimes, other markers of poor nutrition are seen on blood tests as a result of malabsorption. In ulcerative colitis, blood tests show similar signs of inflammation and anemia as in Crohn's disease. Generally, ulcerative colitis is not associated with malabsorption, so serum screening for nutritional deficiency is normal. Since chronic infections can mimic some of the symptoms of IBD, stool samples can differentiate the two: in IBD there is no evidence of bacterial or parasitic infection.

In a small percentage (fewer than 20 percent) of individuals, your child's doctor may not initially be able to make the distinction between ulcerative colitis and Crohn's disease. The term "indeterminate colitis" is often used until a more specific diagnosis can be made.

How do I treat inflammatory bowel disease?
Whether your child has ulcerative colitis or Crohn's disease, the experience of having a chronic illness can be quite overwhelming. He will be absent from school frequently, which can also be challenging. You and your family will have to educate your child's peers, teachers and other family members to help avoid embarrassment and reinforce that your child need not be treated differently. You can find support through your pediatrician, gastroenterologist and the local chapter of the Crohn's and Colitis Foundation of America (www.ccfc.org).

Crohn's Disease. No treatment is a cure. Your child's treatment is aimed at controlling symptoms, improving nutrition and promoting normal growth and puberty. Your child's doctor will choose his therapy based on the severity and location of gut inflammation. Nutrition is important and your child should be encouraged to eat a balanced diet. If his growth is poor, he can have easily digested liquid (elemental) nutrition as a supplement, often at night via a **nasogastric tube** (gastronomy tube).

If your child's disease is mild, he can take salicylates, such as sulfasalazine and mesalamine (5-ASA), in a pill, enema or suppository. If he has more extensive inflammation, he can take a course of steroids, such as prednisone or budesonide, by enema, pill or intravenously. Steroids are potent medications and chronic steroid use causes a long list of side effects. So, the challenge in treating his Crohn's disease is to minimize steroid use. He might end up taking other powerful drugs that affect inflammation such as azathioprine, methotrexate and infliximab. Sometimes, a course of antibiotics (metronidazole or ciprofloxacin) can also be useful in controlling symptoms.

In some instances of Crohn's disease, the inflammation can be so severe that he might have to be admitted to hospital for bowel rest, intravenous nutrition and intravenous steroids. Occasionally, he might need surgery. When individuals with Crohn's disease develop a narrowing (or stricture) of a portion of the intestine, surgical removal of the narrowed region can be helpful.

If his colon is involved, it is known that there is a slightly increased risk of colon cancer as he enters adulthood. For this reason, your child should have ongoing monitoring by a gastroenterologist.

Ulcerative Colitis. Mild ulcerative colitis can be treated with the salicylates mesalamine (5-ASA) or sulfasalazine. Moderate disease can be treated with steroids. More severe disease may require admission to hospital, blood transfusion, bowel rest and intravenous nutrition. Sometimes, potent immune system modulators, such as cyclosporine and azathioprine may be used to reduce steroid use.

In severe disease that does not respond to steroids or where children flare repeatedly when weaned off steroids, your child might require surgical removal of the colon. Colectomy (removal of the colon) may require two different surgical procedures, but it can provide a cure.

If your child does not undergo colectomy, he will have an increased risk of colon cancer as he reaches adulthood. It is recommended that anyone who has had ulcerative colitis for more than 10 years should undergo routine surveillance colonoscopies.

Intussusception

What is intussusception? Intussusception occurs when one part of the bowel, usually the end of

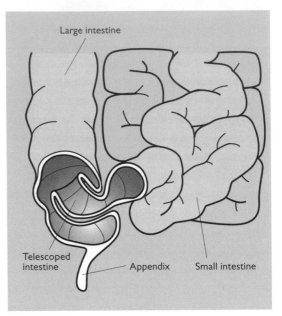

INTUSSUSCEPTION

A condition in which part of the intestine telescopes in on itself, intussusception tends to occur in the area where the large and small intestines meet.

the small intestine, moves into the segment of adjoining bowel (commonly the large intestine) like a telescope. This leads to a blockage of the bowel. It is not common, affecting only two in 1,000 babies.

What causes intussusception? Usually we do not know. It is suspected that a recent viral infection leads to inflammation in the bowel's lymph nodes. These inflamed lymph nodes could then "lead" the first piece of bowel into its neighboring segment. Less often, in about 5 percent of cases, an intussusception occurs because there is an identifiable "lead point" in the bowel. The cause might be in underlying illnesses such as inflammatory bowel disease (IBD), a polyp, Henoch-Schonlein purpura (HSP) or lymphoma (cancer) in the bowel.

What does intussusception look like?
Intussusception occurs in children mostly
between the age of 3 months and 2 years. Your
child will usually have been well. Symptoms tend
to start suddenly, come and go, and get progressively worse. Your child will be sluggish and have
very bad spasms of colicky pain where his knees
are pulled up to his chest. He will be pale, sweaty
and limp, and might vomit. The emesis (what is
vomited up) eventually becomes dark green (bilious). All of these symptoms will alternate with
periods when your child is perfectly well and can
even fall asleep. Eventually, if symptoms continue, the telescoped piece of bowel will get
swollen, and can get permanently stuck. This is
serious, because the bowel can lose its blood supply and die. In the later stages, there might be a
bloody, mucuslike stool that looks like red current
jelly. Your child's stomach might appear bloated
and hard. This is a surgical emergency.

How do you diagnose intussusception? Your
child's doctor may make the diagnosis from
the history you give him, which is classic, and
physical examination. He can also make the
diagnosis from an ultrasound of the belly. He
might order further tests to exclude other serious causes of abdominal pain.

How do you treat intussusception? Your child
needs to be treated urgently in hospital with
an x-ray procedure called an air enema. During
this process, air is pumped into the rectum
with a small tube, using x-ray visualization.
This can reduce or eliminate the intussusception.
If his bowel has burst, or the air enema is unsuccessful at fixing the problem, surgery becomes
necessary. On occasion the problem does not
need treatment because it corrects itself. An
intussusception will recur in 5 percent to 10

percent of cases. With early diagnosis, the
prognosis is excellent.

Lactose Intolerance

What is lactose intolerance? Lactase is an enzyme
found in the small intestine that allows the
human body to digest lactose, the sugar found
in milk and milk products. The amount of lactase
in the small intestine is highest in infancy when
milk is the main food, and then it begins to
fall at about 3 years of age. In some individuals,
lactase activity can drop to a level that may
prevent proper digestion of large quantities of
lactose-rich foods.

Lactose intolerance is the term used to
describe difficulty digesting milk products
because of low lactase activity. It is not a milk
allergy. Lactose intolerance can be either primary, that is, developing without obvious cause,
or secondary, which means that it results from
some disease.

Primary lactose intolerance happens when
the level of lactase production gradually declines
to a degree that prevents the digestion of all the
lactose consumed. It is more common in certain
ethnic groups, particularly people of Asian and
African ancestry and, as such, can run in families.
However, children or adults from any background can develop lactose intolerance. It can
develop at any age in childhood, adolescence
or adulthood, but rarely develops in infancy.
Except temporarily in premature infants, it is
rare to have a congenital lactase deficiency
evident from birth.

Secondary lactose intolerance is a condition
arising from gastrointestinal infections, such as
a stomach flu (see Gastroenteritis, pages 97–98),
or inflammatory bowel disease (see pages 371–74)

that leads to a decrease in the lactase activity level of the lining of the small intestine. In the case of gastrointestinal infection, the intolerance is a temporary condition and gets better after the lining of the small bowel heals.

What does lactose intolerance look like? In primary lactose intolerance, symptoms vary from one child to another. Lactose that cannot be digested travels through the intestines and causes more water to be expelled in stools, thereby making them loose. Bacteria in the intestine can digest the lactose, producing gas, which can cause cramps, bloating and flatulence. Most children develop symptoms 30 minutes to 2 hours after eating foods with a lot of lactose, such as a glass of milk. However, since lactose is found in many different foods, it is sometimes difficult to correlate symptoms with the ingestion of lactose. Some children have enough lactase to digest some lactose-containing foods, like cheese or yogurt, but have more symptoms with high-lactose products, particularly a glass of milk. Children with primary lactose intolerance grow well and have good energy levels. Blood tests that screen for nutritional deficiencies, such as anemia or low serum albumin are normal in children with isolated primary lactose intolerance.

Your child's doctor might recommend temporarily removing milk products from your child's diet and observing the symptoms. If they lessen, the doctor might suspect a diagnosis of primary lactose intolerance. However, the diagnosis is best made by a breath hydrogen test, which is a noninvasive test that involves measuring the amount of hydrogen that is breathed out of the lungs. If the hydrogen in your child's breath rises after he eats or drinks lactose, this suggests lactose intolerance.

If your child develops secondary lactose intolerance after a gastrointestinal infection, he was likely healthy prior to the stomach flu. After the fever and vomiting settle and the initial diarrhea improves somewhat, cramps and looser stools reoccur when he drinks milk or eats milk products. This settles after a few days or weeks as the cells that line the gastrointestinal tract regenerate.

The child with inflammatory bowel disease might have symptoms due to lactose intolerance as part of the other symptoms seen with the underlying disease. In that case, he might be fatigued and grow poorly.

How do I treat lactose intolerance? Lactose intolerance is not life-threatening. If secondary lactose intolerance occurs after an infection, temporarily removing milk products from your child's diet and slowly reintroducing them after the diarrhea settles will help. Doctors might suggest using a soya or lactose-free formula for a brief period if your baby is still dependent on milk as a major source of nutrition.

Primary lactose intolerance and secondary lactose intolerance related to inflammatory bowel disease involve long-term changes in your child's diet. The goal of treatment is a happy child who enjoys his food and does not suffer any more symptoms.

- The first step involves you and your family learning how to read ingredients to identify milk products in foods.
- The second step involves everyone getting acquainted with the types of lactose-free products and lactase replacements that are available. Lactose-free milk, nondairy cheese and lactose-free ice cream are available in grocery stores.

	PRIMARY LACTOSE INTOLERANCE	SECONDARY LACTOSE INTOLERANCE (INFECTION)	SECONDARY LACTOSE INTOLERANCE (INFLAMMATORY BOWEL DISEASE)
CAUSE	Decreased lactase activity	Decreased lactase activity	Decreased lactase activity
RELATED CONDITION	None	Gastrointestinal infection	Inflammatory bowel disease
GROWTH	Good	Good	May be impaired
DIAGNOSIS	Hydrogen breath test	Based on history	Hydrogen breath test
TREATMENT	Lactose-free diet or replacement	Temporary avoidance of lactose	Lactose-free diet or lactase replacement

- Your child could use chewable lactase replacements that are available without a prescription and usually found in the drugstore aisle with other digestive medications. He could chew these lactase pills before eating or drinking regular milk products to aid his digestion and prevent symptoms.

- Once symptoms are controlled and he is happier, you can slowly reintroduce small amounts of lactose, to identify which foods and what volumes of lactose he can digest without suffering any symptoms. Yogurt, cottage cheese and hard, aged cheeses may be easier to digest. It is important that his nutritional need for calcium is met. In some cases, he might have to take calcium supplements.

If lactose intolerance is diagnosed and a well-balanced, lactose-free diet is instituted or lactase enzyme pills are used, your child with lactose intolerance can remain healthy and symptom-free.

Pancreatitis

What is pancreatitis? The pancreas is an organ in the abdomen that has two important functions.

First, it secretes the hormones insulin and glucagon that are both involved in controlling the body's blood sugar level. The pancreas also plays a major role in digestion: it excretes enzymes into the small bowel that digest nutrients. Pancreatitis is the term used to describe an inflamed pancreas. It is a serious condition that can have a variety of causes. Frequently, pancreatitis is caused by an initial blockage of the ducts that drain the pancreatic enzymes. As a result, these digestive enzymes remain within the pancreas, become activated and begin to damage the pancreas itself.

Pancreatitis is not common in children and when it occurs, the cause is sometimes elusive. However, some of the known triggers in children include:

- abdominal trauma,
- infections,
- certain medications,
- gallstones,
- cystic fibrosis,
- inflammatory diseases,
- congenital abnormalities of the pancreas,
- conditions causing high serum calcium.

What does pancreatitis look like? You might have taken your child to see his doctor because of abdominal pain and vomiting. Typically, the pain is steady and localized in the upper abdomen. However, if your child is too young to tell you what is wrong, irritability might be the only sign. He might have a fever. Some children with pancreatitis will have a distended belly that is tender to touch. If he has been vomiting, he might be dehydrated. Depending on what caused the pancreatitis, he could have other symptoms.

Your child's doctor will order certain tests to help confirm the diagnosis.

- He might find elevated levels of pancreatic enzymes (for example, amylase) present in the blood.
- When associated with gallstones, liver enzyme tests are also abnormal.
- If the function of the pancreas is seriously affected by inflammation, the blood glucose may be elevated and the calcium levels are abnormal.
- An ultrasound and CT scan of the abdomen are also very useful in the diagnosis and evaluation of pancreatitis.

How do you treat pancreatitis? Your child will be treated in the hospital for the underlying cause, to control pain and to maintain adequate nutrition while the pancreatic inflammation gets better. Most children need a one- to two-week period of bowel rest during which nothing is eaten. This means a nasogastric tube must be inserted through his nose down to the stomach to drain the stomach and relieve abdominal distension. He will be given intravenous narcotics to control pain and intravenous nutrition. Your child's blood will be tested frequently to monitor blood sugar, calcium and pancreatic enzyme levels. Often repeat scans are also performed to monitor the inflammation of the pancreas. When the inflammation appears to have settled, oral nutrition can slowly be reintroduced. The vast majority of children make an excellent recovery without recurrences if the underlying cause is dealt with.

Pyloric Stenosis

What is pyloric stenosis? Pyloric stenosis (PS) is a condition caused by a thickening of the muscle that produces a narrowing at the outlet of the stomach, the "pylorus," where it empties into the small bowel. Because of the blockage, food cannot leave the stomach. No one knows for sure what causes it. There are probably many factors, including inherited and environmental ones.

What does pyloric stenosis look like? Pyloric stenosis is a relatively common condition seen more frequently in firstborn male infants. There might be other people in the family who had PS. The babies are usually fine at birth. Symptoms tend to start around 2 to 4 weeks of age, but could begin as late as 3 months of age. The hallmark of this condition is progressive, persistent and projectile vomiting. "Projectile" means forceful vomit that travels a few feet through the air. It can be intermittent, or happen after every feeding but goes on for weeks. As the blockage gets worse over time, the vomiting worsens. The color of the vomit is usually the color of the breast milk or formula. This is different from some of the conditions that cause blockages lower down in the intestines where the vomit is dark green (bilious). In PS there is not usually any associated fever, which is more suggestive of an infection such as a stomach flu.

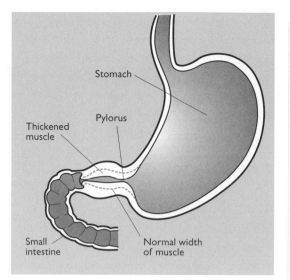

PYLORIC STENOSIS

In pyloric stenosis, the pylorus is narrowed as a result of thickening of the surrounding muscle.

Typically your baby is very hungry, but throws up when he feeds, and does not gain weight well. Ultimately he will become dehydrated with fewer wet diapers, a sunken soft spot on his head, dry mouth and sluggishness. There are many other possible causes of nonbilious vomiting in this age group. The main condition to consider is gastroesophageal reflux (see pages 367–70). In this common problem, stomach contents reflux back up into the esophagus and mouth.

How do you test for pyloric stenosis? Your child's doctor will order an ultrasound of the baby's abdomen, the test of choice, that will show the long, thickened pylorus. If this confirms the diagnosis, no further imaging is required. He might order a barium swallow if necessary. In this test your baby drinks a nontoxic white, chalky substance (barium) to outline his stomach. Under x-ray examination, it also shows the long, narrowed stomach outlet. These x-rays can also exclude some of the other causes of vomiting.

How do you treat pyloric stenosis? Your baby will have to have surgery to treat the PS. This small operation involves relieving the obstruction by splitting the thickened muscle of the pylorus. The procedure is called a "pyloromyotomy" and is performed through a tiny incision or laparoscope. Any dehydration and salt abnormalities in the blood are treated with intravenous fluids before the operation. A nasogastric tube will be placed through your child's nose to empty the stomach of its contents. The babies are usually in the hospital for a few days but are back to normal within two to three days. The surgery will cure the PS and is well tolerated with no long-term problems.

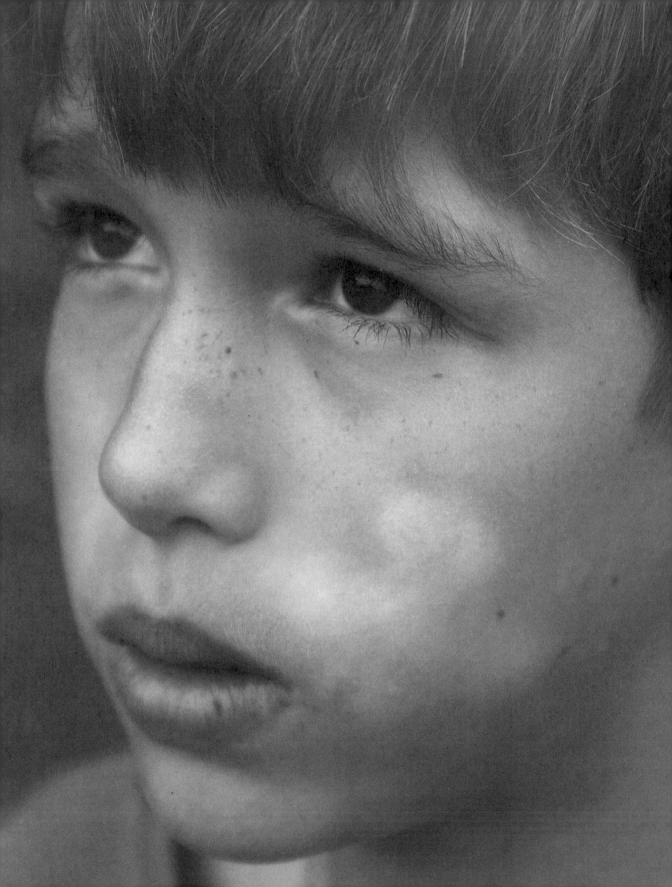

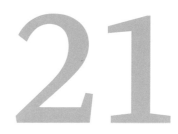

Skin Conditions

Acne

What is acne? Acne is a skin condition that affects 80 percent of teenagers and young adults. This means that just about everybody gets it as part of growing up. How badly your child gets it will dictate how it should be treated.

To better understand what to do about acne, it helps to know a bit about how it develops. Acne is the result of the increased production of sebum, the oily moisturizing fluid secreted by the skin. This increase is triggered by elevated levels of the masculinizing hormone androgen that tends to increase with puberty. Puberty is also associated with the presence in the hair follicle of bacteria, called *Propionibacterium acnes*, that leads to redness and inflammation. In addition, abnormal shedding of the superficial layers of the skin leads to plugging of the hair follicles. This produces the various types of pimples, such as whiteheads (closed comedones) or blackheads (open comedones).

Acne lesions, particularly comedones, can precede the onset of puberty by one to two years. However, acne in very young, prepubertal children should always be investigated. Typically acne lasts throughout puberty. Occasionally, acne lesions may persist into adulthood.

What does acne look like? Whiteheads and blackheads are the most common manifestations of acne. Typically, they occur on the forehead, around the nose and on the chin; however, the rest of the face and the upper trunk can also be affected. Red raised lesions (**papules**) and pus-filled lesions (**pustules**) can coexist with comedones. In severe cases cysts and abscesses that lead to scarring can develop.

How do I treat acne? The goals of acne treatment are to improve your child's appearance and prevent scarring. Skin care is important for all acne patients no matter how severe their acne is. Your child should wash her face once or twice a day with a mild soap or an acne cleanser. She should be careful to not overwash because of the potential for irritation. A child with acne should avoid oil-based creams, sunscreens or makeup. Diet modifications are not necessary, although some teenagers notice that certain foods will increase their acne lesions. Picking at the lesions is strongly discouraged because it leads to inflammation and increased likelihood of scarring.

Acne treatment depends on the severity and type of lesions. Mild acne refers to a limited number of lesions, primarily consisting of comedones, with a few papules and pustules. This type of acne is best managed with topical treatment. Your teen can use benzoyl peroxide preparations that are essentially antiseptics alone or mixed with antibiotics to reduce the inflammation due to *P. acnes*. Chemicals called retinoids, usually vitamin A acid, thin the scaly layer of the skin and, hence, reduce plugging of hair follicles. They are used either alone or mixed with antibiotics for milder acne. It is important to recognize that all acne treatments need to be used consistently for several weeks before you will notice an improvement.

Moderate acne consists of multiple, scattered, inflammatory lesions, namely papules and pustules. This type of acne is usually treated more aggressively due to the increased risk of scarring. Your child's doctor or dermatologist will recommend oral antibiotics, usually a tetracycline, for up to one year. Response to therapy is not quick: failure of the treatment should not be judged before two to three months of treatment. Hormones, in the form of the birth control pill, are another option for girls with this type of acne. If your child's acne does not respond to either of these medications she should be considered for treatment with an oral retinoid.

If your child has severe acne, which means there are many cysts and multiple inflammatory lesions, she will be treated with isotretinoin (Accutane). Although very effective for acne treatment, there are risks associated with its use that should be carefully discussed with the physician. The most significant of these risks is the possibility of having a malformed child for girls who become pregnant while on isotretinoin. Therefore, all sexually active females require two forms of contraception (in case one fails) while taking that drug as well as for two months after she finishes taking it.

Your teen will also have to have monthly blood tests to monitor for other rare medical complications (liver damage, increased lipids) that are reversible once the medication is discontinued. The link between depression and isotretinoin is still not clear; however, if your child is taking it, you should be on the watch for mood changes.

Alopecia (Hair Loss)

What is alopecia? Hair loss is divided into localized scalp hair loss, called patchy alopecia, and diffuse hair loss ranging from thinning of all the hair to total hair loss. The most common variety of patchy alopecia seen in children is alopecia areata. This type of alopecia is presumed to be the result of the immune system attacking the hair follicles leading to hair loss. It can occasionally recover spontaneously; however, most cases require treatment. Other causes of localized hair loss are trauma or scarring, fungal infection and traction on the hair as a result of tight braiding or the child pulling or twisting her hair. Diffuse alopecia is less commonly seen. In children the most common type is thinning of the hair. Infections, fever and emotional trauma leading to an increase in the number of hairs that are lost daily are responsible for hair thinning, typically noticeable several months after the initiating event. Other causes of diffuse alopecia include aggressive hair styling, straightening, perming of the hair and medical conditions, such as thyroid disease and lupus.

It is entirely normal for babies to lose their hair within a few weeks of birth and it can sometimes take months before it grows back. Infants often have bald patches over the back of their head from rubbing their head while lying down.

What does alopecia look like? Alopecia areata can result in single or multiple patches of the scalp that are totally devoid of hair. Your child's underlying skin is normal and the hair follicles are easily visible. A fungal infection can look like patches with sparse hair associated with scaling of the skin or with a black dotted appearance due to sharp breaking of the infected hairs close to the roots. Inflammatory forms of fungal infection will result in scarring alopecia, which is sometimes irreversible. Traction alopecia looks like thinning of the hair at the site of the braids. Diffuse alopecia can be unrecognized for a few months. Your or your child might have noticed an increased amount of hair on the pillowcase or her brush, leading in time to overall thinning or widening of the parts. Gently pulling the hair will recover at least 10 hairs.

Male pattern alopecia is very unusual in children, occurring mainly in adolescent boys with a familial tendency to baldness. When it does develop, there is the typical thinning of the crown area or receding hairline that adult males display.

How do you treat alopecia? Treating your child's alopecia depends on its cause.

- Alopecia areata is treated with high-potency topical corticosteroids. The success rate is about 50 percent to 60 percent after several months. The success rate is less in very large affected areas. Occasionally your child's alopecia might improve spontaneously without treatment, sometimes years after it began.
- Traction alopecia or hair pulling is reversible once the hair is not traumatized.
- Alopecia induced by fungal infection improves with antifungal treatment.
- Scarring alopecia as a result of trauma or inflammatory fungal infection is irreversible.

- Diffuse thinning of the hair improves after several months.
- Hair loss that occurred because of some systemic disease will improve with correction of the underlying illness.

Bacterial Skin Infections

IMPETIGO, FOLLICULITIS, BOILS

What are bacterial skin infections? Bacteria are small, invisible germs that exist almost everywhere. Some of them are constantly present on the skin as "good bacteria" and prevent infection with more aggressive, "bad bacteria." Skin infection occurs when the skin is exposed to either a high load of "bad bacteria" or the integrity of the skin is damaged, for example, if your child has scratches, cuts or eczema. The most common bacteria causing skin infection are *Staphylococcus aureus* and *Streptococcus pyogenes*.

- When infection is superficial and not centered around the hair follicles it is called **impetigo**.
- If the infection is around a hair follicle, the infection is called folliculitis. This is usually the result of obstruction of the hair follicle from creams, moisturizers or from direct contact with the bacteria pseudomonas (hot tub folliculitis).
- An infected hair follicle can accumulate pus under pressure and create an abscess or boil.

Bacterial infections can be spread from person to person. Some children are carriers of staphylococcus and streptococcus, usually in their nasal passages or on their skin, for example, in those who have eczema. These children are at higher risk of developing bacterial skin infections.

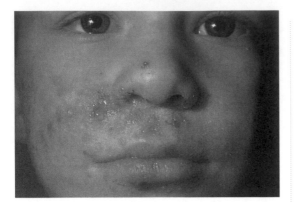

In impetigo, the lesions appear as crusted or weeping sores.

What do bacterial skin infections look like?
- Impetigo is pus-filled blisters on a red background. Some of the lesions will ooze yellow, honey-colored material that forms crusts on the skin. Common areas of involvement are the lips, below the nose and in the folds around the nose. Occasionally the bacteria will produce a toxin that will lead to large blister formation (bullous impetigo).
- Folliculitis is pus-filled pimples that surround a hair follicle. They are scattered on the body and typically affect areas with hair follicles. Boils or abscesses are single lesions that are raised, painful and pus-filled with a hair follicle opening in the middle. They can break open spontaneously and drain a large content of creamy yellow material.

How do you treat bacterial skin infections? All bacterial infections are treatable. If only small areas are infected, your child's doctor might suggest topical antibiotics. When large areas of the body are affected and the child is unwell, she will recommend an oral or intravenous antibiotic. This is particularly true for young infants, who are at higher risk of getting the infection into their bloodstream if left untreated. Children with recurrent boils should be checked to see if they carry the offending bacterium in their nose. If the child or any family members are chronic carriers of infection, antibiotics applied daily into the nostrils can eliminate the bacterium in one month.

Canker Sore (Aphthous Ulcer)

What is a canker sore? Aphthous ulcers are painful ulcers affecting the lining of the mouth or edges of the tongue. Canker sores are quite common in toddlers and children and are not serious, although they can be very painful. They are not contagious. There is no known cause for these ulcers but a long list of potential causes has been suggested; for example, trauma, stress, nutritional deficiencies, infections, menstruation, or allergic or toxic drug reactions. Canker sores sometimes run in families.

What does a canker sore look like? Canker sores usually start off as red bumps that develop into painful whitish gray ulcers with a raised red inflamed edge. The ulcers look like a small crater and can vary in size from tiny (1/10 inch/2 mm) to quite large (bigger than 2/5 inch/10 mm). They may appear singly or in crops. Toddlers might dribble and refuse to eat because of the pain. They tend to take a few days to as long as a couple of weeks before they settle down.

How do I treat a canker sore? The ulcers cannot be "cured" but the symptoms can be treated. You should avoid feeding your child acidic and spicy food and drinks. You can try to relieve the pain with a local anesthetic gel, which is generally available from the pharmacy without a prescription. Don't expect miracles from these gels. Older children might use antiseptic mouthwashes or salt water for oral hygiene.

If the ulcers haven't settled after 10 days or recur frequently then you should consider taking your child to her doctor. Sometimes she may recommend an anti-inflammatory topical steroid cream to hasten healing.

Cold Sores (Herpes Simplex Infection)

What are cold sores? Herpes simplex type 1 (HSV-1) viral infections are very common. It is estimated that over 90 percent of adults show evidence of having had a previous herpes infection. Often the infection starts in childhood through contact with oral secretions or open lesions of an infected person. Cold or fever sores are the most common manifestations of herpes simplex. Affected children have blisters on their lips. The first episode might be associated with fever and similar blisters that affect the gums and tongue. Other sites can also be involved, for example, eyes and other areas of the skin or fingers (herpetic whitlow). Most children are not very sick and the infection clears spontaneously or with treatment. However, newborns, children with a suppressed immune system or an immuno-deficiency and children with eczema are unable to handle the infection and can become very sick.

What do cold sores look like? Typical herpes lesions consist of grouped blisters on a red background. Mouth sores are shallow white ulcers surrounded by a rim of redness. Occasionally the infection can lead to significant swelling (edema). This is particularly true for the herpes infection affecting the fingers (whitlow), where the stretching of the tissues from the swelling leads to significant pain. Herpes lesions resolve with crusting that tends to peel off with no long-term scarring.

How do you treat cold sores? Most uncomplicated herpes infections, particularly the ones affecting the lips, require no treatment. Topical antiviral agents are usually not helpful unless you begin the treatment at the first sign of the infection. Systemic antiviral medication is necessary for children with widespread disease, newborns or children with an abnormal or suppressed immune system. Children with sores in the mouth might refuse to eat due to the pain. Occasionally young children require admission to hospital for pain control and fluid therapy to prevent dehydration.

Recurrences of HSV-1 infection are very common, because the virus stays dormant in the nerve endings and tends to flareup from time to time. Colds, fever or excessive sun exposure are common triggers for virus reactivation and then the reappearance of blisters or sores. A different type of herpes virus (HSV-2) causes genital lesions. Genital herpes due to HSV-2 in children should raise the suspicion of sexual abuse. The exception is an infant born to a mother with a history of, or active, genital herpes infection.

Contact Dermatitis

What is contact dermatitis? There are two types of contact dermatitis. The first type is called irritant contact dermatitis and can occur in anybody. It is usually caused by chemicals; for example, soaps, detergents and cleansing agents. Irritant contact dermatitis clears up after you stop using the offending agent. The second type is an allergic reaction (allergic contact dermatitis) and occurs only in susceptible individuals. The most common causes of allergic contact dermatitis in children are poison ivy and nickel. Allergic contact dermatitis due to henna has recently become more common with the current henna tattooing fad.

What does contact dermatitis look like? The appearance of contact dermatitis depends on the severity of the reaction. In most cases, your child will have background redness. In severe cases, she will also have raised, bumpy lesions and blisters. All cases of contact dermatitis reactions are extremely itchy.

- Poison ivy dermatitis usually makes itself known by a burninglike sensation prior to development of the rash. Typically, the lesions are in a linear, brushed pattern at the site of the contact, which is usually skin not covered with clothes.
- Nickel dermatitis is commonly seen at the site of metal fasteners in the middle of the chest and abdomen in infants or around the belt line in older children. Depending on the offending agent, your child's rash will clear up within a few days to a few weeks after contact is stopped.

Occasionally, there is a residual hyperpigmentation that can last for months after the rash is gone. This is particularly true for reactions to henna tattoos.

How do I treat contact dermatitis? Treatment of contact dermatitis depends on its severity. Mild forms of the disease will clear up after you stop using the offending agent and with the application of a mild to moderate topical corticosteroid. Severe cases, particularly if your child has poison ivy dermatitis, require systemic steroids for a few weeks in order to prevent recurrences.

Diaper Rash (Diaper Dermatitis)

What is diaper rash? The most common cause of diaper rash is irritation of the baby's skin due to contact with urine and feces. Almost every infant has at least one episode of diaper rash before she is toilet trained. Despite the recent advances in the technology of diaper manufacturing, diaper area irritation persists. Besides irritant dermatitis, there are other causes of diaper rash, such as yeast (candida) infection, seborrheic dermatitis and bacterial infection. Psoriasis is another rare cause of diaper rash in infancy.

What does diaper rash look like? The appearance of the rash is very typical of its cause.

- If your child has contact, or irritant dermatitis, she will have various degrees of redness around the anus (perianal area). The area between the groin folds will not be affected, as it is protected from contact with the diaper contents by rolls of fat. The redness can progress to shallow ulcerations that are extremely painful.
- Yeast infection looks red with powderlike flaking at the edges. It primarily affects the perianal area. Small, similar lesions, called "satellite lesions," are usually found away from the perianal area.
- Bacterial infections, usually due to streptococcus and staphylococcus, typically are small pus-filled lesions on a red background. Occasionally the lesions progress to large

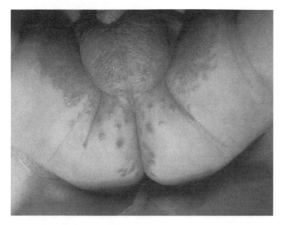

DIAPER RASH

In this photo, the irritated skin in the diaper area has become secondarily infected with yeast (Candida albicans).

blisters that slough off and leave a raw red background.
- Psoriasis is areas of intense red coloration with thick, white scaling overlying it.

How do I treat diaper rash? Treatment of diaper rash depends on its cause. Prevention of the rash is the best method of dealing with contact or irritant dermatitis.

- What is important is what you take off the skin rather than what you put on it. You will need to change your child's diaper frequently and cleanse the area thoroughly. Avoid fragrances and alcohol-based wipes to prevent diaper area irritation. Once your child has a rash, apply generous layers of zinc-oxide-based protective creams to help control contact diaper rash. When irritation does not clear up on its own, a mild corticosteroid preparation prescribed by your child's doctor is likely to get the job done.
- Yeast infection is treated with an antifungal topical preparation that may be combined with corticosteroids.

- Bacterial infections can be more serious. You will have to take your child to see her doctor, especially if she appears sick. Treatment with oral antibiotics tends to be very effective.

Eczema (Atopic Dermatitis)

What is eczema? Eczema or atopic dermatitis is a chronic skin condition that affects around 15 percent to 20 percent of children. Children with eczema have very dry, itchy skin that they scratch. It is the end result of the interaction of many factors such as a genetic predisposition, environment (hot humid weather, dry cold temperatures, **allergens**, etc.) and the persistent presence of bacteria on the skin. Eczema can have a big impact on the affected child and her family because it can interfere with regular activities and normal growth and sleep patterns. Eczema is a condition that lasts for years and typically has a waxing and waning course. It will flare up during certain months of the year. Atopic dermatitis is often the first sign of an allergic tendency (atopy) that refers to the presence of eczema, **allergic rhinitis** and asthma.

What does eczema look like? The severity of eczema is very variable. Some children have mild disease characterized by dry, itchy patches and minimal redness. More severely affected children have widespread areas of redness, skin breakdown because of scratching and crusting. Due to constant inflammation of the skin, affected children will develop areas of thickening of the skin that looks almost leathery (lichenification) and premature wrinkling. When eczema becomes infected with bacteria, the affected areas are intensely red

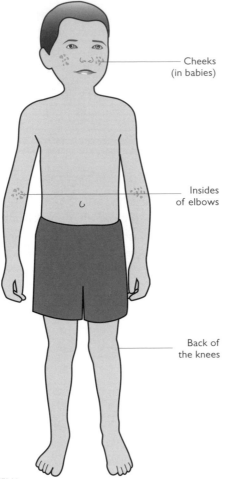

Cheeks
(in babies)

Insides
of elbows

Back of
the knees

ECZEMA

In children aged 4 years and over, the areas shown here are those most often affected by eczema. The rash tends to affect sites at joints where there are folds of skin.

and can have a pussy discharge. Infection with herpes virus can lead to widespread blistering (eczema herpeticum). Different areas of skin are affected at different ages. Eczema is often first noticed on the cheeks in infants, from where it tends to spread to the extensor surfaces (outside of the elbow and knee). Older children tend to have it on the flexor surfaces (for example, the inside of the elbow and knee).

How do I treat eczema? There is no cure for eczema. Current treatments are helpful in controlling the flare-ups. The most important aspects of treating your child's eczema consist of avoiding potential environmental allergens and irritants, dealing with the dryness of the skin, preventing scratching and treating the inflammation (redness). Environmental control is very important. You should keep your child's bedroom cool and humid. In addition, you should not use harsh detergents, bleaches and softeners, and wool clothing to help decrease the skin irritation and prevent scratching.

You will need to control the dryness. Your child should bathe frequently, at least daily and even up to three times a day, in lukewarm water (hot water will lead to more itching). Add an emulsifying agent (an oil that mixes with the water) to the bath to help keep the skin moist. However, your child should not stay in the bath longer than 10 minutes. Follow her bath with the application all over the body of a nonper-fumed moisturizing ointment, like petroleum jelly, for smaller children or a moisturizing cream for older children and teenagers.

Your child's doctor will prescribe an anti-inflammatory agent to apply to the affected areas only. The anti-inflammatory agents available are various preparations of corticosteroids and newer immune system modifying preparations, such as tacrolimus and pimecrolimus. Mild to mid-potency topical corticosteroids are safe for long-term use on the skin and are currently still the first line of therapy. The newer agents are as effective as the mild to mid-potency topical corti-costeroids but are reserved as alternative therapy for resistant cases due to the uncertainty of their long-term safety and high cost.

Your child can get relief from the itch by tak-ing antihistamines. Itching can become a habit that is hard to control. Redirect your child's attention to a different activity and use a moisturizer on the itchy areas.

Treating a child with atopic dermatitis is a very frustrating and demanding experience. However, most children outgrow their eczema by their teen years. Involving the child in the treatment plan is helpful in the long run. Your should not treat your child with eczema any differently than your other children because of her skin condition.

Fungal Skin Infections

TINEA CORPORIS AND CAPITIS, RINGWORM, ATHLETE'S FOOT

What are fungal infections? Fungi are microorganisms that are commonly found on the skin. They multiply and cause disease when the proper growing conditions are available. Fungal infections are generally named tinea.

- When tinea is found on the body it is called tinea corporis and because it usually has a ringlike appearance it is commonly known as ringworm.
- Tinea affecting the foot is called tinea pedis or athlete's foot.
- Fungal infection on the scalp (tinea capitis) is the most common fungal infection in children.

Fungal infections tend to spread easily from person to person.

What do fungal infections look like? What it looks like depends on the location of your child's infection.

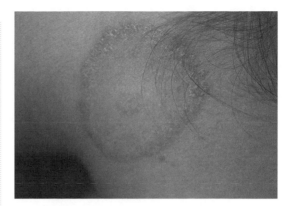

RINGWORM

Note the red, scaly margins that are characteristic of ringworm (tinea corporis).

- Tinea capitis looks like patches of hair loss with a black dot appearance (due to broken, infected hairs), scaly and itchy patches or a large, tender **kerion** (a boggy mass of inflammation with multiple openings that drain pus). Usually, tinea capitis is accompanied by swollen lymph glands on the back of the scalp.
- Tinea corporis can be found anywhere on the body as one or multiple lesions. It is usually mildly itchy and looks like ringlike lesions with a red, scaly border and clear center. They tend to expand outward from the border.
- Athlete's foot appears as red, softened areas in the spaces between the toes. They are associated with an itchy or burning sensation. Affected nails become yellow-green and grow thick. If left untreated, the growth of your child's toenail can be permanently affected.

How do you treat fungal infections? Treatment depends on the type of fungus and the location of the infection. If your child has tinea on the scalp and nail infections, she wil require oral antifungal preparations. Tinea on the body and on the foot responds to topical applications of antifungal creams.

Head Lice (Pediculosis)

What are head lice? Lice are insects that live on the surface of the skin and feed by sucking blood from the skin. The infecting lice cause intense itching due to irritation from their saliva. Lice eggs are deposited on the hair shafts and are called nits. Lice infestation is very common and is spread by close contact. They have the ability to jump from one child to the other and can live for a short time away from the human body.

What do head lice look like? Visible, crawling lice are easy to spot. They are dark grayish. In addition to intense itching, the presence of the louse is associated with small red bumps (**papules**) or wheals on the scalp. Nits are light gray and hold fast to the hair shaft, which differentiates them from dandruff. They look like miniature cocoons attached to a branch. The persistence of lice is usually related to the inability to kill all the eggs.

How do I treat head lice? Pediculicides, or lice killers, are effective in treating lice, provided they are correctly used. You will have to apply permethrin 1 percent shampoo, the most common treatment, and leave it on your child's head for 10 to 15 minutes. This is followed by rinsing the hair and combing it with a nit comb. When you see a lot of nits, it is usually good to use an occlusive preparation (for example, petroleum jelly, mineral oil, thick hair gel) and leave it on for 12 hours to suffocate all of the nits. In addition, you will have to wash all combs, bedding, clothing and towels carefully. The whole process needs to be repeated after one week. If your child is in school or day care, you should inform them in case other children are also affected.

Ingrown Toenail

What is an ingrown toenail? Ingrown toenail is the condition that occurs when the side of the toenail cuts into the flesh beside the nail. This usually happens to the big toe at the side corners. Ingrown toenails are relatively common in children and are prone to recurrence. Both improper nail trimming and poorly fitting shoes can predispose children to this problem.

What does an ingrown toenail look like? Ingrown toenails hurt. There will be a red painful swelling at the corner of the affected toe. Your child might have a yellowish pussy discharge from the area. If the condition persists for a while, it can develop granulation tissue, which is a dark red piece of fleshy tissue with a moist crusted surface.

How do I treat an ingrown toenail? It is better to prevent ingrown toenails than to treat them. You should cut the nails with a straight border, instead of a curve, to prevent ingrown toenails. Teach your child to cut the same way and to look for the corners of the nail. They should be visible and not buried into the soft tissue at the side of the nail. Fit your child with shoes that are neither too tight, causing banging of the nail into the front of the shoe, or too loose, so that the foot slides forward too easily inside the shoe. Make sure your child tells you when she has grown out of her shoes.

Once present, treat an ingrown toenail by soaking the toe in warm water for 20 minutes a couple of times a day. Apply an antibiotic ointment to the area. Have your child wear a shoe that does not cause pressure on the toenail. If this is not effective or there seems to be a pussy discharge with redness moving down the toe, take your child to see her doctor who may prescribe a course of antibiotics. If this fails or the

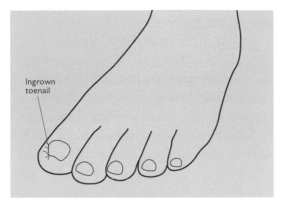

INGROWN TOENAIL

The side of the toenail cuts into the flesh beside the nail, usually affecting the big toe.

problem keeps on coming back, there is a surgical procedure, called a wedge resection, that should cure the problem. This involves removing the edge of the toenail that is "ingrown" together with the nailbed underneath.

Moles (Nevi)

What are moles? Moles, or nevi, are pigmented skin lesions that can be present at birth (birthmarks) or appear later in life as a result of sun exposure.

Pigmented birthmarks, also known as congenital nevi, are very common. Most of them cause problems only due to their cosmetic appearance. Very few have any medical significance—there is little risk of them changing into skin cancer. This risk is related to the size of the lesion. Smaller nevi, usually smaller than 1/5 inch (0.5 cm) in diameter, do not pose an increased risk of becoming malignant. There is a 1 percent to 5 percent risk of malignant transformation of medium-sized lesions, between 1/5 and 4 inches (0.5 and 10 cm) in

diameter, during your child's lifetime. Large or giant nevi, measuring more than 4 inches (10 cm) in diameter, pose more than a 5 percent risk of becoming malignant. The cause of congenital nevi is unknown.

Acquired nevi tend to appear within the first 10 years of life in response to sun exposure. The risk of malignant change in regular nevi is less than 1 percent over a lifetime. However, the risk of skin cancer arising from the lesions is higher in children who have more than 50 nevi on their body, have moles that measure more than 1/5 inch (0.5 cm) in diameter and a family history of skin cancer.

What do nevi look like? Moles, or nevi, have darker pigmentation than the rest of the skin. Most nevi are a few millimeters in diameter and tend to grow as the child grows. A normal nevus is less than 1/5 inch (0.5 cm) in diameter, has a regular color throughout and regular smooth borders. Congenital nevi are uneven and a darker color than acquired nevi and develop dark, coarse hair in them. Congenital nevi will grow with the child. A dysplastic nevus is a nevus with an increased risk of becoming malignant. These nevi are usually larger than 1/5 inch (0.5 cm), have multiple colors and uneven edges. You and your child's doctor will have to monitor them regularly.

How do you treat moles? Most moles do not need to be surgically removed. Medical reasons for removing a mole are:

- signs suggestive of malignant potential, and
- dysplastic nevi in the presence of a positive family history of skin cancer, particularly melanoma.

Your child's doctor should examine her skin as part of her annual health maintenance visits. Close-up photographs of the larger, atypical nevi are helpful in monitoring changes. You should inspect the moles every three months. If your child's moles develop any of these features, you will have to take her to her doctor:

- changes in color or texture,
- rapid changes in size,
- irregular outline,
- bleeding or pain at the site.

However, the most important management step in looking after your child's moles is to make sure she avoids too much sun and wears sun protection.

Pityriasis Rosea

What is pityriasis rosea? Pityriasis rosea is a relatively common skin condition more often seen in older children and adolescents. It is rarely diagnosed in children under 2. The disorder is felt to be a reaction on the skin to a viral infection, particularly herpes virus types 6 and 7. Affected children rarely feel sick. However, the rash can be very itchy and can last up to six weeks.

What does pityriasis rosea look like? The first stage of the disease consists of a single patch, commonly located on the trunk and less often on the neck and extremities. The patch appears as a coin-shaped lesion, measuring about 1/2 inch (1 to 2 cm) in diameter with a salmon-red background and some very fine scaling at the edge. This patch is called a "herald patch" because it occurs one to two weeks before, and thus heralds the next stage of the disease. The second stage of the disease shows up as

many smaller patches with a similar appearance arranged in a "Christmas tree" distribution often along the ribs on the trunk. Occasionally, children can have more widespread lesions including on the face. This stage lasts two to four weeks. In most of the cases, the rash clears up with no skin changes. In dark-skinned children, pigmented areas that last several months can result.

How do I treat pityriasis rosea? Pityriasis rosea is a self-resolving condition. However, mild corticosteroid creams can help fade the lesions and improve the itching. A short course of oral antibiotics, such as erythromycin, has been shown to be successful in shortening the duration of the rash. Children are not contagious and the rash does not generally recur.

Psoriasis

What is psoriasis? Psoriasis is a noninfectious skin disease with a strong genetic component that typically starts in childhood. It is a lifelong condition characterized by flare-ups and remissions. Psoriasis features an accelerated turnover of the skin cells, which produces an accumulation of multiple layers of skin. The result is the formation of a characteristic psoriatic scale.

In children, infections, particularly streptococcal ones, are the trigger for the appearance of psoriatic lesions. This form of psoriasis shows up as drop-shaped lesions and is called the guttate variant. Children with the guttate variant and no affected relatives have a self-limited form of the disease that clears up in a few months.

What does psoriasis look like? Psoriasis has red patches with thick, silvery, overlying scale. Psoriatic lesions are not itchy and can be found

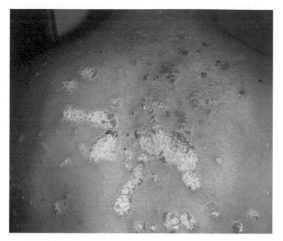

PSORIASIS

Psoriasis with red, patchy lesions covered in a thick silvery scale.

anywhere on your child's body. Her scalp, extremities and groin are typical affected areas. Persistent, nonpainful, redness around the anus should raise the suspicion your child has psoriasis. Her nails are usually also affected and will have dotlike pits, lose their shine, thicken and lift off the nail bed and have a yellowish discoloration.

How do you treat psoriasis? Psoriasis is difficult to treat. Depending on the severity of your child's condition, there are various treatment options. Your child's doctor might prescribe topical treatment using corticosteroid preparations, vitamin D derivatives that thin the scale or a combination of the two. Occasionally tar preparations are added to enhance the anti-inflammatory effect of the topical corticosteroids. If your child's disease is widespread she might have light therapy, which has been used with some success. Rarely, severely affected children will require powerful oral medications in order to control the disease.

Scabies

What is scabies? Scabies is a common, highly contagious skin disease caused by an almost invisible organism, the "itch mite" (*Sarcoptes scabiei*). The mite reproduces on the surface of the skin and the impregnated female burrows into the skin where she lays her eggs. Most people with scabies start to have severe itching and typical skin lesions four to six weeks from the contact. During this period, it is possible to spread the disease to other people. Scabies mites spread rapidly through minimal contact or through sharing of towels or linens. Transmission through animals such as dogs and cats is very unlikely as the mites can only reproduce on human beings.

What does scabies look like? Your child with scabies will have itchy red skin lesions typically in the webs between the fingers and around the wrists. These lesions are red bumps or threalike lines with a tiny hole at the end. After a few days other areas become involved with an increased number of lesions in the armpits, groin area and belt line. Children in the first year of life can have lesions on the neck and face as well as pus-filled lesions on the palms and soles.

How do you treat scabies? Scabies is a highly contagious disease that requires treatment of the whole family even if they are not itchy. Permethrin 5 percent cream or lotion is an effective treatment option. You will need to apply the lotion or cream and rub it in from the neck down if your child is over 1 year of age, with particular attention to web spaces and skin folds. If your child is younger than 1 year and has lesions on her face and neck, you will need to include these areas as well. Leave the lotion on for 12 hours and wash it off in the morning. Another treatment a week later is recommended. You will have to wash all clothing, bedding and towels thoroughly and dry it at high temperatures. The itch can persist for two to four weeks even after effective treatment. Your child's doctor might also prescribe a topical corticosteroid and an antihistamine to help control the residual symptoms.

If your baby is under the age of 6 months, and/or your are pregnant, you will require other skin treatments in order to avoid the risk of neurological problems, which is a potential side effect of the medication.

Sunburn

What is sunburn? The sun emits a spectrum of waves, some short and others very long. Some of these waves are not harmful for the human body, such as the visible light that has an intermediate length and is made up of the rainbow colors. The shortest waves are ultraviolet waves B (UVB) and A (UVA). UVA and UVB are the rays responsible for most of the damage to the skin. Unfortunately, their effect, sunburn, is not noticed until redness and pain develop several hours after exposure.

A number of variables can affect the degree of sunburn. The length of sun exposure and the time of the day when exposure occurs (maximum damage happens between 10 a.m. and 2 p.m.) are obviously important and relatively controllable factors. Location, the proximity to the equator and the altitude above sea level, and the color of the skin (lighter skin is more susceptible to sun damage) are less so. It is estimated that 20 to 30 minutes of sun exposure are needed to cause redness in a light-skinned individual. These figures

are significantly lower for children and especially babies. The skin damage related to sunburn consists of premature aging of the skin and an increased incidence of skin cancer.

How do I avoid sunburn? Protection from sun damage is possible. You should keep your baby inside whenever possible during the maximum radiation exposure between 10 a.m. and 2 p.m. Your older child should be protected daily from sun exposure. She needs to wear a hat and protective clothing, and you have to apply sunscreen to exposed skin. When you know you are going to be out in the sun for a while, you will need to reapply sunscreen every two hours and after swimming. In addition, your child can wear sunscreen-impregnated clothing that covers a large portion of the body. A variety of sunscreens especially formulated for children are currently available on the market. Most of them are designed for children over 6 months of age. Babies younger than 6 months should be covered with protective clothing and have zinc oxide cream or titanium dioxide sunblock applied to exposed areas if sun exposure cannot be prevented.

How do I treat sunburn? In cases of mild sunburn, cold wet compresses or even a cool bath can be helpful. Use a soft towel to pat rather than rub your child dry. A light, fragrance-free moisturizer can be applied to the affected skin. Ibuprofen or some other anti-inflammatory can be taken by mouth to relieve the discomfort.

If your child has severe blistering and pain then it would be wise to consult your health care provider. And of course, keep her out of the sun while she is sunburned.

Vascular Anomalies

What are vascular anomalies? Vascular anomalies, commonly called birthmarks, are reddish lesions derived from blood vessels that are typically noticed at, or shortly after, birth. There are two types of vascular birthmarks. Hemangiomas, also called strawberry birthmarks, are a benign overgrowth of blood vessels. They can be present at birth but more typically appear as a red mark or patch within the first few weeks of life. Vascular malformations or stains are abnormal blood vessels that are always present at birth. The cause of vascular anomalies is not known. Very rarely, there will be a family history of similar problems.

What do vascular anomalies look like? Hemangiomas are soft, bright red patches or lumpy lesions of various shapes and sizes. They tend to feel a bit warmer due to increased blood supply to the affected area. Hemangiomas commonly appear on the head and neck; however, they can develop anywhere on the body. When your child is crying or has a fever, the size and discoloration can become more prominent. The appearance of vascular malformations depends on the type of blood vessel that is affected and the depth of involvement. For example, abnormal superficial capillaries, the smallest caliber blood vessels, look like red blotches on the skin, called port wine stains. Deeper, bigger vessel involvement can look like bluish or flesh-colored, raised lesions on the skin. Vascular anomalies are occasionally associated with overgrowth of the underlying tissues, particularly when present on an extremity. This is explained by the presence of abnormal blood vessels not only in the skin, but also in the deeper structures, such as muscle and bone. Typically, hemangiomas progress in three

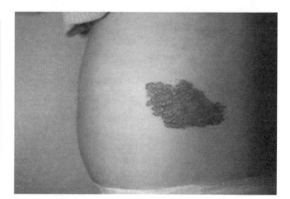

HEMANGIOMA

Hemangiomas are often referred to as "strawberry" birthmarks.

stages. The first consists of rapid growth, out of proportion with the rest of the body. It is not unusual to see it doubling and tripling in size within a few weeks. This stage can last up to six or seven months. The second stage is characterized by stagnation in growth, but changes in the color from a bright red to purple or gray. This stage usually lasts until your child is 18 months to 2 years of age. The last stage of the disease is the regression phase and consists of the lesion shrinking. The rate of shrinkage is variable. On average, 10 percent of hemangiomas disappear per year. This means that 90 percent to 100 percent of hemangiomas clear up by the time your child is 9 or 10 years old. Maturing hemangiomas flatten out, assume a purple-gray discoloration and are the same temperature as surrounding skin. Eventually the lesions disappear completely without leaving any marks on the skin. However, in some cases, residual changes such as loose, wrinkled skin or mottled discoloration of the skin with spiderlike blood vessels can occur.

Vascular malformations can occur anywhere on the body. The "angel kiss" and "stork bites" are variants of vascular malformations that show up on the mid-forehead and the nape of the neck, respectively. They are extremely common, occurring in almost 50 percent of children. The forehead lesions tend to disappear in the first two years of life, while the lower scalp lesions can persist. Most other vascular malformations do not disappear, although the color can fade slightly in the first year of life. Increased discoloration and texture of the lesion can be noticed around puberty.

How do you treat vascular anomalies? Most hemangiomas go away without treatment. However, 10 percent of the lesions will require treatment because they cause a disturbance of function or distort your child's facial structures. Hemangiomas around the eyes are a typical example of functional impairment, either because they obstruct her vision or because they cause pressure on the eyeball.

The most accepted treatment is with oral corticosteroids. Laser treatment is usually of limited benefit due to the inability of the laser to penetrate more than 1 to 2 millimeters from the surface of the skin. In addition, laser treatment requires several sessions with anesthesia depending on the size of the lesions. Laser treatment is a good option for residual discoloration in some cases after spontaneous or medically induced shrinkage of the lesion. Your child might have to have surgery if spontaneous shrinkage has been incomplete and the location allows for a good aesthetic result. This procedure is usually performed before your child becomes aware of her appearance, around the time she starts school. You have to consider your child's best interests before making any decision about treatment. The risks and benefits of any procedure should be carefully discussed with your child's

physician, remembering that 90 percent of the lesions go away on their own leaving no sign.

Treatment of vascular malformations depends on the type of blood vessel, size, location and the functional and aesthetic implications. Port wine stains can be successfully treated with laser therapy. Deeper, larger lesions can be treated with injections that close off the abnormal vessels (**sclerotherapy**) or with surgery. Treatment options are tailored to each child.

Vascular anomalies present a challenge to families, particularly when your child's face is affected. You need to work with your child's doctor and any other consultants to be realistic about your expectations and make informed decisions.

Warts and Mollusca

What are warts and mollusca? Warts and mollusca are related skin problems caused by viruses. These two conditions are very common in childhood and are very contagious.

Warts can be present anywhere on the body but the typical areas affected are the hands and feet, particularly the soles. The latter are called plantar warts. Warts can also occur near the anus and genitals: these might be due to a slightly different virus from the one causing warts elsewhere on the body.

Mollusca are smallish bumps that can be single or multiple, and are considered extremely contagious. It is felt that children spread the lesions by scratching the existing ones, carrying the virus under the nails, and touching new skin areas. Most adults have been exposed to the virus during their childhood; therefore, the risk of mollusca lesions spreading to an adult is very low.

What do warts and mollusca look like? Warts can be flat or they can stick out from the surface of the skin and have a rough appearance. They are usually skin-colored. Warts can bleed if traumatized. Mollusca lesions are dome-shaped, skin-colored lesions that measure a few millimeters in diameter. They are usually not painful or itchy. Occasionally, children with **atopic dermatitis** will develop mild redness and itching around the mollusca lesions.

How are warts and mollusca treated? There are many different treatments for warts. Unfortunately, most of the treatments have a limited success rate. The most common methods employed in treating warts cause local destruction of the abnormal skin, either by freezing or chemical irritation. The warts can be frozen with liquid nitrogen that leads to blister formation and elimination of the virus. Unfortunately, this method requires several treatments and is usually associated with significant discomfort. Therefore, it is rarely recommended for young children. The other common treatment consists of topical applications of salicylic acid preparations. Either commercial salicylic acid drops or salicylic acid paste under a bandage that seals the treatment in are used. You will have to continue this treatment for several days.

More recently, there has been some limited success with the use of duct tape alone or in combination with other therapies. It is not known how duct tape works. It is important to remember that most warts last for several years. Eventually the body's immune system eliminates the virus. Therefore, when looking at treatment options it may be appropriate to choose the least traumatic option.

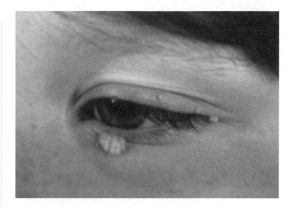

WARTS
Warts around the eye.

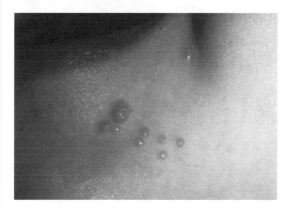

MOLLUSCA
Multiple dome-shaped mollusca lesions.

Mollusca lesions also eventually disappear but, unfortunately, last for several months. In some cases, no intervention is a reasonable option. For children with only a few lesions, scraping off each lesion is curative. Irritant treatment with solutions such as cantharidin is beneficial in most cases and is well tolerated by children. The application of cantharidin results in a small blister that clears up in a few days with clearance of the lesions. Only a physician can apply this treatment. Other treatments, such as liquid nitrogen, can also be tried.

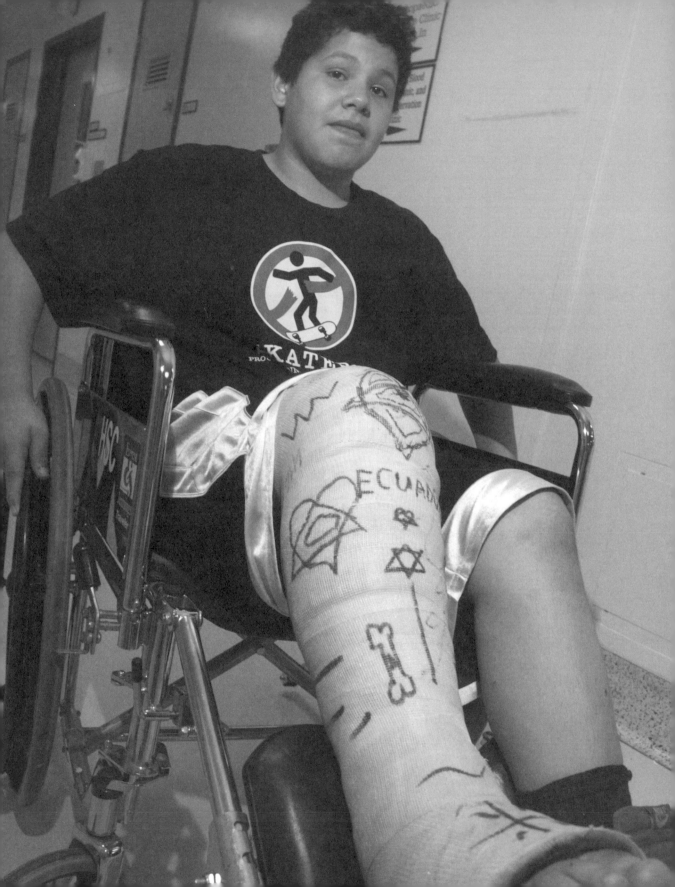

Accidents and Emergencies

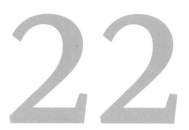

Preventing Accidents

Most parents are afraid that one day their child might become sick with some serious disease such as cancer or meningitis. What many parents do not realize is that after early infancy, accidents and injuries are the greatest threat to their child's well-being. In the United States, injuries accout for about 4,000 deaths and millions of emergency department visits annually in children under the age of 15.

What are the most common injuries in children?
In the first year of life, choking and suffocation are the most common causes of death due to injury, while falls are the most common reason for hospitalization as a result of injury for both infants and older children. In older children, motor vehicle accidents (MVAs) are the major cause of death due to injury. Half of the victims are pedestrians and about 20 percent are cyclists. Boys are more likely to be injured from almost all of the different causes.

Many of these accidental deaths and injuries are preventable.

There are some times when you can predict that there will be a higher than normal risk of injuries. For example, when your children are developing a new skill such as climbing or walking, injury could result if you or their other caregivers are not prepared for this by childproofing the environment. If your children are not familiar with their surroundings (for example, visiting a home with a swimming pool) injuries are more likely to occur.

How can injuries be prevented?

Motor Vehicles
- Babies in the first 9 to 12 months (under 20 pounds/9 kg) should be placed in a rear-facing infant car seat in the back seat. After this, children up to the age of 4 or 5 years (20 to 40 pounds/9 to 18 kg) can use a forward-facing car seat. Older children (over 40 pounds/18 kg) up to the age of 8 or 9 should be switched to a booster seat, once again in the back seat of the car.
- Children under the age of 7 should not cross the street without close adult supervision, and those under 10 should not cross major streets. You still need to teach older children not to run out from behind parked cars and to watch carefully for approaching cars.
- All bicyclists should receive training in road safety and wear a helmet. Wearing a properly fitted helmet will reduce the risk of fatal head injury by 85 percent. In communities that have

introduced mandatory bicycle helmet legislation, head injuries from bicycle accidents have been reduced by half. Children should not ride after dark unless they have front and rear lights and wear reflective clothing. You need to set the example for your child.

Falls

- Never leave your young child alone, even for a second, when he is on a high surface; for example a changing table or bed.
- Do not use baby walkers because many children have suffered serious injuries from falling down stairs or grabbing the handles of pots containing hot liquid.
- Install gates at the top and bottom of the stairs when your infant is about to start crawling.
- Supervise your children under 5 years closely in the playground and only use those playgrounds that are designed for preschool children, because the equipment is smaller and developmentally appropriate. Sand, wood chips and synthetic surfaces tend to be soft and are therefore good playground surfaces.
- Ensure your children wear a helmet, knee pads, elbow pads and wrist pads when in-line skating. Similar safety gear is recommended for scooter riders. Children should get off the scooter to cross the street and go down steep hills.
- Have your children wear proper fitting safety equipment, for example helmets or padding, when playing sports such as skiing or hockey.

For information on prevention of burns, drowning, ingestions and choking, see individual sections on these topics.

How can I prepare myself for emergencies? It is important to be prepared for possible accidents and injuries by having a first-aid kit at home and in your car. It is also recommended that anyone responsible for taking care of children should take a course in basic lifesaving procedures. Do not wait for an emergency to happen—learn first aid techniques now! These courses are available through many community agencies, and can prepare you to deal with life-threatening problems such as choking, severe bleeding, breathing stoppage (**apnea**) or circulatory failure. Learn to do cardiopulmonary resuscitation (CPR); it can save a life if a child has stopped breathing as a result of choking, drowning or asphyxiation due to strangulation or smoke inhalation. Brain cells begin to die within minutes of being starved of oxygen, so starting CPR as soon as possible after a child's heart stops can make a big difference.

Animal Bites

What are animal bites? Children can be bitten by a variety of animals, as well as other children. About 90 percent of bite injuries are from dogs, cats or humans. It is estimated that American children incur 4.7 million dog bites, 400,000 cat bites and 250,000 human bites annually.

The majority of dog bites occur in children between the ages of 6 and 11 years. Approximately two-thirds of these attacks occur around the home and 75 percent of the biting animals are known to the children. Half of the attacks are said to be unprovoked. Boys seem more prone to dog bites and girls to cat bites. Up to 5 percent of dog bites will become infected and 20 percent to 50 percent of cat bites become infected. If there are no signs of infection by three to four days then infection is unlikely to occur.

What does an animal bite look like? Most injuries are either scratches or puncture wounds. Claw wounds should be regarded the same as bites because the claws can contain saliva and germs. The deeper the wound, for example, as when the skin is punctured, the higher the rate of infection compared with superficial lacerations. You should be concerned by any increase in the extent of the surrounding redness or swelling. If you see red streaks moving upward from the wound, this indicates an infection.

How do I treat animal bites? Again prevention is important. Teach your child:

- not to play with unfamiliar animals;
- not to put his face near a dog; and
- not to stay alone with dogs even if he is very familiar with them.

Large dogs, such as rottweilers, pit bulls or German shepherds, are more likely to cause serious injury or death, but any dog is capable of injuring a child so care must always be taken around them. Teasing and tormenting increases the risk of a friendly animal attacking a child.

Wash all bite wounds adequately. If possible, cleanse and flush the wound under a faucet for at least 5 to 10 minutes. Then, apply an antibiotic ointment. Bandages and pain relievers are optional.

The specific treatment required will depend on the circumstances of the attack, particularly the type of animal involved.

- Small indoor pet rodents like gerbils and hamsters pose no risk of rabies and the bite seldom becomes infected. Your child will rarely need medical attention.
- Wild rodents such as squirrels, mice and chipmunks are also considered rabies-free but can cause other types of infections.
- Most human bites are from toddlers and they usually do not penetrate the skin. If your child's skin is not broken, you don't have to take him to see a doctor. Simple cleansing and a hug will do.
- Whenever rabies is a possibility, such as bites by raccoons, foxes, bats or unprovoked attacks by an unknown animal, your child will need to be seen by a doctor.

All bites, particularly dog, cat and human bites with significant damage to the skin or underlying tissues, such as puncture wounds, should be assessed by a physician. Whether your child's doctor prescribes antibiotics to prevent infection depends on the location and nature of the wound. Usually, oral antibiotics, such as amoxicillin-clavulanic acid, are prescribed. Your child's doctor will have to decide if he needs stitches. The need is variable and must be assessed from case to case. Although the risk of **tetanus** from an animal bite is extremely rare, you should be sure to have your child's immunization records with you if you go to an emergency room rather than his own doctor.

The other risk following cat bites is cat scratch disease. This consists of enlarged lymph nodes above the area of the bite/scratch, as well as a prolonged fever. The glands in the armpit (axilla) are the most likely to be infected. Kittens are more often the culprits than adult cats. Total recovery is the usual outcome.

Pets add immeasurably to a child's life. Although animal bites are a concern, you should not let that possibility stand in the way of obtaining a pet.

Ankle Injuries

What are ankle injuries? Ankle injuries are the most common **acute** athletic injury. The majority of these ankle injuries are sprains rather than fractures. This means that the supporting tissues that connect the bones, called ligaments, are damaged rather than the bones themselves.

You probably know that the ankle is the important joint that connects the leg to the foot. It is made up of two long bones in the lower leg, the tibia and fibula, which are attached by supporting ligaments to the talus, a larger bone in the foot.

Ankle sprains usually happen when the foot inverts or "turns under," and the athlete comes down with his full weight on the outside of the ankle. This stretches the ligaments of the ankle

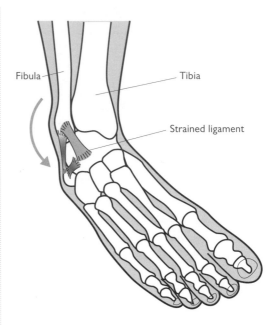

SPRAINED/STRAINED ANKLE
Sprains usually happen when the foot "turns under," stretching the ligaments of the ankle joint.

joint and can even tear them, causing a sprained ankle. If the injury is severe enough, the ends of the fibula or even the outer foot bone (the fifth metatarsus) can break off, resulting in a fracture. Much more rarely, the ankle will turn out (evert), which damages the inner, or medial, ligaments and usually produces a fracture.

Ankle injuries can occur with any sport or activity but are more likely to occur with jumping sports such as basketball or gymnastics. They also commonly occur when activities occur on an uneven playing field.

What do ankle injuries look like? The child knows that he has "gone over" on his ankle and this is followed by pain, swelling, discoloration and an inability to bear weight and walk normally. The more severe the sprain, the looser and less

R.I.C.E.: THE INITIAL TREATMENT OF SPRAINED ANKLES

"R" for REST: your child should refrain from weight-bearing if standing causes any pain. Older children can use crutches, if necessary.

"I" for ICE: Use ice packs for 20 to 30 minutes every two hours (when awake) until the pain at rest disappears.

"C" for COMPRESSION: Wrap an elastic bandage around the ankle for two to three days.

"E" for ELEVATE: Keep your child's ankle raised above the level of the heart for one day. You can place a pillow under the ankle.

stable the joint will be. Although x-rays are not necessary for all ankle injuries, if your child has swelling and is unable to bear weight, you should take him to an emergency department to get x-rayed.

How do I treat an ankle injury? For the first two or three days, sprained ankles should be treated with Rest, Ice, Compression and Elevation or "R.I.C.E."

You can give your child pain relief in the form of acetaminophen or ibuprofen. When the pain and swelling have cleared up, your child might begin exercises and physiotherapy to strengthen the ankle. It takes a prolonged period of time for an ankle to fully recover and recurrences are common. Wearing an ankle brace until all swelling subsides and for sports activities for a few months will reduce the chance of reinjury. Your child should avoid prolonged immobilization to

minimize stiffness and muscle weakness, although fractures and severe sprains will require a cast.

Bee and Wasp Stings

What are bee stings? Bees and wasps usually "sting" in self-defense (or to subdue prey) by injecting venom through a stinger at the end of their bodies.

What do bee stings look like? Generally, insect stings by honeybees, yellow jackets and hornets produce similar reactions. The particular reaction of any child is governed by his sensitivity, the number of attacking insects and his age. Depending on the child's reaction, a sting can vary from a small red itchy raised spot to a larger hive that can measure over an inch (or several centimeters) in diameter. There can be swelling, pain or itchiness at the site of the sting. Local reactions can be quite significant but are not a major concern. For example, if a hand was stung, resulting in extensive swelling of both the hand and arm, this would still be considered a local reaction.

The major concern in insect stings is the development of a severe, generalized (systemic) allergic response. This is called an anaphylactic, or hypersensitivity, reaction. **Acute** hypersensitivity reactions cause swelling of the lips or tongue, difficulty breathing or a choking sensation in the throat. The first symptom is frequently a tingling sensation around the mouth or face. This is a true emergency.

How can I prevent a bee sting? Prevention is extremely important. There are several simple strategies to avoid bees and other stinging insects.

- Don't let your child walk outside in bare feet.
- Stay away and keep your child away from any nests or locations where you see many flying insects gathering at one spot.
- At picnics and when eating outdoors, don't let your child drink from opened beverage cans that have been sitting around. Bees frequently fly into sweet drink containers.
- Keep all food covered.
- Cover garbage cans and keep them away from eating areas.
- Avoid strong perfumes and hair sprays—they attract stinging insects.
- Avoid brightly colored clothing or clothing with flowery patterns as they also attract insects.
- Mosquito repellents are of no value in preventing stinging insects, although they should be used to prevent mosquito bites. More information about mosquitoes and repellant use is in Chapter 3.

What should I do about a bee sting? Following a bite from a stinging insect, wash the area with soap and water. In the case of honeybees, remove the stinger as quickly as possible; it is best removed by a gentle scraping motion. Treat local reactions with ice or cold compresses to decrease the swelling. You could give your child oral antihistamines to decrease the reaction and relieve the itch but do not use antihistamine cream. Acetaminophen or ibuprofen will provide pain relief, if needed.

If your child has a generalized reaction to a sting, he should be given an injection of epinephrine (adrenaline) and prednisone by mouth, if available, as well as an oral antihistamine. Transport him quickly to the nearest hospital even if he seems to be improving because relapses may occur.

A GENERALIZED REACTION TO AN INSECT STING IS AN **EMERGENCY!**

Give an oral antihistamine and injectable adrenaline, if available, and go immediately to the nearest hospital even if the child seems initially to have recovered.

If you know your child is susceptible to systemic reactions, you must have a plan to respond to these situations. Once a child has experienced an anaphylactic reaction to bees, you should have an injectable adrenaline dispenser available at all times. Your child should also wear a medical alert bracelet to identify the problem. Fortunately, only about one child in five who suffers an initial systemic reaction from a stinging insect will have a similar response with subsequent stings. Desensitization injections (allergy shots) to the specific stinging insect have an over 95 percent rate of success of preventing a future anaphylactic reaction. Talk to your child's doctor about this if your child has had a life-threatening reaction.

You will have to educate your child's teacher and other caregivers about his reaction to stings and have the medication available wherever he goes.

Choking and Aspiration

What is choking and aspiration? Children and even young babies are capable of putting things in their mouth that can cause them to choke. Aspiration is what happens when the object goes down the windpipe into the airway instead of down the esophagus into the stomach. Most foreign bodies

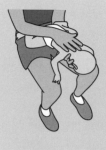

1. Give 5 back blows
Lay baby facedown with head low along your forearm. Support head and shoulders on your hand and give 5 blows with the heel of your other hand between the shoulders.

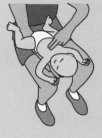

2. Give 5 chest thrusts
Turn baby's face up along your other arm, holding the head in your hand. Place 2 fingers 1 finger's breadth below the nipple line. Give 5 sharp downward thrusts.

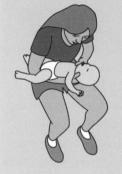

3. Check Mouth
Look in baby's mouth. Do not put your finger in unless obstruction can be seen. Give rescue breaths. Repeat steps 1–3 until obstruction is cleared.

HOW TO HELP A CHOKING BABY

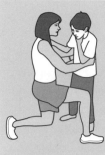

1. Recognize a choking child
Ask the child, "Are you choking?" If the child can speak or cough, do not interfere. If he is unable to speak or breathe, go to step 2.

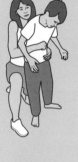

2. Stand or kneel behind child
You may have to kneel behind child. Wrap your arms around child. Position a fist, thumb-side in, above navel, but well below breastbone.

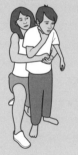

3. Give abdominal thrusts (Heimlich maneuver)
Grasp fist with other hand. Give inward and upward abdominal thrusts. Repeat thrusts until obstruction is relieved.

HOW TO HELP A CHOKING CHILD

that are aspirated are expelled rapidly by a reflex cough. But, if your child does not clear the object, his airway can plug and the event immediately becomes life-threatening. Choking is one of the leading causes of death from injury in the first year of life. Smaller objects can lodge in one of the branches of the airways, which although not fatal can cause significant problems that can persist for a long time before being diagnosed.

What do choking and aspiration look like? If your child is choking, he may appear unable to

breathe, speak or even cry. He will clutch at his throat. He might even start to turn red in the face followed by a dusky blue, particularly around the mouth. If the foreign body gets stuck in his voicebox (larynx), his cough can be croupy or hoarse and can be fatal if not dealt with appropriately. If the foreign body gets aspirated into the airways in the lungs, then it might show up as cough and wheezing after the episode of choking. The emergency doctor might order x-rays of his chest to help decide whether a foreign body has been aspirated into the lungs.

What can I do?

Emergency measures. If your child is able to speak or cough, it might be better not to interfere. Calmly encourage him to cough the object out. Keep watching, obviously, to make sure that he is breathing adequately. If this doesn't seem to be working and he is genuinely choking, you can lay your baby face down over your forearm or across your lap with his head down and give 5 short sharp blows with the heel of your hand between his shoulder blades. (See illustration on page 405.) If this doesn't help, turn him over so he is face up and place two fingers just below the nipple line in the middle of the chest and give five sharp downward thrusts. You should then look in his mouth for any obvious sign of obstruction that might be easy to remove. After going through the process as described, if he is not breathing, get someone to call 9-1-1 or your emergency number, and start rescue breathing prior to repeating the sequence.

If your child is over the age of 1 year, kneel or stand behind him, depending on his height, wrap your arms around him and with a fist, thumb-side inward, covered with your other hand, press sharply inward and upward above the child's belly button. (See illustration on page 405.) This is meant to mimic a forceful cough and is known as the "Heimlich maneuver." It can be done five times every three seconds, and can be continued with increasing force until the object is dislodged. Check inside his mouth for something that has come out and can be easily removed. If at any time your baby or child becomes unconscious, have someone call 9-1-1 immediately and you, or someone familiar with CPR, would need to check the child's airway, breathing and circulation and start resuscitation with mouth-to-mouth respirations and chest compresions if appropriate.

Preventative measures. Prevention of choking and aspiration are crucial.

- Keep small choking hazards and toys with small or loosely attached parts far out of reach of young children; this can be especially challenging when he has older siblings.
- Check that food is appropriate for your child's ability to chew and swallow.
- Check new toys to make sure they are age appropriate.

Cold-induced Injuries: Hypothermia and Frostbite

What are cold-induced injuries? Children are at greater risk from cold exposure than adults because they lose heat from their skin more rapidly. Furthermore, children love the outdoors, are often unaware of the cold and tend to be reluctant to leave their winter games and come inside. Unfortunately, this can lead to overexposure. Because of the growing involvement of children in winter sports such as skiing, skating and snowmobiling, children's cold-related injuries have increased.

Hypothermia is the condition that exists when bodily functions are impaired because the core body temperature is too low. This occurs at a body temperature of about 95°F (35°C) or less. Frostbite occurs when cold exposure is severe enough to damage tissue, especially the skin and the layers just under the skin.

What do cold-induced injuries look like? The initial body response to heat loss is shivering, which really is the body's attempt to generate warmth through exercise. When hypothermia begins there is a slow onset of fatigue, lethargy and apathy.

As the core temperature drops there is increased mental confusion and decreased heart rate.

Frostbite will most likely occur in exposed areas. Your child's cheeks, toes, ears, fingers, chin and nose are especially susceptible. Initially the symptoms consist of tingling, stinging or itchiness that go on to numbness in the affected areas. This progresses and the area then becomes white, cold and numb.

Cold-induced fat inflammation (panniculitis) is actually a fairly common problem. Typically, it occurs in a toddler's cheeks when they are excessively exposed to the cold and wind. It begins with reddish lesions on the cheeks and then firm lumps develop in the cheeks under the skin. These last two to three weeks and then slowly disappear. However, there is a tendency for them to recur with further cold exposure.

What do I do about cold-induced injuries?
Prevention is the highest priority. You should be aware of the length of time your children are outside especially when it is colder and windier than usual. Layering of clothing is the method that will best provide warmth and still permit the removal of layers when necessary. Thirty percent of heat loss occurs through the head and therefore a warm hat is extremely important. A scarf or neck-warmer will also help prevent heat loss. Generally mittens are warmer than gloves but they tend to limit dexterity and risk being discarded during play. It is also important that boots are waterproof and large enough to permit adequate circulation. Wet clothing increases the risk of heat loss as does the wind. Encourage your children to wear dry, wind-resistant garments.

When your child appears excessively chilled, the best treatment is to try to prevent further heat loss. Remove his wet clothing quickly and replace with dry, warm clothing. Then transport

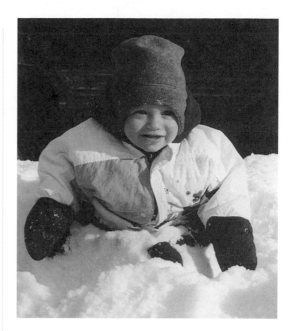

him to warm shelter. If there is any alteration in your child's level of consciousness, you will need to take him to an emergency department for evaluation.

The treatment of suspected frostbite consists of warming not just the involved regions but the whole child. Do not rub the affected area, as that can cause blistering. Do not apply snow or ice. Don't apply direct heat or break any blisters that might have formed. If, upon warming, his skin color does not appear warm and flushed, take him immediately to an emergency department for a medical assessment.

Cuts and Lacerations

Children frequently sustain minor injury including cuts and lacerations. You must decide whether the injury is something you can treat yourself or whether professional help is necessary. Most will heal by themselves. If your child has any loss of function, such as numbness or losing the ability to bend or straighten a joint fully, you need to have a physician examine the laceration.

How do I treat cuts and lacerations? Any bleeding must be stopped. Apply direct pressure with clean gauze or even clean paper tissues, if nothing else is available. If you have rubber gloves available, wear these before coming into direct contact with blood. Lacerations of the scalp, face and mouth frequently bleed a lot. This is due to the large blood supply to these areas. However, because of this, infection is not usually an issue. If your child has cut his tongue or lips from his own teeth during a fall, he won't usually require stitches.

The most important factor in minimizing scarring is to ensure the wound is clean. You need to determine whether there is a foreign body in the cut. These might include bits of sticks or stones and gravel. A foreign body will increase the risk of infection. To eliminate or minimize bacterial contamination, irrigate a potentially dirty wound with sterile water or a cleansing solution. After the wound is cleaned, keep it dry.

Most wounds benefit from being closed to give the body the best potential for healing and to decrease scarring. Closure of a laceration involves getting the wound edges close together. The closer the wound edges are held together the thinner the scar will be. Because of cosmetic concerns, the amount of separation you might tolerate on the face is different than on the scalp or back. Tissue adhesives have proven to be an effective method of wound closure in simple lacerations. They have the benefit of ease of use, less pain and less time to apply. If your child has a deep wound, you might have to take him to an emergency room for stitching to obtain the best

result. Generally, the time interval between the laceration and the repair should be as short as possible: lacerations should be sutured within 6 to 8 hours of injury. The length of the laceration only determines the number of stitches or staples that will be necessary. They generally take 7 to 14 days to heal, although those on the face heal more quickly.

Make sure you take your child's immunization record with you to the emergency room because his **tetanus** status must always be checked. A tetanus booster is required every 10 years although after a potentially contaminated laceration a booster should be given after five years. To avoid sun damage to fresh new skin, during the summer after the stitches have been removed and the scar is fresh, you should apply sunscreen.

Dental Trauma

What is dental trauma? Unfortunately, injuries to children's teeth are a very common occurrence. Approximately 50 percent of youngsters will sustain some type of dental injury ranging from minor chipping to a completely knocked out (avulsed) tooth. Dental trauma can happen to the primary "baby" teeth as well as a child's permanent ones.

The most commonly injured primary teeth are the incisors, which are positioned in the front of the mouth. The aim of treatment in the preschool child is to prevent further injury to the underlying developing permanent teeth. Treatment objectives should be based on this and heroic efforts to save a baby tooth might not be advisable.

In cases of dental trauma in a child with mixed dentition (some primary and some permanent teeth), the loss of a tooth might or might not interfere with the eventual alignment of the permanent teeth. The age of your child and the specific tooth are factors determining whether your dentist will advise space-maintaining procedures.

Dental injury in the permanent or mixed dentition can take a number of different forms. This can include everything from insignificant chipping to a more serious fracture that can expose the nerve and blood vessel in the center of the tooth, to a completely avulsed tooth. Injury can also include the tooth being forced upward, downward or to the side. A tooth that has been knocked out might appear to be the most dramatic injury however it might still be salvageable. The most crucial factor determining whether the tooth can be saved is time.

What do I do about dental trauma? Although falls are the most common cause of dental injury in preschool and slightly older children, sports accidents account for the majority of dental injuries in teenagers. Mouth guards will prevent oral injuries when used in sports. Evidence shows that custom-made mouth guards are superior to stock ones.

You should take your child with loosened teeth and minor chips to his dentist. He will assess the degree of damage and blunt any sharp edges. Obviously, while a tooth remains loose, your child should avoid hard food.

Consider a secondary tooth that has been knocked out as a dental emergency. It should be held by the "tooth" and not the root. You or your child can gently rinse the tooth in water and place it back in the tooth socket. Your child should keep the tooth in place with finger pressure or by biting on a gauze pad. Take your child to a dentist immediately. If it is not possible to replace the tooth in the child's mouth, place the tooth in milk (not water or saline). Pack the container in ice, and head off to the dentist immediately.

Drowning

How common is drowning? Drowning is the second most common cause of death by unintentional injury in American children aged 1 to 14 years. Males represent around 80 percent of all water-related fatalities. This is especially prevalent in the age groups 1 to 4 years and 15 to 24 years. Toddlers commonly drown in swimming pools at home. Older adolescent males often drown in natural bodies of water frequently in association with risk-taking behavior, alcohol or drug use.

Survival for more than 24 hours is termed near-drowning, regardless of whether the victim later dies or recovers. Small children are especially vulnerable to near-drowning and are at high risk of brain damage. The number of near-drowning victims outnumbers the number of drowning victims. This frequently occurs when children are resuscitated following a "water-related" accident.

What factors can contribute to drowning? Alcohol is involved in 25 percent of drowning fatalities. Flotation devices are an important safety feature but in one study only 12 percent of victims in boating accidents were wearing a personal flotation device. Many drownings and near-drownings happen to children who fall into a swimming pool when they are unsupervised.

How can drowning be prevented? Swimming pool submersions are especially preventable. Seven percent of drownings are swimming pool related.

Most pool submersions occur at the child's own home and nearly half occur within the first six months of pool exposure. Brief lapses (less than five minutes) in supervision account for most of these.

- *Never* leave your child unsupervised near a pool or in the bathtub, even if he is wearing a personal flotation device.
- You must have self-closing and self-locking gates and fences.
- Remove toys from the pool area at the end of swim time.
- *Never* swim in an unsupervised location.
- Learn CPR (cardiopulmonary resuscitation) and make sure that anyone supervising your child near water has this knowledge.

Bathtub drowning occurs predominately in children under 2 years of age. Parents should not overestimate the coordination of an "older" infant. Children with epilepsy and other mental or motor disabilities are at increased risk of drowning in a bathtub and should shower in a nonglass cubicle.

You can prevent boating accidents by having everyone in the boat wear personal flotation devices. Boat safety programs are very beneficial. All passengers in a boat must understand simple rules of boating, such as avoiding overcrowding, avoiding alcohol and not standing up in small boats. Water safety education courses have significantly decreased the number of water-related fatalities. It is important that everyone in your family take these programs, but they must be followed to be effective.

If a drowning or near-drowning incident occurs, your child is more likely to be successfully helped if you know CPR and can begin resuscitation before paramedics arrive.

Foreign Bodies in the Eye

A number of objects of varying shapes and sizes can get into your child's eye. Usually these are small but irritating. The commonest foreign bodies are dust, dirt, sand and cosmetics. Occasionally, chemicals can get under the eyelids and irritate or even damage the eye.

What do foreign bodies in the eye look like? Typically, there is sudden discomfort or pain that causes the child to complain of "something in my eye." Often, the object lodges under his eyelid and he will have increased discomfort when he moves his eye. Your child might appear to blink excessively and find it difficult to keep the eye open. His eye will tear more and the white part of the eye, the sclera, can quickly become red. Frequently, the foreign body is easily visible, either when you look directly in the eye or when you retract the lid gently.

How do I treat foreign bodies in the eye? Smaller particles are often flushed out naturally by tears. If your child's symptoms persist at all or if the object is not totally removed, take your child to his doctor or to an emergency room. Many foreign bodies can be removed by irrigation with a salt solution or by gently wiping them with a cotton-tipped applicator. A drop of a local anesthetic in the eye can make it easier to remove the foreign body. If necessary, the doctor examining your child will put a drop of a special solution containing fluorescein in his eye to outline any scratches. He will use a special light to help him see these scratches. Local antibiotic drops or ointment might also be required to prevent infection. If a liquid chemical has caused the problem, first flush the eye with water for at least a few minutes and then take the child to the emergency department.

Fractures

What are fractures? A fracture or broken bone occurs when the force applied to the bone is greater than it can withstand. Fractures are extremely common throughout childhood and are one of the most frequent reasons for a child to be seen in the emergency department.

There are features of children's growing bones that are unique, making their fractures different than an adult's. For example, children have bones that are less dense than adults. This means that children, especially toddlers, can fracture a bone with much less force than needed to break a young adult bone. As well, the sleeve of tissue surrounding the bone is stronger in children. As a result, children's bones can bend or buckle rather than completely fracture through the entire width of the bone. These are called "greenstick" fractures because of their resemblance to a bent tree branch. Finally, because children's ligaments are relatively stronger than their bones, a fracture can occur rather than a sprain. Therefore, if a child and an adult have the same injury, the child is likely to fracture a bone whereas an adult will sprain it.

Another feature unique to children's bones is the growth plate. This is the area at the ends of the long bones where new growth occurs. This allows fractures to heal relatively more quickly, and children do not require surgical re-alignment as often as adults in order to promote proper healing. However, injuries to the growth plate area need to be dealt with carefully and sometimes do require surgery to ensure that proper growth is preserved.

Broken collarbones (clavicles) are among the most common fractures in childhood. Typically, they result from a fall on the shoulder or the outstretched hand or in bigger newborns as a result of the birthing process. Most occur in the middle third of the clavicle. More rarely, the clavicle may be fractured closer to the shoulder by a collision of the shoulder into a hard surface, such as the boards of a hockey rink.

What do fractures look like? Pain and swelling of part of a limb after a fall or injury is the most common sign of a fracture. Not infrequently, especially in a toddler, a fracture might not produce any swelling or deformity in the limb but might only be suspected when a young child refuses to walk, bear weight or use his arm. Any of these signs and symptoms could be because of a fracture, and you should take him for medical attention and x-rays of the affected area.

With a broken collarbone, usually children complain of localized pain in the collarbone and are reluctant to lift the affected arm. The area of the fracture is usually tender to touch. Visible swelling and an obvious deformity can be seen.

How do you treat fractures?

Upper limb fractures. A fracture can occur in any of the bones of the forearm (radius and ulna) or in the humerus, the bone of the upper arm. The most common cause of a fracture of the arm is after a fall onto the outstretched arm, for example a fall from climbing-bars. A fracture of the upper arm (humerus) usually results from more severe force. Fractures of the forearm are often dealt with by simple casting, usually for about four weeks. If the fracture has caused the bones to become misaligned, they might need to be reset with or without the need for an operation.

A fracture around the elbow more commonly requires an operation to ensure the bones are aligned properly for adequate healing. After the cast is applied, your child's doctor will review the directions to ensure proper handling of the cast, and signs to watch for that could indicate a problem, for example, more pain than expected and cool and/or pale fingers. Over-the-counter pain medicine is usually adequate for mild injuries. Your doctor will arrange for your child to be seen again over the next several weeks to ensure proper healing is taking place.

In the past, treatment of a broken collarbone consisted of immobilizing the joint with a "figure-eight" bandage wrapped around the shoulders. Recently, the management of a broken collarbone has changed and now your child's arm will be simply placed in a sling for pain relief. Your child's doctor might prescribe pain-relieving medication as well. When the pain improves, your child can remove the sling. As the fracture heals over the next three to six weeks, a visible bump might be noted and this can take months to clear up.

Lower limb fractures. There are two bones in the lower leg, the tibia and fibula, and one in the upper leg, the femur. In general, fractures of the femur occur after more forceful injuries such as a fall from considerable height or in a motor vehicle accident. Fractures of the lower leg are more common and can often result from a lesser force. In toddlers, a fracture of the lower leg bones can occur without an obvious injury or noticeable swelling and might only become apparent after they refuse to bear weight. This is known as a "toddler's fracture."

Fractures of the upper leg are more likely to require surgery to ensure proper healing. A cast is often placed for four to six weeks depending on the type of injury. The type of injury will determine whether and how long your child should avoid bearing weight on the leg.

Head Injuries and Concussions

What are head injuries and concussions? Traumatic brain injury (TBI) happens when a sudden impact to the head damages the brain. The commonest form of TBI is, of course, the concussion. This refers to an event in which there is a brief loss of consciousness following brain trauma. Other forms of TBI include contusions, which refer to bruising of brain tissues, and intracerebral hematomas, in which damage to a major blood vessel causes a clot around the brain.

The American Academy of Neurology (A.A.N.) classifies concussions into three groups:

Grade I: Mild Concussion
This is a "ding injury." There is transient confusion but no loss of consciousness. The symptoms resolve in less than 15 minutes.

Grade II: Moderate Concussion
There is transient confusion. No loss of consciousness. Symptoms or abnormalities last more than 15 minutes.

Grade III: Severe Concussion
This refers to concussions with any loss of consciousness, either brief or prolonged.

Head injuries in children are all too common. Half of all TBIs are due to transportation accidents, including bikes and automobiles. Twenty percent of head injuries are sports-related. In the United States, over 300,000 sports-related brain injuries occur annually. When an athlete has a concussion, there is a significant chance that a second and more damaging concussion will follow that same season.

What do head injuries and concussions look like?
The most common symptom of concussion is headache, which is reported in 85 percent of cases. Other symptoms are confusion, trouble with concentration, drowsiness, unconsciousness, memory loss, dizziness, nausea, weakness and even seizures.

Post-concussive **syndrome** refers to those individuals who develop physical, emotional and/or cognitive (thought processing) symptoms days or even weeks following a TBI. These include decreased mental processing speed, decreased short-term memory and attention span, irritability, fatigue, sleep disturbance, persistent headache and a general "foggy" feeling. If your child has experienced any of these symptoms, he *must* avoid the risk of any further head injury.

How do I treat head injuries and concussions?
Prevention is crucial. Everybody should follow safe preventative practices. These include appropriate, well-fitting equipment where indicated. Helmets are an absolute must for biking, hockey and street skating. Diving into unknown water is an invitation for disaster. A responsible adult who understands the classification and management of concussion should be on the sidelines for all body contact sports.

RETURN TO PLAY GUIDELINES (A.A.N.)

GRADE OF CONCUSSION	SYMPTOMS	RETURN TO PLAY
I	Transient confusion. No loss of consciousness. Symptoms last less than 15 min.	Immediately after abnormalities and symptoms clear.
II	Transient confusion. No loss of consciousness. Symptoms last more than 15 min.	After 1 week free of all symptoms at rest or after exertion.
III	Any loss of consciousness (LOC).	If LOC lasts only seconds: After 1 week if free of all symptoms on exertion. If LOC is prolonged (minutes): After 2 symptom-free weeks.

Your child with even an apparently mild concussion should be monitored for a number of hours. Any clinical deterioration or new symptoms are indications for an immediate hospital assessment. If he loses consciousness, however briefly, you must assume that he has injured his neck; do not remove any helmet, do not administer smelling salts. Rather, call 9-1-1 or your emergency number and have trained people stabilize his neck. Then have the ambulance take the child to hospital. Immediate hospitalization and investigation is also required if your conscious child is suspected of having a skull fracture, has had a seizure or develops weakness or persistent vomiting.

There has been a great deal of discussion regarding when it is appropriate for someone who has had a mild head injury to return to participate in a sport. In general, symptoms that should preclude play at any time are dizziness, slowness in responding to questions, evidence of difficulty concentrating, physical sluggishness and memory loss, especially if there is a loss of memory events before the injury. If your child has *any* symptom, he must not participate in contact sports until all symptoms have resolved. The "Return to Play" guidelines must be observed. These recommendations should be considered the minimum required to allow healing.

Ingestions

What is poisonous around my house? Medicines, both prescription and over-the-counter, are the most common causes of poisoning in infants and young children. However, many other products can be toxic to young children, including household cleaners (for example, bleach), cosmetics (for example, nail polish), plants and garden products (for example, pesticides), alcohol and car products (for example, antifreeze). These poisonous household substances can pose quite a problem because babies and young children are inquisitive and love to explore their environment. One of their main tools for exploration is their mouth, and they frequently will taste and swallow things that do not taste or smell good to adults!

How can I make my home safe?

Dos:
- Keep medicines stored in bottles with child-resistant caps, but remember that some children can still open them.
- Store medicines that can be poisonous to children (this includes vitamins and herbal medicines that contain compounds like iron) in locked or inaccessible cabinets.
- Install safety latches on cupboards.
- Leave medicines and other products in their original container (a child might think antifreeze stored in a pop bottle is pop!).
- Teach children the meaning of warning labels (for example, poison, corrosive, explosive, flammable).
- Learn the names of poisonous houseplants and what they look like (for example, dieffenbachia, poinsettia). Do not have them in your home.
- Read labels before using poisonous products (for example, oven cleaner, pesticide).
- Keep the number of your local poison information center handy. The American Association of Poison Control Centers (1-800-222-1222) has excellent tips about safety and poisons.

Insect Bites

Mankind does not occupy the planet alone. We share it with literally billions of insects and, therefore, insect bites will become an inevitable part of your child's life. In some parts of the world, this has immense consequence: malaria, for example, transmitted by a mosquito bite, kills thousands of children annually in tropical areas. In North America, although some serious problems can sometimes occur, the great majority of stings and insect bites merely result in an irritating annoyance.

What do insect bites look like? The commonest insect that bites children is the mosquito. Initially, there may be a transient, round area of swelling (wheal) at the site of the bite. In a day or two, an itchy bump (**papule**) develops that children find impossible not to scratch. As a result, the tops of the papules can become crusted. Occasionally, a secondary infection ensues that produces the late onset of redness and swelling.

Often, the actual bites are unnoticed initially, although the bite of a horsefly is hard to miss. A small central bite mark may be seen at the site of a raised red papule. Numerous bites may appear as an irregular "rash" on your child's body; crawling insects can leave a series of bites in a trail, or at preferred sites like the back of the neck. If there is a strong reaction to the bites, the local lymph nodes might enlarge.

Of course, there are many other insects that bite children: spiders, tics, flies and lice are the most common. Stings also occur frequently, sometimes with serious consequences: this problem is discussed elsewhere (see Bee and Wasp Stings, pages 403–404).

How do I treat insect bites? Once again, prevention is best. Insect repellents reduce the number of bites and should be worn when a child is playing outdoors, particularly in a setting where insects are plentiful. Insect repellents containing DEET are generally safe for children but authorities recommend certain precautions:

- DEET should not be used in infants under 6 months of age.
- The concentration of DEET in the repellent should be less than 10 percent. This will give about two to three hours protection.
- Children 6 to 24 months should receive only one application a day and those 2 to 12 years should have no more than three applications daily.
- Citronella (5–15 percent) is a natural repellent but its effectiveness is short-lived—only about 20 minutes. Its value is therefore limited. Newer repellents using 2 percent soybean oil are proving to be more effective.
- Other common-sense precautions, such as using netting when young infants are outdoors in buggy situations, limiting outdoor play at sunset or when it is damp, and wearing protective clothing when camping obviously will help reduce the number of insect bites.

When insect bites do occur, as they inevitably do, treat the symptoms. You can apply soothing lotions, such as calamine. Their effect might be limited but at least they give the appearance that some relief is being offered. It is more helpful to cut your child's fingernails closely so he scratches less, reducing the possibility of secondary infection. If your child is unable to sleep because of itching and discomfort, you can give him an antihistamine at bedtime.

Generally, it isn't necessary to call the doctor when insect bites occur. However, if there is spreading redness at the site of a bite, fever, muscle pain, cramping or any signs of a more generalized reaction, seek medical attention.

Knee Injuries

What are knee injuries? Many of the most troublesome injuries in sport involve the knee. Adolescents, for whom sports are frequently a huge part of life, are more likely to incur serious knee injuries than younger children.

The knee is supported by tough bands of rubbery tissue called ligaments. Two ligaments run along the sides of the knee, the medial collateral on the inside of the knee and the lateral collateral on the outside. These provide sideways stability. Inside the knee joint is the anterior cruciate ligament (ACL). It connects the front of the tibia to the back of the femur at an angle and stabilizes the center of the knee from excess twisting and front-to-back displacement. There are also two layers of cartilage, called the medial and lateral menisci, between the upper and lower leg that cushion the knee and stabilize the thighbone on the lower leg.

Most injuries to the knee are injuries to the ligaments and menisci rather than fractures (breaks) of the bone. These tears and strains can occur in combination and are not necessarily single isolated injuries. The medial collateral ligament tends to be strained by a sideward force on the outside of the knee. Injuries to the ACL, the most common serious ligamentous injury, occur with twisting injuries of the knee when it is straight and the foot is anchored on the ground. This can happen with contact in sports but can also occur with a sudden twisting motion of the leg when the foot sticks to the ground, for example, when cleats are stuck in the ground or a gymnast's shoe doesn't allow him to pivot. Menisci also can tear after forceful twisting or during a squat. Patellar (kneecap) fractures can happen after a direct frontal blow to the knee, such as a fall onto the pavement.

What do knee injuries look like? Usually, your child or teen can identify a sudden traumatic event or activity that produces immediate pain.

- Medial collateral ligament injury: the child might report a tearing sensation followed by pain and swelling on the side of the knee. There can be instability with movement to the side if the damage is severe.
- ACL injury: the child might feel a "pop" in the knee. Typically there is swelling and pain in the knee and the child might be unable to walk because the knee "gives way." Children with ACL injuries might be able to bear weight, walk and run but are unable to change directions or jump.
- A meniscus tear can also be associated with an initial pop followed by swelling and restricted joint movement. A torn meniscus can cause a locking or catching sensation in the knee.

Plain x-rays of the knee will not show damage to ligaments and cartilage; they only exclude a broken bone. The doctor caring for your child will do a physical examination and probably order an MRI to define this injury. Occasionally, the exact nature of a damaged knee can only be determined by direct inspection of the joint using an arthroscope (a telescope placed into the knee joint) in a simple day- surgery procedure.

What do I do about a knee injury? Initially, the knee should be treated with "R.I.C.E.": Rest, Ice, Compression, Elevation, (see page 403). Have your child sit or lie down with a pillow placed

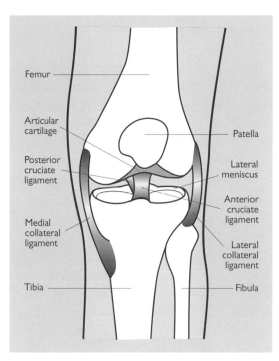

ANATOMY OF THE KNEE
The knee is supported by tough bands of rubbery tissue called ligaments.

under his knee (Rest and Elevation). Ice packs should be applied for 30 minutes every three hours for two days or at least until the pain and swelling resolve (Ice). An elastic wrap should be applied to the knee to limit swelling (Compression).

All but the most minor knee injuries are significant and require a medical assessment. This will require examination of the knee plus routine x-rays of the joint. They may even require MRI and arthroscopy to delineate the problem. Surgery will be required to mend a torn ACL, but trauma to the collateral ligaments seldom requires surgery. Conservative therapy including rest, progressive exercises and limitation of activity may be all that is required for many knee injuries depending on the amount of physical activity your child intends to pursue.

Nasal Injuries

What are nasal injuries? Children frequently injure their noses. This typically results from a fall or direct blow to the face during an organized sport or when just playing around. Children's noses are quite different from adult ones. Their nasal cartilage—the projecting tissue of the front of the nose—is softer and more compliant. Rather than crack, it bends more easily with trauma. The impacting force is spread across the middle of the face causing swelling of the nose and adjacent parts of the cheeks. Still, when enough force is involved, the nasal cartilage will crack or become detached from the bony framework of the nose, which is the upper portion of the nose. The septum, the cartilage that divides the nostrils, is also very susceptible to injury.

What do nasal injuries look like? Typically, your child's nose looks swollen and his nostrils might bleed. In the first few days, it can be difficult to assess whether or not a fracture has occurred. Usually, it is just the cartilage that is injured and cartilage does not show up on an x-ray. Because of this x-rays are not often helpful. It takes three to four days for the swelling to settle before parents can say whether their child's nose has been changed by the trauma, and it won't be too late to have the nose fixed if that is necessary.

What do I do about nasal injuries? The first step is always to prevent more swelling; gentle pressure with ice will help. Apply ice wrapped in a towel for 15 minutes at a time followed by removing the ice for an equal interval. Take your child to the doctor as soon as convenient to have the nose examined and ensure there has been no injury to the septum. If the cartilage has been broken and

the nose is not straight, your child might require surgery to realign his nose. The procedure is very brief and does not require an incision. If you think your child's nose looks crooked after an injury, it probably is broken and should be seen by a physician. If the trauma was significant, your child's doctor might order x-rays to evaluate not just the nose but also the facial bones.

Pulled Elbow

What is a pulled elbow? The formal name for a pulled elbow is dislocated radial head. In this condition, the head of the radius, which is one of the long bones between the wrist and the elbow, pulls out from the ligament that holds it in place. This occurs when there is a sudden tug on the arm when your child is holding his elbow straight. Often this happens when someone is holding your child's hand as he falls. It can also occur if your child is lifted suddenly by the hands. It does not take much force to dislocate the elbow; often it is the sudden jerking of the arm that produces the dislocation. Pulled elbows are most likely to happen in toddlers.

What does a pulled elbow look like? When the radial head is dislocated, your child refuses to use his arm and it looks limp. Attempting to move the elbow usually results in crying.

How do you treat a pulled elbow? Usually the elbow can be fixed by merely rotating the forearm from a palm up to a palm down position while applying slight traction to the wrist and then returning the wrist to the palm up position. This simple maneuver is usually successful and

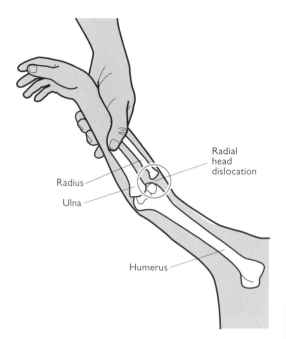

PULLED ELBOW

A sudden tug on the arm when the child's elbow is straight can dislocate the head of the radius.

Radial head dislocation

Radius

Ulna

Humerus

produces an instant cure. Thus, it is one of the most rewarding conditions for physicians to treat. X-rays are seldom necessary. It is important to understand the mechanism of the injury—pulling on a toddler's forearm—to prevent another episode. Fortunately, by 4 years of age, the elbow matures so that radial head dislocation no longer occurs.

Scalds and Burns

What are scalds and burns? Scalds are injuries that result from contact with a hot object or hot liquid. They are most commonly seen in children under 3 years of age. Burns are the consequence of direct flame exposure. These are commonly seen in children older than 2 years

who are playing with matches, fire and flammable materials. Burns are usually more serious.

What do scalds and burns look like? Burns are categorized by the depth of their damage to the skin.

- First-degree burns involve only the superficial layers. They are characterized by redness, swelling and local pain, similar to mild sunburn. These usually heal in a few days.
- Second-degree burns are deeper and are characterized by pain and blistering. They generally heal in 7 to 14 days.
- Third-degree burns are deeper and involve the full thickness of the skin. They will require skin grafting.

How do I treat scalds and burns? Obviously, prevention is most important.

- Do not allow your children to play with matches.
- Lock up all flammable materials safely.
- Watch toddlers constantly when they are near open flames, such as campfires.
- Stoves, hot oven doors and even the glass screen of a fireplace often cause burns to little hands. So is the hot steam that emanates from a vaporizer.
- You must always watch for spilled hot liquids.
- Scald injuries from hot water in bathtubs remains a major concern. Lower the setting of your hot water tank to 120°F (55°C) to reduce the chance of scalds.
- Install smoke detectors and plan routes of escape from your home in case of fire to reduce risks.

If your child has a minor burn, place it immediately under cold running water, if available. Otherwise, cover the area with a clean cloth cooled with water. Do not apply butter and other greasy medications in the initial treatment of the burn. Only a doctor should break blisters.

Pain relief is important: don't hesitate to give acetaminophen or ibuprofen if your child appears to be in pain. First-degree burns should be left exposed but deeper burns should be dressed with fine mesh gauze impregnated with petroleum jelly or antibiotic ointment. Change the dressings every few days. It is important to use sunblock on skin that has been damaged by a burn after it has healed. This should be continued for a year.

Shoulder Injuries

SHOULDER DISLOCATION

What is shoulder dislocation? The shoulder is said to be dislocated when the ball of the upper arm bone (head of the humerus) comes out of its socket near the shoulder blade. This usually happens during a fall on an outstretched arm with the arm being forced upward and backward. Shoulder dislocations are uncommon in children: they become more frequent in adolescent athletes involved in sports with contact or associated with falls, such as skiing.

What does shoulder dislocation look like? When the shoulder is dislocated, your teenager will complain of severe shoulder pain and will be unable to use the affected arm. He (boys are five times more likely than girls to dislocate their shoulder) might also complain of generalized

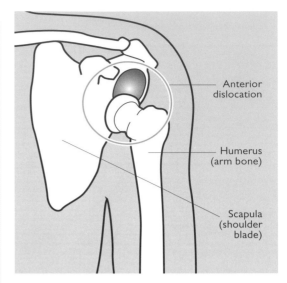

SHOULDER INJURIES
The shoulder is dislocated when the head of the humerus comes out of its socket.

weakness of the entire arm. The outside of the shoulder appears flatter than the round contour of the healthy arm. The top of the humerus can be felt in the underarm.

How do I treat shoulder dislocation? This injury requires medical attention immediately. It is optimal if the dislocation can be fixed by a qualified person within one hour. In the meantime, place the limb in a sling and offer acetaminophen or ibuprofen for pain relief. Some children dislocate their shoulder several times and require surgery to prevent recurrences.

SHOULDER SUBLUXATION

What is shoulder subluxation? Sometimes, during vigorous overarm activity, the head of the humerus momentarily pops out of the socket and then returns to its proper position. This is called a subluxation of the shoulder and is more likely to occur in athletes who participate in racquet sports or strenuous throwing.

What does shoulder subluxation look like? The athlete will usually notice a sensation of the shoulder joint popping out and then back in again. There is brief but severe shoulder pain, particularly if his arm is brought across his chest. For a while, the arm can feel numb.

How do I treat shoulder subluxation? When a shoulder subluxation occurs, offer oral pain relief, such as ibuprofen. Ice the shoulder for 10 to 15 minutes each half hour and get it checked by a physician or other qualified individual. After a few days, you can apply heat and your child can begin shoulder strengthening exercises gradually and carefully. Unfortunately, the problem tends to recur and your child might need surgery to tighten the structures that secure the shoulder joint.

SHOULDER SEPARATION

What is shoulder separation? This refers to shoulder injuries that tear or stretch the ligaments that hold the shoulder together. Most commonly, the ligament connecting the collarbone (clavicle) to the shoulder blade is the one involved. Shoulder separations result from a fall onto the tip of the shoulder or a direct blow to the shoulder, such as when a hockey player slams into the boards.

What does shoulder separation look like? Depending on the degree of the injury, there is localized shoulder pain at the tip of the clavicle. This pain is worsened by attempting to lift the shoulder. More severe tears are also associated with swelling and the presence of a deformity created by the outer end of the collarbone sticking up.

How do I treat shoulder separation? Place your child's arm in a sling, apply ice intermittently, give oral pain relievers and get the shoulder examined by an experienced health care provider. Further treatment will depend upon the degree of injury. Your child will recover from mild strains in 7 to 10 days. Severe injury might require months of rehabilitation. Rarely, surgery will be needed to return the elite athlete to full function.

Slivers

It is one of life's annoying realities that kids get slivers. For that matter, so do their parents. So it is worthwhile to learn how best to manage slivers.

What are slivers? The variety of foreign objects that can become imbedded in a child is potentially limitless. In reality, the most common objects to cause slivers are wood, glass and metallic splinters. Some splinters, such as wood and thorns, can easily become infected and promote quite an inflammatory reaction. Others, like glass or metal, are more inert. Slivers can be large or small, superficial or deep, lie horizontally or vertically and be easy to remove or clearly difficult to do so.

What do slivers look like? Most slivers are visible and can be adequately assessed just by looking at them. Some imbedded objects, like a needle or thorn in the foot, may only be noticed because a toddler starts limping. In the emergency department, certain foreign bodies (metal, glass) are usually visible on simple x-rays and others, like a piece of wood deep in a wound, may not be detected except by an ultrasound examination.

How do I treat slivers? Generally, slivers should be removed. A common exception is the situation in which numerous, tiny fragments of wood are superficially, and painlessly, imbedded in the skin: removal would cause more trouble than the splinters. Clean the area involved with antiseptic and the tiny fragments will eventually come out with the normal shedding of the skin.

Most slivers can be removed at home. Seek medical assistance if the splinter is deep, looks infected or if you aren't sure that your child has had a **tetanus** shot in the preceding five years. Also, it's a good idea to get help if you don't think you'll be able to remove the splinter easily, or if you try but find removal more difficult than anticipated.

Usually, splinters can be removed using tweezers and a needle that have been sterilized with alcohol.

- First, wash the area thoroughly and apply some antiseptic solution.
- Firmly grasp the exposed end of the sliver with the tweezers and pull it out along the angle of entry.
- If the splinter is just below the skin, a light feathering stroke with the needle will often expose the sliver so that it can then be removed with tweezers.
- Horizontal, shallow splinters can be removed by stroking the overlying skin along the long axis of the sliver with a needle, or sharply pointed blade, exposing the fragment and then flicking it out.

Sometimes you must be creative. Plant spines that might be crushed by tweezers or fiberglass pieces can often be removed by applying some wax hair remover, if available, and then peeling off the fragments.

Once the splinter has been removed, wash the area again and apply an antiseptic or antibiotic ointment. It's also wise to periodically check the wound for a few days to make sure an infection hasn't developed.

Glossary

ABSENCE SEIZURES a brief staring spell during which the child is unresponsive with no speech or movement, sometimes accompanied by flickering of the eyes.

ACELLULAR not consisting of whole cells. Acellular vaccines, such as PERTUSSIS, contain only fragments of bacteria cells that are able to trigger an immune response by the body, leading to immunization.

ACUTE of a sudden onset.

AGRANULOCYTOSIS a very low number of NEUTROPHILS (white blood cells).

ALLERGENS various substances that trigger an allergic reaction.

ALLERGIC RHINITIS also called "hay fever." A type of allergy leading to inflammation of the nasal passages. Symptoms may include congestion, runny nose, cough, sneezing and itchy nose or eyes.

AMBLYOPIA a permanent impairment of vision caused by lack of use of the eye. This may be due to various conditions, such as cataracts or STRABISMUS.

ANAPHYLACTIC a life-threatening allergic reaction consisting of swelling of the lips or tongue, difficulty breathing or swallowing, URTICARIA and abdominal pain.

ANENCEPHALY complete or near complete underdevelopment of the brain, and sometimes skull.

ANEURYSM a balloonlike widening of an artery.

ANOVULATION failure of the ovaries to release eggs.

ANTIBODY also called "immunoglobulin." A protein made by B-lymphocytes, a type of white blood cell that helps fight infections.

ANTINUCLEAR ANTIBODY abnormal antibodies to the nucleus inside our cells.

ANTIPYRETICS medications used to control fever.

APLASTIC CRISIS severe anemia in a patient with an underlying blood disorder, such as sickle cell disease or thalassemia major, following exposure to some infections or drugs.

APNEA the absence of breathing for periods of at least 10 to 15 seconds. (See also OBSTRUCTIVE SLEEP APNEA.)

ARTERIOVENOUS MALFORMATION a malformation of the blood vessels (consisting of a complex tangle of arteries and veins).

ARTHROGRYPOSIS skeletal abnormalities that consist of stiff joints with limited range of movement resulting in deformities.

ASPIRATION PNEUMONIA an infection of the lungs due to the inhalation of food or other objects into the lungs.

ASTIGMATISM an inability of the eye to focus on all parts of an object at the same time, usually caused by an irregularly shaped cornea.

ATAXIA TELANGIECTASIA a rare inherited disease consisting of immune system abnormalities, poor coordination and dilated blood vessels on the skin and eyes.

ATLANTO-AXIAL SUBLUXATION a loss of stability in the top two bones of the neck that can predispose to spinal cord injury.

ATOPIC DERMATITIS also called "eczema." A chronic skin condition, of variable severity, characterized by dry, red and itchy patches of skin.

ATOPY a tendency to develop allergies.

AUTISM SPECTRUM DISORDERS: autism, pervasive developmental disorders and Asperger's syndrome, a group of similar developmental conditions characterized by difficulties or delays in the areas of communication, socialization, play and behavior.

AUTOMATISMS semipurposeful actions such as lip smacking, chewing movements of the mouth and picking or pulling at clothing.

AUTOSOMAL pertaining to chromosomes or genes that are not the sex-linked, or X and Y chromosomes.

AXILLA the underarm (armpit).

BACTEREMIA also called "blood poisoning." A bacterial infection in the blood.

BALLOON ANGIOPLASTY dilation of an obstructed artery using a balloon catheter.

BALLOON VALVULOPLASTY a minimally invasive procedure for treating STENOSIS of a heart valve. A wire that contains a balloon is introduced into the narrow valve, and then inflated to open up the narrowing.

BILIRUBIN a naturally occuring breakdown product of hemoglobin, which is found in the red blood cells and is responsible for carrying oxygen. If it becomes excessive in the blood it will lead to a yellowish (jaundiced) skin and eye color.

BLEPHARITIS inflammation of the edges of the eyelids caused by irritation from skin conditions, infections or allergic reactions. The skin around the lashes is often red, itchy and scaly, and there may be a loss of eyelashes from frequent rubbing.

BLEPHAROSPASM a tendency to squeeze the eyelid tightly closed; sometimes seen in glaucoma.

BLINDED TRIAL when either a real medication or a sugar pill (a placebo) are given and the child and observers are unaware of which is being taken at that time. Parents and children may evaluate the effectiveness and side effects unaware whether the placebo or the real drug is being consumed, thus allowing for an unbiased evaluation.

BRADYCARDIA an abnormally slow heart rate for age.

BRONCHIECTASIS enlarged, damaged bronchial tubes.

BRONCHIOLITIS a viral infection that causes swelling and increased mucus in the small airways of the lungs, that tends to occur in infants under 2 years of age. Symptoms typically include fast, heavy breathing, and wheezing.

CAPUT a self-resolving soft and squishy swelling over the top part of the newborn's head, often more prominent if a "vacuum" has been used in the delivery.

CECOSTOMY TUBE a tube that is inserted into the CECUM by a surgeon or radiologist, to assist with the evacuation of stool from the bowel.

CECUM part of the large intestine.

CELIAC DISEASE A condition where the small intestines are unable to tolerate gluten, a protein found in barley, wheat, rye and possibly oats. Symptoms may include poor appetite and weight gain, abdominal pain, vomiting or loose stools.

CELLULITIS an infection of the skin and underlying soft tissues.

CEPHALOHEMATOMAS soft, mushy swellings, usually over the side of the skull caused by bruising from the pressure of the birth canal against the baby's head. Sometimes they may become quite hard, but they always disappear, although this may take a few months.

CEPHALOSPORINS a class of antibiotic medications.

CEREBROSPINAL FLUID (CSF) a fluid that surrounds the brain and spinal cord.

CHALAZION a discrete, firm, nontender bump within the eyelid.

CHICKEN POX a very common and contagious viral illness caused by the varicella-zoster virus. It is characterized by an itchy rash consisting of small fluid-filled vesicles on a red base.

COARCTATION a narrowing or obstruction (typically of the aorta, the body's main artery).

COBB'S ANGLE the degree of curvature on a spinal x-ray in a child with scoliosis.

COMEDONES also called "pimples." They may be whiteheads (closed) or blackheads (open).

CONJUNCTIVITIS also called "pink eye." Inflammation of the thin layer covering one or both eyes, caused by infection, allergies, chemicals or irritants. Symptoms include redness of the whites of the eye, itchiness and discharge.

COXSACKIE a common virus that may cause many illnesses, including "hand, foot and mouth disease," MYOCARDITIS and ENCEPHALITIS.

CRANIOSYNOSTOSIS an abnormality resulting in premature fusion of the different bones of the skull, which can impair the ability of the skull and the brain to grow properly.

C-REACTIVE PROTEIN a nonspecific marker of inflammation in the blood, which may be an indirect sign of infection.

DEBRIDEMENT a surgical procedure in which infected areas of skin and soft tissue are removed, which is sometimes necessary to control infection.

DEFORMATIONAL PLAGIOCEPHALY see POSITIONAL PLAGIOCEPHALY.

DIASTOLE the phase of the cardiac cycle when the atria are emptying and the ventricles are filling (getting ready to pump blood out to the lungs and the rest of the body).

DORSAL GANGLIA the location in the sensory nerve where the varicella-zoster virus, the cause of chicken pox, remains inactive following an acute infection.

DOUBLE PNEUMONIA an older term referring to infection in both lungs.

DOWN'S SYNDROME a genetic condition resulting from three copies of chromosome 21, instead of the normal two. The result is a combination of typical physical features, with developmental and cognitive problems.

DUODENAL ARTESIA a cause of small bowel obstruction, occurring more frequently in Down's syndrome, that requires surgical repair.

DYSPLASIA the abnormal development or growth of organs, tissues or cells.

EDEMA swelling or puffiness.

EFFUSION a collection of fluid in an abnormal location (e.g., around the lungs, in the middle ear or in a joint).

ELECTROENCEPHALOGRAM (EEG) a tracing of the electrical activity in the brain usually used to look for evidence of seizure activity.

ELECTROMYOGRAM a tracing of the electrical activity of a muscle, sometimes useful in the assessment of low muscle tone or weakness.

EMBOLISM when a blood vessel is suddenly blocked by a clot or other particle.

ENCEPHALITIS an infection of the brain that is usually caused by viruses. It may lead to swelling of the brain with disruption of normal brain function that can result in headaches, seizures and changes in behavior, personality or consciousness.

ENCEPHALOCELE a hole in the skull caused by incomplete bone closure, which allows brain tissue to protrude through it.

ENCEPHALOPATHY a fluctuating level of consciousness with many potential causes.

ENDOSCOPY a small flexible tube placed through the mouth and gullet into the gastrointestinal tract, which allows for direct observation and tissue sampling to look for abnormalites. This is usually done with the child under anesthetic.

ENTEROVIRUSES a family of viruses that includes COXSACKIE, echo and polio viruses. Most infections with this family of viruses are mild and transient; however, some may cause serious disease.

EPICANTHAL SKIN FOLDS a fold of skin that partially covers the inner corner of the eye, which can be normal but is also seen in some conditions (e.g., Down's syndrome).

EPIGLOTTITIS a serious infection of the throat near the voice box that makes it difficult for a child to swallow and breathe.

EPIPHYSES the ends of the long bones where childhood bone growth occurs.

EPISTAXIS a nosebleed.

ERYTHROCYTE SEDIMENTATION (ESR) A non-specific marker of inflammation in the blood that may be an indirect sign of infection.

EXANTHEM SUBITUM also known as "roseola" or "sixth disease." A viral infection caused by human herpesvirus 6 that occurs in young children and leads to high fever and irritability for three to four days, followed by a spotty rash lasting hours to days.

FONTANELLE also called a "soft spot." Two areas on the skull of a newborn, one at the top and the other toward the back, where the bones have not yet fused together.

FRAGILE X SYNDROME a common genetic cause of developmental delay or learning and behavioral problems that predominantly affects males. Those affected may have a slightly longer face with a prominent jaw and large ears, and large testicles in older boys.

FUNDOPLICATION a surgical procedure in which the top of the stomach is wrapped around the bottom of the esophagus to prevent vomiting. It is used to treat severe cases of gastroesophageal reflux disease (GERD) that do not respond to medications.

GENERALIZED TONIC CLONIC SEIZURE a common type of seizure in which the child will suddenly lose consciousness and develop stiffening of the arms and legs (tonic phase) followed by rhythmic jerking (clonic phase) of the whole body.

GIARDIA LAMBLIA a parasite that may infect the small intestine or biliary tract, causing watery diarrhea and abdominal pain.

GLIOMA a type of tumor arising from brain or spinal cord tissue.

GLOMERULONEPHRITIS inflammation of the kidneys often presenting with blood and protein in the urine.

GRANULOMA a small mass of tissue resulting from chronic inflammation; one of the body's responses to infection.

GYNECOMASTIA extra breast tissue in males that often develops at puberty.

HANEN PARENT TRAINING a parent training course offering early language intervention and learning resources, available for parents of children with multiple disabilities.

HEMIPLEGIA weakness on one side of the body.

HEMORRHAGIC STROKE a sudden disruption of the blood supply to the brain resulting from bleeding from one of the brain's blood vessels. Damage to brain cells and neurologic injury, including motor and speech difficulties, may ensue.

HEPATOPORTOENTEROSTOMY also called the "Kasai procedure." The surgical treatment for biliary atresia in which the blocked bile ducts are removed and the liver is connected directly to the intestines to permit the flow of bile.

HERPANGINA painful fluid-filled blisters and ulcers in the back portion of the mouth caused by infection with COXSACKIE virus.

HIRSCHSPRUNG'S DISEASE an uncommon condition leading to severe constipation as a result of faulty development of the nerve supply to the large bowel.

HISTAMINE a chemical released in the body as part of an allergic reaction. Histamine release is responsible for many allergic symptoms including hives, itching and wheezing.

HIV VIRAL LOAD a test that measures the number of copies of the virus in HIV-infected patient's blood. It is used to determine if the virus is under control and to see how well the medications are working.

HORDEOLUM also called a "stye." A painful, but self-resolving, localized bacterial infection of the edge of the eyelid appearing as a red lump that may have a yellow head of pus around the base of the eyelash.

HYDROCELE a common cause of an enlarged scrotum in male infants resulting from a collection of fluid surrounding the testicle. Most disappear shortly after birth.

HYDROCEPHALUS an abnormal excessive accumulation of spinal fluid in and around the brain, sometimes requiring a shunt for drainage.

HYPEROPIA also called "farsightedness." It occurs when the image of an object becomes focused behind the retina of the eye causing close objects to appear blurred.

HYPOGAMMAGLOBULINEMIA a disorder caused by low levels of immunoglobulins in the blood, due to abnormalities or deficiencies in B-lymphocytes, resulting in susceptibility to recurrent infections with specific germs.

HYPOGLYCEMIA low blood sugar.

HYPOTONIA lower than normal resting muscle tone causing the child to seem floppy with decreased control of movements.

HYPOXIC SPELLS also called "Tet spells." Sudden onset, cyanotic (blue) episodes associated with fast breathing, irritability and crying seen in children with tetralogy of Fallot.

IDIOPATHIC THROMBOCYTOPENIC PURPURA a bleeding disorder that occurs when the immune system destroys its own clotting cells (platelets) leading to bruising and petechiae, tiny spots caused by bleeding into the skin.

IMMUNE GLOBULIN see IMMUNOGLOBULIN

IMMUNOGLOBULIN also called "antibodies." Proteins made by B-lymphocytes, a type of white blood cell that help fight infection.

IMPETIGO a superficial skin infection. It commonly occurs around the lips and nose, and appears as pus-filled blisters on a red background, sometimes with honey-colored or reddish crusts.

INCUBATION PERIOD the interval between the time that the infection is first acquired and when the symptoms start to appear.

INTUSSUSCEPTION the telescoping of a piece of intestine into the next part of the bowel which then becomes stuck, leading to acute episodes of abdominal pain and perhaps bloody stools. It most commonly occurs between the ages of 6 months and 3 years.

ISCHEMIC STROKE a sudden disruption of the blood supply to the brain resulting from a thrombus or embolus. Damage to brain cells and neurologic injury, including motor and speech difficulties, may ensue.

KERION a fungal infection on the scalp that appears as a boggy reddish mass with multiple openings that drain pus.

KOSTMANN SYNDROME also called "congenital agranulo-cytosis." A severe cause of reduced neutrophils, starting from birth.

KYPHOSCOLIOSIS a front-to-back and side-to-side curvature of the upper spine.

KYPHOSIS the forward curve of the spine in the thorax, or chest region.

LEUKOTRIENE ANTAGONISTS newer anti-inflammatory medications for the treatment of asthma that do not contain steroids.

LICHENIFICATION areas of thickening of the skin that looks almost leathery, often seen in children with chronic eczema.

LIPOGRANULOMA a collection of fat, oil and other tissue resulting from the obstruction of an oil producing gland, for example, a "chalazion" in the eyelid.

LOCKJAW see TETANUS.

LOW-GRADE FEVER a mildly elevated temperature, less than 101.3°F (38.5°C), usually associated with an infection, which is often caused by a virus.

LUMBAR PUNCTURE a test used to diagnose meningitis or encephlitis, in which a needle is placed in the lower back, below the point that the spinal cord ends, and a small amount of cerebrospinal fluid (CSF) is removed to send to the laboratory.

LYMPHADENITIS inflammation or swelling of a lymph gland, usually caused by an infection in the area drained by the lymph gland.

MACROCEPHALY a large head, measuring greater than the 97th percentile on a standard head circumference growth chart.

MENINGES the protective three-layer covering of the brain and spinal cord.

MENINGITIS an infection of the fluid and membranes (meninges) that cover the brain and spinal cord.

MICROCEPHALY a small head, measuring less than the third percentile on a standard head circumference growth chart.

MILIARY TUBERCULOSIS a form of tuberculosis, more common in infants and children, where the infection spreads in the bloodstream to other areas outside of the lung.

MOLDING a process whereby the bones within the skull have shifted to allow the baby's head to descend through the birth canal, resulting in a temporary "cone head" shape.

MOSAICISM a cause of genetic diseases that occurs when the individual has two different cell types from a single fertilized egg; one cell "line" may not contain the correct number or structure of chromosomes.

MULTIMERS proteins that are made up of two or more parts, for example, those that make up the von Willebrand clotting factor.

MYELIN the protective covering around nerves.

MYOCARDITIS inflammation of the heart muscle, typically as a result of a viral infection.

MYOCLONIC SEIZURE brief, often symmetric jerking movements of the muscles.

MYOPIA also called "nearsightedness." It occurs when the image of an object is focused in front of the retina causing distant objects to appear blurry.

NASOGASTRIC TUBE a tube passed through the nostril into the stomach, which can be used to provide nutrition, fluids or medications.

NEBULIZER a device that changes liquid medication, such as albuterol (Ventolin) or epinephrine, into a mist that may then be inhaled by the child through a mask.

NECROTIZING FASCIITIS also called "flesh-eating disease." An uncommon but life-threatening bacterial infection that affects the skin, the fat just below the skin and a layer below the fat called the fascia.

NEUTROPENIA an abnormally low number of neutrophils in the blood leaving the body susceptible to bacterial and certain fungal infections.

NEUTROPHILS a type of white blood cell that serves as the major defense against bacterial and certain fungal infections.

NON-DISJUNCTION when the chromosomes of a cell do not separate equally during meiosis, the natural process of cell division, leading to unequal genetic material in the resulting pair of cells.

OBESITY the excessive accumulation of fat, rather than excessive weight. This is often defined as a body mass index (BMI) at or above the 95th percentile in children aged 2 to 20 years.

OBSTRUCTIVE SLEEP APNEA partial or complete blockage of the upper air passages during sleep, which causes abnormal breathing and sleep patterns. It may lead to daytime sleepiness, behavioral and attention problems, growth problems or heart problems.

ORAL REHYDRATION SOLUTION (ORS) liquids that contain an appropriate mixture of water and salts which are used to replace fluid loss from diarrhea and/ or vomiting. Also called oral electrolyte solution and oral rehydration salts.

OSGOOD-SCHLATTER DISEASE a painful condition affecting the "tibial tubercle," the bump on the shinbone just below the knee. It is caused by overuse and typically affects active preteen and teenage boys.

OTITIS MEDIA WITH EFFUSION a nonpainful condition that typically follows an ear infection (acute otitis media) in which fluid collects behind the tympanic membrane, or eardrum, and usually clears within three months.

OTOPLASTY a cosmetic procedure used to improve the appearance of protruding ears by repositioning the ear cartilage closer to the head, so that they do not stick out.

PANNICULITIS inflammation of fat that occurs with excessive exposure to cold and wind and leads to the formation of a firm lump under the exposed area.

PAPULE a small (less than 2/5 inch or 1 cm), raised lesion on the skin.

PAROTID GLANDS glands in the cheeks that produce saliva.

PAUCIARTICULAR ARTHRITIS joint inflammation in which four or fewer joints are affected.

PERICARDITIS inflammation of the sac that surrounds the heart, seen in some infectious or rheumatological conditions.

PERIORBITAL the area of skin and soft tissue surrounding the eye, including the eyelids.

PERTUSSIS also called "whooping cough." An infection of the airways caused by a bacteria, *Bordetella pertussis*, that leads to violent coughing spasms and can go on for weeks or months.

PETECHIAE pinpoint bleeding spots in the skin that look like small red-purple dots.

PHAGOCYTOSIS the process by which neutrophils engulf and destroy foreign material, including bacteria.

PHENOTYPE the observable features of a child that are determined by both genetics and environment.

PHENYLKETONURIA a metabolic disease in which an enzyme deficiency leads to an excessive buildup of amino acids, resulting in significant brain damage if left untreated. This disease is screened for in the newborn period.

PHONOLOGICAL AWARENESS the process of recognizing, processing and using the sounds that make up language; the primary problem in children with a specific reading disability.

PHOTOPHOBIA an abnormal sensitivity of the eyes to light, seen classically in children with meningitis.

PLASMAPHERESIS a blood cleansing technique, similar to dialysis.

PLATELETS small blood cells that are necessary for normal clotting.

PLEURA the lining around the lung.

PLEURAL EFFUSION a fluid collection around the outside of the lungs that may lead to difficulty breathing or chest pain.

PLEURITIS inflammation of the lining of the lung, or pleura, seen in some infectious and rheumatological diseases.

POLYARTICULAR JUVENILE RHEUMATOID ARTHRITIS (JRA) joint inflammation in which five or more joints are affected.

POLYDIPSIA the act of drinking excessively.

POLYURIA the act of passing increased amounts of urine.

POSITIONAL PLAGIOCEPHALY also called "deformational plagiocephaly." The asymmetric flattening of the skull that occurs when an infant displays a preference for keeping the head turned one way or the other.

PROPHYLACTIC THERAPY a medication taken to prevent the occurrence of, rather than treat, a disease.

PROPTOSIS an abnormal pushed forward or bulging out of the eyes.

PSEUDOHYPERTROPHY a term used to describe the calf muscles of a child with Duchenne muscular dystrophy, where the muscles appear large, but they are in fact very weak.

PURPURA another name for a bruise.

PUSTULES small (less than 2/5 inch or 1cm) pus-filled blisters on the skin.

PYELONEPHRITIS an infection of the kidney.

PYLORUS the part of the stomach that empties into the small bowel.

REFERRED PAIN pain felt in one part of the body that originates in another.

RHEUMATOID FACTOR POSITIVE (RF+VE) JRA joint inflammation accompanied by the presence of a marker (rheumatoid factor) in the blood; closely resembles adult rheumatoid arthritis.

RHINITIS inflammation of the nasal passages that may result from allergen exposure or infection, and typically results in a congested or runny nose.

ROSEOLA also known as "exanthem subitum." A viral infection caused by human herpesvirus 6 that occurs in young children and leads to high fever and irritability for three to four days, followed by a spotty rash lasting for hours to days.

SCLEROTHERAPY injection of a material that is irritating to the blood vessels and is helpful to close up abnormal blood vessels.

SEDIMENTATION RATE see ERYTHROCYTE SEDIMENTATION RATE (ESR).

SELECTIVE SEROTONIN REUPTAKE INHIBITORS (SSRIS) a family of drugs used to treat depression or anxiety by raising serotonin levels in the brain.

SEPTICEMIA a very serious bacterial infection of the blood (blood poisoning), causing low blood pressure or "shock."

SINUSITIS inflammation of the air-filled cavities, or sinuses, in the face.

SPINA BIFIDA a condition resulting from the incomplete closure of the spine early in pregnancy. The protective covering of the spine, the meninges, or the spinal cord itself protrudes through the skin, typically leading to weakness and lack of sensation below the level of the affected spinal cord.

SPINAL MUSCULAR ATROPHY a rare inherited condition of nerve degeneration that leads to weakness and low muscle tone.

SPLENIC SEQUESTRATION a potentially life-threatening complication of sickle-cell disease in which the spleen becomes engorged with blood, leading to pallor, pain in the upper left part of the abdomen and shock.

SPLENOMEGALY an abnormally enlarged spleen.

STANDARD DEVIATIONS a mathematical term used to describe an "acceptable" amount of distance from the average. On growth charts, for example, anyone above or below three standard deviations from the average is considered outside the normal range.

STENOSIS narrowing.

STRABISMUS also called "crossed eyes" or "squint." A misalignment of the eyes.

STREPTOCOCCAL PHARYNGITIS also called "strep throat." Inflammation of the tonsils, leading to fever and a sore throat, caused by infection with the bacteria group A streptococcus.

SUDDEN INFANT DEATH SYNDROME (SIDS) the sudden and unexpected death of an apparently healthy baby in the first year of life, which remains unexplained after a comprehensive investigation.

SUTURES where the bones of a baby's skull meet.

SWOLLEN GLANDS enlarged lymph nodes that are most commonly felt in the neck, underarm or groin, but may be found throughout the body. Most commonly resulting from infection, they may also rarely occur in rheumatologic and malignant conditions.

SYMPATHECTOMY the surgical cutting of the sympathetic nerves.

SYNCOPE a fainting spell.

SYNDROME a combination of signs and symptoms that characterizes a specific diagnosis.

SYNOVITIS inflammation of the lining surrounding a joint, which usually occurs as a result of an infection or a rheumatologic condition.

SYSTOLE the phase of the cardiac cycle when the heart pumps blood from the two ventricles to the lungs and the rest of the body.

SYSTOLIC MURMUR an extra heart sound that is heard with a stethoscope when blood courses through the heart during the pumping phase, or systole. Though they are most often heard in normal hearts, they may occasionally indicate an underlying heart problem.

TACHYCARDIA an abnormally fast heart rate for age.

TETANUS a serious infection caused by bacteria that live in soil, dust and manure, which all children should be vaccinated against.

THELARCHE the development of breast tissue.

THROMBOCYTOPENIA an abnormally low number of clotting cells, called "platelets," in the bloodstream.

THROMBUS a blood clot.

TRACHEITIS inflammation of the windpipe, or trachea, usually as a result of a viral infection. Often called "croup." It typically causes a barky cough and can interfere with breathing.

TRANSCUTANEOUS ELECTRICAL NERVE STIMULATION (TENS) a method of treating pain in which a low-voltage electric current is passed across the skin.

TRANSIENT SYNOVITIS a self-resolving condition, primarily affecting the lining of the hip joint, which typically follows a viral infection. Affected children usually refuse to walk or limp due to the pain.

TRANSLOCATION when part of a chromosome attaches to another chromosome and hitches a ride into the newly created egg during meiosis, or cell division. The result is extra genetic information from the additional chromosome piece in the new cell, which may or may not lead to problems.

TRISOMY 21 see DOWN'S SYNDROME.

TURNER SYNDROME a genetic condition in which girls have only one x-chromosome (normally they have two), causing nonfunctioning ovaries and other physical abnormalities.

TYMPANIC MEMBRANE the eardrum.

URTICARIA also called "hives." A skin rash characterized by itchy, red, raised lesions.

UVEITIS inflammation of the uvea, or front half of the eyeball.

VARICELLA see CHICKEN POX.

VARICOCELE a common condition in which the veins supplying the testicle swell with blood, typically presenting as a painless lump above the testicle; feels like a "bag of worms."

VEGETATIONS clumps of bacteria or fungi that are attached to a heart valve and are seen as part of a serious infection called infective endocarditis.

VENTRICULOPERITONEAL (VP) SHUNT a special tube that is surgically inserted into the brain to divert some of the excess cerebrospinal fluid (CSF) from the ventricles to the abdominal cavity.

VESICLES small (less than 2/5 inch or 1cm) fluid-filled blisters on the skin.

VESICOURETERAL REFLUX a condition in which urine flows backward from the bladder to the ureters and/or kidneys.

VOIDING CYSTOURETHROGRAM (VCUG) a test requiring placement of a catheter into the bladder and insertion of a small amount of dye. An x-ray is then taken while the child urinates; it is the recommended way of diagnosing vesicoureteral reflux.

VOLVULUS a very rare but serious cause of abdominal pain caused by the twisting of the small intestines on its stalk.

VOMITUS the medical term for the contents that are expelled when a child vomits.

VON WILLEBRAND DISEASE the most common inherited disorder that affects the blood's ability to clot properly, in which von Willebrand factor, a protein that helps platelets stick to damaged blood vessels, is either too low or not functioning properly.

WALKING PNEUMONIA a colloquial term used to describe a milder infection in the lungs, in a child who does not require hospitalization and remains active and fairly well.

X-LINKED AGAMMAGLOBULINEMIA also called "Bruton's agammaglobulinemia." An often fatal disease characterized by the lack of all or most of antibody production, resulting in frequent severe infections.

Acknowledgments

We would like to thank a number of individuals whose efforts made this book possible:

To our expert contributors for their enthusiasm and efforts that made this book a reality.

To Key Porter Books, specifically Linda Pruessen and Ruth Chernia, for editorial guidance and enthusiasm.

To the wonderful administrative and support staff at Sick Kids, including Heidi Falckh, Robert Teteruck (for his wonderful photographs), Sarah Ahmed and Tiziana Altobelli. Also to Chris Forrest for allowing us to use some of his photographs.

To John Lightfoot, for providing the illustrations that help make everything clear.

To Current Medicine LLC for graciously allowing the use of some of their images.

To Shelley and Lynn for helping with reading and listening to the various drafts of this book.

And finally, to our families, for tolerating our late nights at the computer.

—JF and NS

Photo Credits

Every reasonable effort has been made on the part of the Publisher to credit the photographs and images appropriately. Information enabling the Publisher to rectify any erroneous or omitted credit is welcome.

Photographs on pages 2, 12, 16, 55, 62, 80, 132, 148, 160, 182, 190, 197, 203, 204, 209, 212, 222, 244, 260, 286, 312, 322, 330, 346, 362, 380 and 398 appear courtesy of the Hospital for Sick Children's Graphics Department.

Photographs on pages 100, 105, 114, 124, 214, 316, 320, 321 and 384 appear courtesy of Current Medicine, LLC.

Photograph on page 66 appears courtesy of Coranne Lipford.

Page 144: MyPyramid for Kids poster, U.S. Department of Agriculture, Food and Nutrition Service, September 2005. Reproduced with the permission of the USDA, 2006.

Page 232: Photograph appears courtesy of Corbis Canada.

Page 296: Photograph appears courtesy of Stock Connection.

Pages 134, 135 and 137: Charts reproduced with the permission of the National Center for Health Statistics, 2000.

All photographs not listed here supplied by the authors.

Index